Atherosclerosis 2.0: From Molecular Mechanisms, Pathophysiology to Novel Therapeutic Approaches

Atherosclerosis 2.0: From Molecular Mechanisms, Pathophysiology to Novel Therapeutic Approaches

Guest Editor

Antonio Barbato

MDPI

Basel • Beijing • Wuhan • Barcelona • Belgrade • Novi Sad • Cluj • Manchester

Guest Editor
Antonio Barbato
Department of Clinical
Medicine and Surgery
University of Naples Federico II
Naples
Italy

Editorial Office
MDPI AG
Grosspeteranlage 5
4052 Basel, Switzerland

This is a reprint of the Special Issue, published open access by the journal *International Journal of Molecular Sciences* (ISSN 1422-0067), freely accessible at: https://www.mdpi.com/journal/ijms/special_issues/U5W7P23110.

For citation purposes, cite each article independently as indicated on the article page online and as indicated below:

Lastname, A.A.; Lastname, B.B. Article Title. *Journal Name* **Year**, *Volume Number*, Page Range.

ISBN 978-3-7258-7152-0 (Hbk)
ISBN 978-3-7258-7153-7 (PDF)
https://doi.org/10.3390/books978-3-7258-7153-7

Cover image courtesy of Antonio Barbato

Contents

About the Editor

Antonio Barbato

Antonio Barbato is a physician-scientist specializing in Internal Medicine and cardiovascular research. Trained at the University of Naples Federico II, he contributed to landmark epidemiological studies, including the Olivetti Prospective Heart Study, investigating genetic and metabolic predictors of cardiovascular disease. His early work focused on the association between gene polymorphisms and hypertension, advancing his expertise in medical database management and statistical analysis.

He earned a PhD in Clinical Pathophysiology and Experimental Medicine from the University of Naples Federico II, during which he analyzed data from the Olivetti Heart Study and the Wandsworth Heart & Stroke Study. As a research fellow at St. George's Hospital, University of London—supported by the "*S. Campus*" scholarship from the Italian Society of Hypertension—he studied ethnic differences in blood pressure salt sensitivity and managed high-risk cardiovascular patients.

His current research explores molecular and clinical mechanisms underlying the bone–heart axis in cardiovascular pathogenesis.

Dr. Barbato has authored more than 150 scientific publications, including 73 full-length articles in peer-reviewed international journals.

Preface

Atherosclerosis is a common condition associated with vascular aging. However, several factors can influence this process, resulting in increased cardiovascular risk even at a young age. In addition to well-known factors (e.g., hypertension, dyslipidemia, diabetes, and excess body weight), several emerging factors associated with atherosclerosis that could potentially explain residual cardiovascular risk are examined and discussed in this reprint.

This Special Issue on atherosclerosis reports the most recent scientific evidence available on the topic and to present reviews of the current literature on the role of emerging factors in the development of atherosclerosis, as demonstrated by both experimental and clinical studies. This will provide a broad body of data from which to identify potential new targets for cardiovascular risk reduction.

Antonio Barbato
Guest Editor

International Journal of *Molecular Sciences*

MDPI

Editorial

Special Issue "Atherosclerosis 2: From Molecular Mechanisms and Pathophysiology to Novel Therapeutic Approaches"

Antonio Barbato

Department of Clinical Medicine and Surgery, University of Naples Federico II, 80131 Naples, Italy; abarbato@unina.it

Atherosclerosis is a chronic inflammatory disease that affects medium- and large-sized arteries and remains a leading cause of global morbidity and mortality [1]. It is characterized by the accumulation of lipids, inflammatory cells, and fibrous tissue in the arterial wall, leading to the formation of atherosclerotic plaques [2]. In addition to well-known factors (e.g., high blood pressure, dyslipidemia, diabetes, and excess body weight), there are several emerging factors associated with atherosclerosis, such as inflammation, endothelial dysfunction, intestinal microbiota alteration, uric acid, vitamin D, or miRNA expression, which could potentially explain the residual cardiovascular risk [3].

This Special Issue integrates key findings from recent original investigations and review articles to present a multifaceted view of the current landscape in atherosclerosis research. A brief introduction to the main innovations and limitations emerging from this Special Issue is provided below.

The foundation of vascular health lies in the endothelium, and its phenotype can vary based on anatomical location. Frolov, A. et al. [4] employed a multi-omics approach to compare endothelial cells from the human coronary artery (HCAEC) and the internal thoracic artery (HITAEC), the latter being a common graft in coronary bypass surgery. They identified significant molecular heterogeneity: HCAECs exhibited a profile oriented toward extracellular matrix construction, while HITAECs showed greater pro-inflammatory activity. Intriguingly, despite these molecular differences, no specific protein markers were found that functionally distinguished the two cell types in vitro. A notable limitation included the inability to compare the proteomic data under laminar flow and static conditions, as the amount of total protein extracted from endothelial cells cultured in flow chambers was insufficient.

Endothelial dysfunction is a critical early event in atherosclerosis, often driven by factors like angiotensin II (Ang II). The molecular mediators of this process are under intense investigation. Dutka, M. et al. [5] demonstrated using a knockout mouse model that osteoprotegerin (OPG) is an essential factor for the development of Ang II-induced endothelial dysfunction. The novel observation that the absence of OPG exerts a protective effect suggests that OPG functions not merely as a biomarker but as an active mediator of the pathological process, as its deficiency is associated with reduced levels of pro-inflammatory cytokines within the vascular wall following Ang II stimulation. However, the translation of these findings to humans requires caution due to the complex regulation of OPG in human physiology.

Beyond biochemical stimuli, hemodynamic forces are central in determining sites of atherosclerotic plaque development. Cho, M. et al. [6] utilized a partial ligation mouse model of atherosclerosis and computational fluid dynamics (CFD) to analyze wall shear stress (WSS). Their innovative contribution was analyzing the standard deviation of time-averaged WSS as a new metric to correlate the heterogeneity of shear stress with plaque progression and inflammation. This approach provides a more nuanced understanding of hemodynamics than mean WSS alone, though the model primarily focuses on shear stress, neglecting other contributing biological factors.

As atherosclerosis progresses, circulating monocytes infiltrate the subendothelial space and transform into lipid-laden foam cells, a hallmark of the disease. Henni Mansour, A.S. et al. [7] provided a detailed characterization of different experimental models of these "foamy" macrophages. Their novel analysis, using flow cytometry and two-photon Excited Fluorescence (TPEF) imaging, revealed that foam cells generated with oxidized LDL (Mox) exhibit a more inflammatory and dysfunctional profile than those generated with acetylated LDL (Mac). Furthermore, they showed that this pro-inflammatory state could be partially reversed with antioxidant and cytokine treatments, offering a potential pathway for therapeutic intervention. The inherent limitation, however, is that these in vitro models cannot fully capture the complexity of the plaque microenvironment in vivo.

The search for novel molecular players continues with Kathuria, I. et al. [8] identifying nidogen-2 (NID2), a basement membrane protein, as a harmful factor that promotes both hepatosteatosis and atherosclerosis in a mouse model. To study the effect of NID2 overexpression, Apoe−/− mice were used in this study. One group of Apoe−/− mice, designated as controls, received an intraperitoneal injection of saline, while another group was administered a single dose of a recombinant AAV expressing the human *NID2* gene under the ubiquitous cytomegalovirus promoter, to induce NID2 overexpression. The novelty of this study is to link NID2 overexpression to the inhibition of AMP-activated protein kinase (AMPK) activation in the liver, a key regulator of energy metabolism. A significant limitation was that NID2 was overexpressed systemically in this mice model, making it difficult to isolate the specific contribution of liver versus vascular cells to the observed atherosclerotic phenotype.

Translating molecular findings into clinical practice is the goal of the work of Iusupova, A.O. et al. [9], who conducted a clinical study analyzing microRNAs and inflammatory proteins in patients with different phenotypes of coronary artery disease. Their key finding was that miRNA-145 serves as an independent predictor of ischemia with non-obstructive coronary arteries (INOCA), highlighting its potential as a valuable diagnostic biomarker to distinguish this challenging patient group. The study's conclusions are tempered by a relatively small sample size and a focus on a limited panel of biomarkers.

Several recent reviews have synthesized broader areas of research. Sohn, M. and Lim, S. [10] performed a systematic review with meta-analysis on the antiplatelet agent cilostazol, confirming its efficacy in reducing major adverse cardiovascular events (MACE), particularly stroke, with a lower bleeding risk than aspirin. They caution, however, that the evidence base is predominantly from East Asian populations, limiting generalizability.

Theofilis, P. et al. [11] provided a comprehensive overview of coronary plaque erosion, an important alternative mechanism of acute coronary syndrome distinct from rupture. Their review integrates the latest on molecular mechanisms (e.g., neutrophil involvement), advanced intracoronary imaging diagnostics such as optical coherence tomography or intravascular ultrasound–near-infrared spectroscopy, and emerging conservative treatment strategies.

Exploring the link between systemic inflammation and accelerated atherosclerosis, Kasher, M. et al. [12] reviewed evidence for glycoprotein acetyls (GlycA) as a novel biomarker. This study included original genetic analyses, suggesting GlycA is a causal mediator linking the inflammation of rheumatoid arthritis to atherosclerosis, partly through shared lipid pathways. However, the origin of genome-wide association studies (GWAS) data from European cohorts may affect the generalizability of these genetic findings.

Finally, Getz, G.S. & Reardon, C.A. [13] reviewed the site specificity of atherosclerotic lesions, drawing largely on murine studies. They present an updated synthesis moving beyond hemodynamics alone to include the roles of genetics, adaptive immunity, and perivascular adipose tissue.

Conclusions and Future Directions

The current research landscape reflects a multi-pronged and increasingly sophisticated approach to understanding atherosclerosis. The integration of multi-omics, advanced imaging modalities, and large-scale genetic data is driving a critical shift from correlational observations toward establishing causal pathways. Despite these significant advances, several knowledge gaps persist, representing major difficulties in the effective management of the disease [14].

A recurring theme across contemporary research is the challenge of translating findings from simplified in vitro systems and animal models to the complex reality of human pathophysiology [15]. While essential for mechanistic discovery, these models often fail to capture the full spectrum of the disease's heterogeneity. Key areas requiring deeper investigation include the precise molecular mechanisms governing plaque stability, the intricate cellular and metabolic interplay within the plaque microenvironment, and the influence of epigenetic regulators like microRNAs [16]. Furthermore, the impact of demographic factors such as sex and age on disease progression remains incompletely understood, limiting the development of truly personalized diagnostic and therapeutic strategies [17]. Clinically, there is still a pressing need for robust biomarkers for the early detection of vulnerable plaques and for more accurate, non-invasive risk stratification tools. By focusing on these strategic priorities, the scientific community can bridge the existing knowledge gaps and translate research breakthroughs into meaningful clinical innovations that reduce the global burden of atherosclerotic disease.

Conflicts of Interest: The author declares no conflict of interest.

References

1. Björkegren, J.; Lusis, A. Atherosclerosis: Recent developments. *Cell* **2022**, *185*, 1630–1645. [CrossRef] [PubMed]
2. Kong, P.; Cui, Z.Y.; Huang, X.F.; Zhang, D.D.; Guo, R.J.; Han, M. Inflammation and Atherosclerosis: Signaling Pathways and Therapeutic Intervention. *Signal Transduct. Target. Ther.* **2022**, *7*, 131. [CrossRef] [PubMed]
3. Bekbossynova, M.; Saliev, T.; Ivanova-Razumova, T.; Andossova, S.; Kali, A.; Myrzakhmetova, G. Beyond Cholesterol: Emerging Risk Factors in Atherosclerosis. *J. Clin. Med.* **2025**, *14*, 2352. [CrossRef] [PubMed]
4. Frolov, A.; Lobov, A.; Kabilov, M.; Zainullina, B.; Tupikin, A.; Shishkova, D.; Markova, V.; Sinitskaya, A.; Grigoriev, E.; Markova, Y.; et al. Multi-Omics Profiling of Human Endothelial Cells from the Coronary Artery and Internal Thoracic Artery Reveals Molecular but Not Functional Heterogeneity. *Int. J. Mol. Sci.* **2023**, *24*, 15032. [CrossRef] [PubMed]
5. Dutka, M.; Garczorz, W.; Kosowska, A.; Buczek, E.; Godek, P.; Wojakowski, W.; Francuz, T. Osteoprotegerin Is Essential for the Development of Endothelial Dysfunction Induced by Angiotensin II in Mice. *Int. J. Mol. Sci.* **2024**, *25*, 6434. [CrossRef] [PubMed]
6. Cho, M.; Hwang, J.S.; Kim, K.R.; Kim, J.K. Wall Shear Stress (WSS) Analysis in Atherosclerosis in Partial Ligated Apolipoprotein E Knockout Mouse Model through Computational Fluid Dynamics (CFD). *Int. J. Mol. Sci.* **2024**, *25*, 9877. [CrossRef] [PubMed]
7. Henni Mansour, A.S.; Ragues, M.; Brevier, J.; Borowczyk, C.; Grevelinger, J.; Laroche-Traineau, J.; Garaude, J.; Marais, S.; Jacobin-Valat, M.-J.; Gerbaud, E.; et al. Phenotypic, Metabolic, and Functional Characterization of Experimental Models of Foamy Macrophages: Toward Therapeutic Research in Atherosclerosis. *Int. J. Mol. Sci.* **2024**, *25*, 10146. [CrossRef] [PubMed]
8. Kathuria, I.; Prasad, A.; Sharma, B.K.; Aithabathula, R.V.; Ofosu-Boateng, M.; Gyamfi, M.A.; Jiang, J.; Park, F.; Singh, U.P.; Singla, B. Nidogen 2 Overexpression Promotes Hepatosteatosis and Atherosclerosis. *Int. J. Mol. Sci.* **2024**, *25*, 12782. [CrossRef] [PubMed]
9. Iusupova, A.O.; Pakhtusov, N.N.; Slepova, O.A.; Khabarova, N.V.; Privalova, E.V.; Bure, I.V.; Nemtsova, M.V.; Belenkov, Y.N. MiRNA-34a, miRNA-145, and miRNA-222 Expression, Matrix Metalloproteinases, TNF-α and VEGF in Patients with Different Phenotypes of Coronary Artery Disease. *Int. J. Mol. Sci.* **2024**, *25*, 12978. [CrossRef] [PubMed]
10. Sohn, M.; Lim, S. The Role of Cilostazol, a Phosphodiesterase-3 Inhibitor, in the Development of Atherosclerosis and Vascular Biology: A Review with Meta-Analysis. *Int. J. Mol. Sci.* **2024**, *25*, 2593. [CrossRef] [PubMed]

11. Theofilis, P.; Vlachakis, P.K.; Papanikolaou, A.; Karakasis, P.; Oikonomou, E.; Tsioufis, K.; Tousoulis, D. Coronary Plaque Erosion: Epidemiology, Diagnosis, and Treatment. *Int. J. Mol. Sci.* **2024**, *25*, 5786. [CrossRef] [PubMed]
12. Kasher, M.; Freidin, M.B.; Williams, F.M.K.; Cherny, S.S.; Ashkenazi, S.; Livshits, G. Glycoprotein Acetyls Is a Novel Biomarker Predicting Cardiovascular Complications in Rheumatoid Arthritis. *Int. J. Mol. Sci.* **2024**, *25*, 5981. [CrossRef] [PubMed]
13. Getz, G.S.; Reardon, C.A. Insights from Murine Studies on the Site Specificity of Atherosclerosis. *Int. J. Mol. Sci.* **2024**, *25*, 6375. [CrossRef] [PubMed]
14. Libby, P. The changing landscape of atherosclerosis. *Nature* **2021**, *592*, 524–533. [CrossRef] [PubMed]
15. Zhang, Y.; Fatima, M.; Hou, S.; Bai, L.; Zhao, S.; Liu, E. Research methods for animal models of atherosclerosis (Review). *Mol. Med. Rep.* **2021**, *24*, 871. [CrossRef] [PubMed]
16. Xu, S.; Kamato, D.; Little, P.J.; Nakagawa, S.; Pelisek, J.; Jin, Z.G. Targeting Epigenetics and Non-Coding RNAs in Atherosclerosis: From Mechanisms to Therapeutics. *Pharmacol. Ther.* **2019**, *196*, 15–43. [CrossRef] [PubMed]
17. Kerkhof, P.; Tona, F. Sex Differences in Diagnostic Modalities of Atherosclerosis in the Macrocirculation. *Atherosclerosis* **2023**, *384*, 117275. [CrossRef] [PubMed]

International Journal of *Molecular Sciences*

MDPI

Article

Multi-Omics Profiling of Human Endothelial Cells from the Coronary Artery and Internal Thoracic Artery Reveals Molecular but Not Functional Heterogeneity

Alexey Frolov [1], Arseniy Lobov [2], Marsel Kabilov [3], Bozhana Zainullina [4], Alexey Tupikin [3], Daria Shishkova [1], Victoria Markova [1], Anna Sinitskaya [1], Evgeny Grigoriev [1], Yulia Markova [1] and Anton Kutikhin [1,*]

1 Department of Experimental Medicine, Research Institute for Complex Issues of Cardiovascular Diseases, 6 Sosnovy Boulevard, Kemerovo 650002, Russia; frolav@kemcardio.ru (A.F.); shidk@kemcardio.ru (D.S.); markve@kemcardio.ru (V.M.); cepoav@kemcardio.ru (A.S.); grigev@kemcardio.ru (E.G.); markyo@kemcardio.ru (Y.M.)

2 Laboratory for Regenerative Biomedicine, Research Institute of Cytology of the Russian Academy of Sciences, 4 Tikhoretskiy Prospekt, St. Petersburg 194064, Russia; lobov@incras.ru

3 SB RAS Genomics Core Facility, Institute of Chemical Biology and Fundamental Medicine of the Siberian Branch of the Russian Academy of Sciences, 8 Prospekt Akademika Lavrentieva, Novosibirsk 630090, Russia; kabilov@niboch.nsc.ru (M.K.); tupikin@niboch.nsc.ru (A.T.)

4 Centre for Molecular and Cell Technologies, Research Park, Saint Petersburg State University, 7/9 Universitetskaya Embankment, St. Petersburg 199034, Russia; st022665@student.spbu.ru

* Correspondence: kytiag@kemcardio.ru; Tel.: +7-9609077067

Abstract: Major adverse cardiovascular events occurring upon coronary artery bypass graft surgery are typically accompanied by endothelial dysfunction. Total arterial revascularisation, which employs both left and right internal thoracic arteries instead of the saphenous vein to create a bypass, is associated with better mid- and long-term outcomes. We suggested that molecular profiles of human coronary artery endothelial cells (HCAECs) and human internal mammary artery endothelial cells (HITAECs) are coherent in terms of transcriptomic and proteomic signatures, which were then investigated by RNA sequencing and ultra-high performance liquid chromatography-mass spectrometry, respectively. Both HCAECs and HITAECs overexpressed molecules responsible for the synthesis of extracellular matrix (ECM) components, basement membrane assembly, cell-ECM adhesion, organisation of intercellular junctions, and secretion of extracellular vesicles. HCAECs were characterised by higher enrichment with molecular signatures of basement membrane construction, collagen biosynthesis and folding, and formation of intercellular junctions, whilst HITAECs were notable for augmented pro-inflammatory signaling, intensive synthesis of proteins and nitrogen compounds, and enhanced ribosome biogenesis. Despite HCAECs and HITAECs showing a certain degree of molecular heterogeneity, no specific markers at the protein level have been identified. Coherence of differentially expressed molecular categories in HCAECs and HITAECs suggests synergistic interactions between these ECs in a bypass surgery scenario.

Keywords: endothelial cells; endothelial heterogeneity; coronary artery; internal thoracic artery; coronary artery bypass graft surgery; multi-omics; transcriptome; RNA sequencing; global gene expression; proteomic profiling

1. Introduction

Rather than being a simple semi-permeable barrier protecting the blood vessels from thrombosis, lipid retention, and mineral deposition, endothelial cells (ECs) deploy numerous angiocrine factors including cytokines, growth factors, vasoactive substances, and other signaling molecules regulating vascular and systemic homeostasis in a juxtacrine or paracrine manner [1–5]. Single-cell RNA sequencing has demonstrated an organ-specific pattern of EC differentiation [6–9] and molecular heterogeneity between arterial, capillary, venous, and lymphatic ECs [10–15]. Recent advances in single-cell analysis and endothelial differentiation fostered a concept of therapeutic lymphangiogenesis, a treatment implying the guided regeneration of lymphatic networks upon the lymph node dissection to remove or ameliorate lymphoedema [16–18]. Isolation and culture of peripheral blood-derived, endothelial, colony-forming cells, which combine the molecular signatures of arterial, venous, and lymphatic ECs and have a high proliferation rate, significantly improved the development of tissue-engineered vascular grafts [19–23]. Hence, our knowledge of endothelial heterogeneity has been implemented into regenerative medicine and may be valuable for healthcare as soon as clinical trials of pre-endothelialised tissue-engineered vascular grafts or local treatment with autologous cells or angiogenic growth factors show their efficiency.

For >50 years, coronary artery bypass graft (CABG) surgery remains the most frequent cardiovascular intervention [24–27]. As compared with percutaneous coronary intervention, coronary artery bypass graft (CABG) surgery is superior for patients with severe coronary artery disease and those with diabetes mellitus [27–32]. Multiple arterial grafting (MAG), which employs the left internal thoracic artery (ITA) in combination with the right ITA and/or the radial artery as conduits for coronary artery bypass graft (CABG) surgery, is associated with better mid- and long-term outcomes in comparison with single arterial grafting (SAG) which combines the use of the left ITA and saphenous vein (SV) [33–44]. Notably, the superiority of total arterial revascularisation and bilateral ITA grafting to single ITA grafting was arguable [38,45–50], although these CABG techniques were beneficial in patients <70 years of age [40] and in women [51]. To clearly define the efficiency of all MAG modalities, a randomized comparison of the clinical outcome of single versus multiple arterial grafts (ROMA) trial has been initiated, but the results have not been published hitherto [52–54]. A comparison of the two approaches of ITA graft harvesting, the pedicled technique which preserves tunica adventitia and perivascular adipose tissue, and skeletonisation which dissects the ITA without any surrounding tissue, provided inconclusive results, although the former showed better long-term outcomes [55,56] and the latter was associated with lower risk of sternal wound complications [57–59]. The reduced rate of major adverse cardiovascular events accompanying the pedicled technique might indicate an important role of endothelial cells which assemble vasa vasorum and regulate adventitial fibroblasts and perivascular adipocytes by supplying them with context-specific biochemical cues.

The reasons behind the superiority of MAG over SAG might include a higher mechanical competence of anastomoses between the ITA, radial artery, and coronary artery because all of them are muscular arteries with a similar histoarchitecture and diameter [60–69], relatively low (≈25%) collagen content, optimal glycosaminoglycan profile and negligible protease activity in the arterial wall [70–73], quiescent profile of arterial vascular smooth muscle cells (VSMCs) [60,74–83], higher local secretion of vasodilators (e.g., nitric oxide) by ITA as compared to SV [84–91], resistance to oxidative stress [92–94], favourable paracrine interactions between human coronary artery endothelial cells (HCAECs) and human internal thoracic artery endothelial cells (HITAECs) [91], and better vasoreactivity of muscular arteries in response to vasoactive substances [95–99] in conjunction with their anti-thrombotic profile [100,101]. Among these, adequate vasodilation (largely mediated by efficient nitric oxide production without endothelial nitric oxide synthase uncoupling), release of secreted factors into the circulation, and resistance to thrombosis are furnished by ECs. Hence, upkeep of the physiological profile of HCAECs and HITAECs can be considered a key factor to achieve a favourable outcome of CABG surgery in the long term.

Earlier, we documented that HCAECs and HITAECs have mutual benefits if cultured together in vitro, whilst the interactions between arterial and venous ECs are less profitable [91]. To uncover the molecular basis of this phenomenon, we applied an unbiased multi-omics approach, employing RNA sequencing to analyse the transcriptome and ultra-high performance liquid chromatography-mass spectrometry (UHPLC-MS/MS) to perform a label-free proteomic profiling of HCAECs and HITAECs. We hypothesized that HCAECs and HITAECs demonstrate a certain extent of molecular heterogeneity that does not contradict their molecular congruence, defined as the common or synergistically upregulated biochemical pathways and the absence of distinctive functional protein markers.

2. Results

As proteins are central signaling molecules in the human organism and proteome analysis is of major importance for pathophysiology, we first performed label-free proteomic profiling for unbiased and quantitative analysis of proteins expressed in HCAECs and HITAECs. Bioinformatic analysis included denotation of differentially expressed proteins (DEPs, defined as those with a logarithmical fold change ≥ 1 and false discovery rate (FDR)-corrected p value ≤ 0.05) with further drawing of Venn diagrams and volcano plots, and pathway enrichment analysis of observed-versus-expected expression of DEPs within the molecular categories through the established bioinformatic tools (Gene Ontology, Reactome, UniProtKB, and KEGG). Having employed the mentioned workflow, we revealed 244 and 287 proteins (DEPs) upregulated in HCAECs and HITAECs, respectively, whereas 2794 proteins were not differentially expressed between these cell lines (Figure 1 and Supplementary Figure S1).

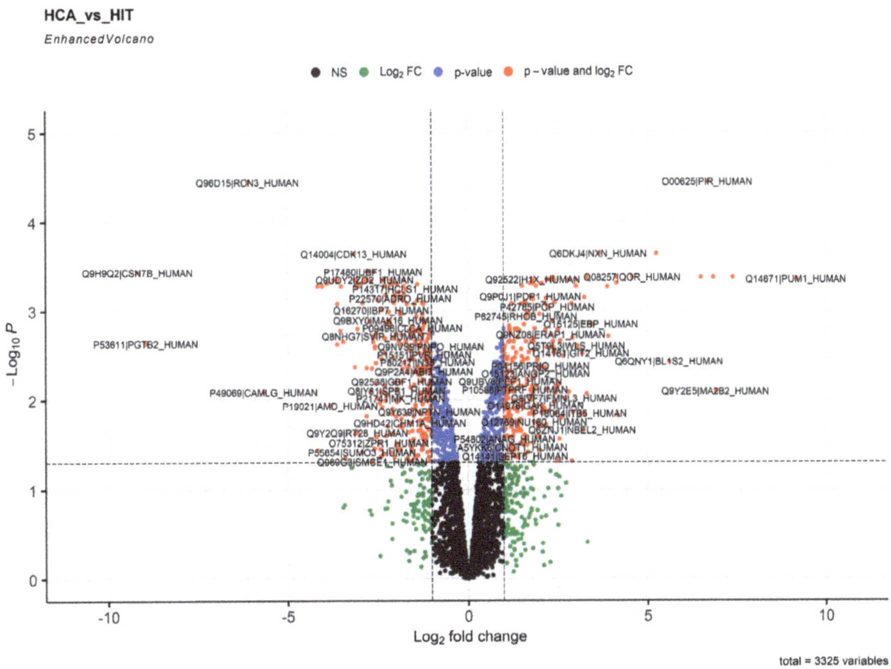

Figure 1. Volcano plot showing the distribution of proteins in the proteome of human coronary artery endothelial cells (HCAECs) and human internal thoracic artery endothelial cells (HITAECs). Gray points depict the proteins with $\log_2$ fold change < 1 and FDR-corrected p value > 0.05. Green points depict the proteins with $\log_2$ fold change > 1 and FDR-corrected p value > 0.05. Blue points depict the proteins with $\log_2$ fold change < 1 and FDR-corrected p value < 0.05. Red points depict the proteins with $\log_2$ fold change > 1 and FDR-corrected p value < 0.05 (DEPs).

Among the molecular categories, both HCAECs and HITAECs overexpressed those responsible for cell attachment to BM, organisation of intercellular junctions, energy generation in mitochondria, and release of EVs (Supplementary Tables S1–S11). However, each of the cell lines also had specific upregulated categories. For instance, HCAECs overexpressed a higher number of proteins accountable for BM formation, collagen synthesis, metabolism of lipids, organic acids, vitamins and carbohydrates, Golgi transporters, and lysosomal and peroxisomal proteins (Supplementary Tables S1–S11), while proteins related to the synthesis of mitochondrial ribosomes, mitochondrial transcription and translation, ribosomal activity, biosynthesis and metabolism of nitrogen compounds, mRNA regulation, synthesis of macromolecules, and formation of elastic fibers were overrepresented in HITAECs (Supplementary Tables S1–S11). Hence, HCAECs and HITAECs exhibited certain molecular heterogeneity.

However, only 12 proteins were overexpressed in HCAECs or HITAECs with a logarithmical fold change > 5 (PUM1, MGST1, MA2B2, A1AT, PIR, FABP4, BL1S2, and DPP4, HCAECs; CSN7B, PGTB2, RCN3, and CAMLG, HITAECs). None of these proteins have been earlier reported as a specific marker of any EC lineage, although dipeptidyl peptidase 4 (DPP4) and adipocyte fatty acid-binding protein (FABP4) are frequently referred to in cardiovascular biology literature.

To better quantify the molecular evolution of HCAECs and HITAECs, we performed transcriptomic profiling under the laminar flow and in the static conditions by means of RNA sequencing. The bioinformatic analysis was the same, with the exception of defining differentially expressed genes (DEGs) instead of DEPs. Under laminar flow, we found 1014 and 849 genes (DEGs with a logarithmical fold change ≥ 1 and FDR-corrected p value ≤ 0.05) upregulated in HCAECs and HITAECs, respectively, whilst 19,228 genes have not been differentially expressed between the cell lines (Figure 2 and Supplementary Figure S2).

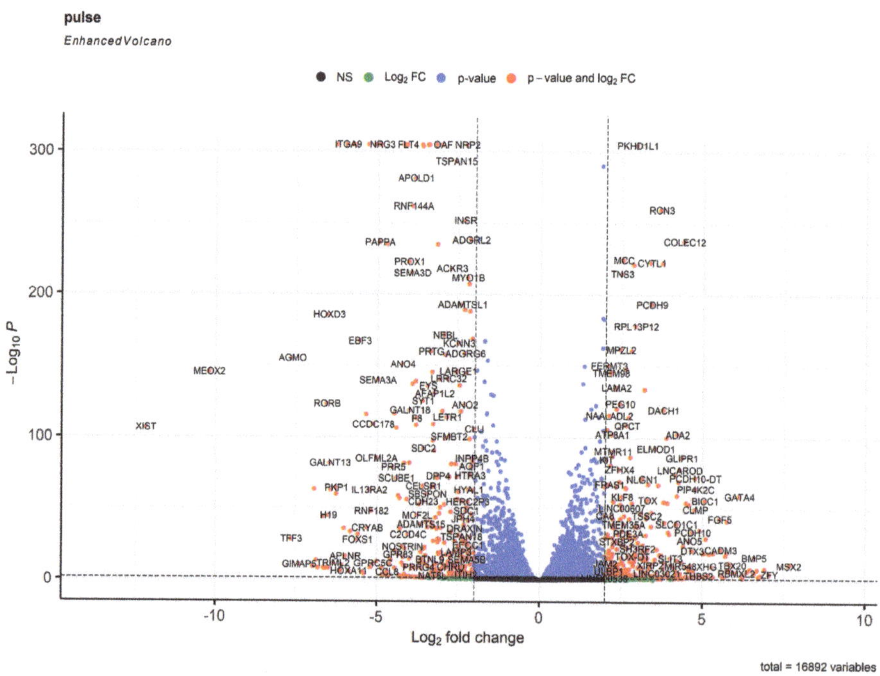

Figure 2. Volcano plot showing the distribution of transcripts in the transcriptome of human coronary artery endothelial cells (HCAECs) and human internal thoracic artery endothelial cells (HITAECs) under laminar flow. Gray points depict the genes with $\log_2$ fold change < 1 and FDR-corrected p value > 0.05. Green points depict the genes with $\log_2$ fold change > 1 and FDR-corrected p value > 0.05. Blue points depict the genes with $\log_2$ fold change < 1 and FDR-corrected p value < 0.05. Red points depict the genes with $\log_2$ fold change > 1 and FDR-corrected p value < 0.05 (DEGs).

The number of DEGs was from 3- to 5-fold higher than DEPs because of post-transcriptional regulation and higher coverage of transcriptomic analysis where the sequencing depth outperforms the protein annotation algorithms after UHPLC-MS/MS. At RNA sequencing, both HCAECs and HITAECs overexpressed genes accountable for the synthesis of collagen and other ECM components, adhesion to the BM, binding to glycosaminoglycans, Ca^{2+}-dependent signaling, organisation of intercellular junctions, secretion of EVs, DNA metabolism and repair, RNA processing, and protein utilisation processes such as ubiquitination and autophagy (Supplementary Tables S12–S22). However, HCAECs were enriched with transcripts responsible for biosynthesis and folding of collagen, organisation of the ECM and BM, assembly of intercellular junctions, binding of integrins to collagen and proteoglycans, and formation of elastic fibers (Supplementary Tables S12–S22), whilst HITAECs had a higher number of transcripts accountable for cytoskeleton organisation, synthesis of glycosaminoglycans, release of EVs, and pro-inflammatory signaling (Supplementary Tables S12–S22).

Under static conditions, we found 729 and 926 genes (DEGs with a logarithmical fold change ≥ 1 and FDR-corrected p value ≤ 0.05) upregulated in HCAECs and HITAECs, respectively, whilst 17,789 genes have not been differentially expressed between the cell lines (Figure 3 and Supplementary Figure S3).

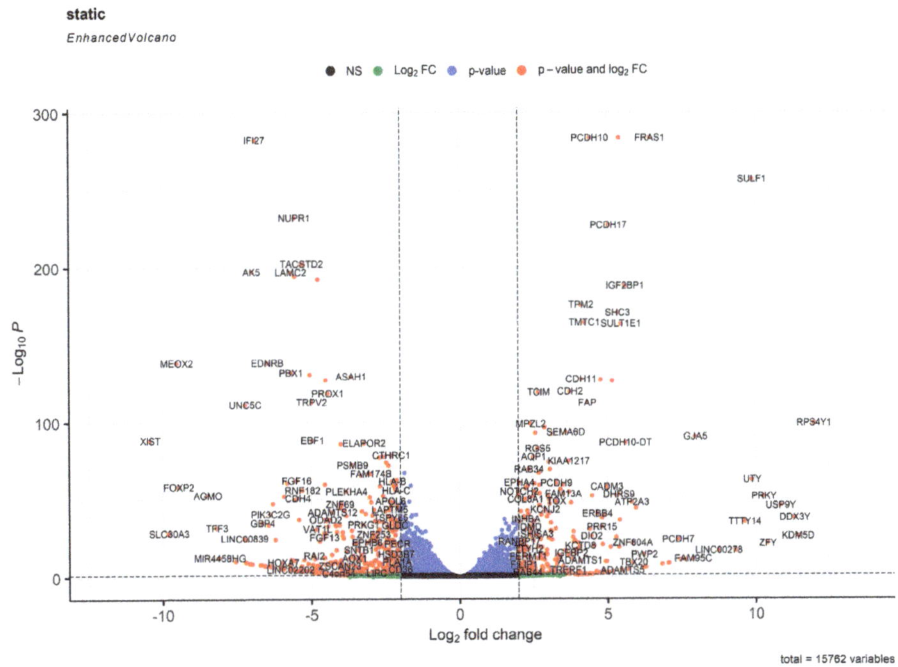

Figure 3. Volcano plot showing the distribution of transcripts in the transcriptome of human coronary artery endothelial cells (HCAECs) and human internal thoracic artery endothelial cells (HITAECs) at static cell culture conditions. Gray points depict the genes with $\log_2$ fold change < 1 and FDR-corrected p value > 0.05. Green points depict the genes with $\log_2$ fold change > 1 and FDR-corrected p value > 0.05. Blue points depict the genes with $\log_2$ fold change < 1 and FDR-corrected p value < 0.05. Red points depict the genes with $\log_2$ fold change > 1 and FDR-corrected p value < 0.05 (DEGs).

Both HCAECs and HITAECs overexpressed genes responsible for synthesis of collagen and other ECM components, adhesion of ECs to the ECM, organisation of intercellular junctions, and release of EVs (Supplementary Tables S23–S33). The expression profile of HCAECs was enriched with transcripts associated with vascular development, production of nitrogen compounds, and proteolysis (Supplementary Tables S23–S33), whilst transcripts related to endosomal and lysosomal compartments, pro-inflammatory response, synthesis of macromolecules, DNA repair, RNA processing and splicing, ribosome biogenesis, and translation were overrepresented in HITAECs (Supplementary Tables S23–S33).

Similar number of DEGs in HCAECs and HITAECs under laminar flow and at static conditions (1863 and 1655, respectively) and their distribution across HCAECs and HITAECs (HCAECs: 1046 DEGs under laminar flow and 729 DEGs at static conditions; HITAECs: 849 DEGs at laminar flow and 926 DEGs under static conditions) testified to the concordance of the results between experimental models and the higher sensitivity (but lower specificity) of RNA sequencing in comparison with proteomic profiling. Taking the results of transcriptomic and proteomic profiling together, both HCAECs and HITAECs demonstrated pronounced expression of genes and proteins responsible for the synthesis of collagen and other ECM components, cell adhesion to ECM and BM components, assembly of intercellular junctions, secretion of EVs, and metabolism of macromolecules (in particular nucleic acids and proteins). When comparing HCAECs and HITAECs, HCAECs had a higher variety and expression of molecular terms attributable for the formation of BM, biosynthesis and folding of collagen, and organisation of intercellular junctions, whereas HITAECs showed molecular signatures of active pro-inflammatory signaling, generation of nitrogen compounds, synthesis of macromolecules, regulation of RNA metabolism, and ribosome biogenesis and activity.

To verify the results obtained from transcriptomic profiling, we performed selective gene expression analysis in HCAECs and HITAECs at the baseline conditions (i.e., in serum-free medium supplied with growth factors) using reverse transcription-quantitative polymerase chain reaction (RT-qPCR). At laminar flow culture, HCAECs demonstrated reduced expression of *ICAM1*, *SELE*, and *SELP* genes which encode cell adhesion molecules for leukocyte adhesion, in line with the downregulation of genes encoding pro-inflammatory interleukins such as *IL6*, *CXCL8*, and *CCL2*, in comparison with HITAECs (Table 1). Intriguingly, *KLF2* and *KLF4* genes showed opposite expressions in HCAECs and HITAECs, which is suggestive of distinct mechanosensitive transcription factors in different EC lines. In accordance with the literature [84–91], *NOS3* gene expression was lower in HCAECs as compared to HITAECs. At static conditions, HCAECs also showed downregulation of the genes for cell adhesion molecules (*VCAM1*, *ICAM1*, and *SELE*) and chemokine genes (*CXCL8* and *CCL2*), although the expression of *IL6*, *CXCL1*, and *MIF* genes was inconsistent between the experiments and expression of *NOS3* gene was also uncertain (Table 1). In terms of relative gene expression, *ICAM1* prevailed over *VCAM1*; *CCL2* and *CXCL8* showed higher expression than *IL6*; and *KLF4* was overexpressed in comparison with *KLF2* (at laminar flow as these factors convey the mechanotransduction signals) in both HCAECs and HITAECs (Table 1). Expression of endothelial-to-mesenchymal transition transcription factors varied across the experiments and was not concordant between the cell lines (Table 1).

Table 1. Reverse transcription-quantitative polymerase chain reaction (RT-qPCR) analysis of the gene expression in human coronary artery endothelial cells (HCAECs) and human internal thoracic artery endothelial cells (HITAECs) cultured at laminar flow or in static conditions. Expression has been normalised for the expression of three housekeeping genes (*GAPDH*, *ACTB*, and *B2M*).

Gene	Flow Culture Chambers (μ-Slide y-Shaped)			Static Conditions Experiment #1			Static Conditions Experiment #2			Static Conditions Experiment #3			Static Conditions Experiment #4		
	HCAECs, ΔCt (Mean ± Standard Deviation)	HITAECs, ΔCt (Mean ± Standard Deviation)	Fold Change (HCAECs to HITAECs)	HCAECs, ΔCt (Mean ± Standard Deviation)	HITAECs, ΔCt (Mean ± Standard Deviation)	Fold Change (HCAECs to HITAECs)	HCAECs, ΔCt (Mean ± Standard Deviation)	HITAECs, ΔCt (Mean ± Standard Deviation)	Fold Change (HCAECs to HITAECs)	HCAECs, ΔCt (Mean ± Standard Deviation)	HITAECs, ΔCt (Mean ± Standard Deviation)	Fold Change (HCAECs to HITAECs)	HCAECs, ΔCt (Mean ± Standard Deviation)	HITAECs, ΔCt (Mean ± Standard Deviation)	Fold Change (HCAECs to HITAECs)
VCAM1	0.0051 ± 0.0004	0.0053 ± 0.0006	0.962	0.0015 ± 0.0004	0.0098 ± 0.0009	0.153	N/D	N/D	N/D	0.0013 ± 0.0002	0.0955 ± 0.0039	0.014	0.0051 ± 0.0002	0.0455 ± 0.0041	0.112
ICAM1	0.0331 ± 0.0021	0.1659 ± 0.0121	0.200	0.0050 ± 0.0003	0.0407 ± 0.0027	0.123	0.0279 ± 0.0132	0.0559 ± 0.0231	0.499	0.0163 ± 0.0079	2.0781 ± 0.7478	0.008	0.0313 ± 0.0096	0.2675 ± 0.1376	0.117
SELE	0.0012 ± 0.0001	0.0265 ± 0.0067	0.045	0.0011 ± 0.0002	0.0481 ± 0.0039	0.023	0.0002 ± 0.00002	0.0219 ± 0.0016	0.009	0.0004 ± 0.0001	0.0942 ± 0.0110	0.004	0.0029 ± 0.0002	0.0939 ± 0.0057	0.031
SELP	0.0010 ± 0.0001	0.0184 ± 0.0028	0.054	0.0025 ± 0.0009	0.0044 ± 0.0011	0.568	0.0899 ± 0.0035	0.0080 ± 0.0037	11.238	0.0127 ± 0.0016	0.0555 ± 0.0099	0.229	0.0321 ± 0.0022	0.0203 ± 0.0011	1.581
IL6	0.0044 ± 0.0004	0.0199 ± 0.0016	0.221	0.0029 ± 0.0007	0.0007 ± 0.0003	4.143	0.0042 ± 0.0003	0.0211 ± 0.0019	0.199	0.0029 ± 0.0002	0.0095 ± 0.0020	0.305	0.0084 ± 0.0009	0.0050 ± 0.0003	1.680
CXCL8	0.0337 ± 0.0009	0.1774 ± 0.0129	0.190	0.0701 ± 0.0045	0.0557 ± 0.0051	1.259	0.0256 ± 0.0029	0.3286 ± 0.0285	0.078	0.0301 ± 0.0028	0.5886 ± 0.0732	0.051	0.1107 ± 0.0063	0.4469 ± 0.0335	0.248
CCL2	0.0112 ± 0.0009	0.2993 ± 0.0247	0.037	0.0279 ± 0.0091	0.2563 ± 0.0137	0.109	0.0614 ± 0.0038	1.0850 ± 0.1059	0.057	0.0543 ± 0.0026	4.3406 ± 0.9546	0.013	0.0920 ± 0.0048	0.9923 ± 0.0732	0.093
CXCL1	N/D	N/D	N/D	0.0763 ± 0.0080	0.0651 ± 0.0061	1.172	0.0984 ± 0.0274	0.2571 ± 0.0556	0.383	0.1074 ± 0.0154	1.6440 ± 0.4153	0.065	0.2617 ± 0.0185	0.2715 ± 0.0439	0.964
MIF	N/D	N/D	N/D	0.2152 ± 0.0231	0.0812 ± 0.0074	2.650	0.4353 ± 0.0956	2.6439 ± 0.1977	0.165	0.1903 ± 0.0117	4.0451 ± 0.5167	0.047	0.4234 ± 0.0139	0.6183 ± 0.0129	0.685

Table 1. *Cont.*

Gene	Flow Culture Chambers (μ-Slide y-Shaped)			Static Conditions Experiment #1			Static Conditions Experiment #2			Static Conditions Experiment #3			Static Conditions Experiment #4		
	HCAECs, ΔCt (Mean ± Standard Deviation)	HITAECs, ΔCt (Mean ± Standard Deviation)	Fold Change (HCAECs to HITAECs)	HCAECs, ΔCt (Mean ± Standard Deviation)	HITAECs, ΔCt (Mean ± Standard Deviation)	Fold Change (HCAECs to HITAECs)	HCAECs, ΔCt (Mean ± Standard Deviation)	HITAECs, ΔCt (Mean ± Standard Deviation)	Fold Change (HCAECs to HITAECs)	HCAECs, ΔCt (Mean ± Standard Deviation)	HITAECs, ΔCt (Mean ± Standard Deviation)	Fold Change (HCAECs to HITAECs)	HCAECs, ΔCt (Mean ± Standard Deviation)	HITAECs, ΔCt (Mean ± Standard Deviation)	Fold Change (HCAECs to HITAECs)
KLF2	0.0047 ± 0.0006	0.0021 ± 0.0002	2.238	0.0018 ± 0.0009	0.0004 ± 0.0001	4.500	N/D	N/D	N/D	N/D	N/D	N/D	N/D	N/D	N/D
KLF4	0.0239 ± 0.0012	0.1268 ± 0.0178	0.188	0.0010 ± 0.0002	0.0005 ± 0.0001	2.000	N/D	N/D	N/D	N/D	N/D	N/D	N/D	N/D	N/D
NFE2L2	0.0618 ± 0.0041	0.0293 ± 0.0010	2.109	0.0866 ± 0.088	0.0523 ± 0.0026	1.656	N/D	N/D	N/D	N/D	N/D	N/D	N/D	N/D	N/D
SNAI1	0.0312 ± 0.0011	0.3193 ± 0.0632	0.098	0.0071 ± 0.0004	0.0121 ± 0.0017	0.587	0.0286 ± 0.0031	0.0381 ± 0.0065	0.751	0.0011 ± 0.0001	0.1209 ± 0.0140	0.009	0.0236 ± 0.0011	0.0237 ± 0.0031	0.996
SNAI2	0.0003 ± 0.00002	0.0002 ± 0.00004	1.500	0.0002 ± 0.00001	0.0001 ± 0.00001	2.000	0.0371 ± 0.0045	0.0025 ± 0.0007	14.840	0.00006 ± 0.00002	0.0043 ± 0.0015	0.014	0.0034 ± 0.0002	0.0001 ± 0.00005	34.000
TWIST1	0.0005 ± 0.0001	0.0001 ± 0.00001	5.000	0.0004 ± 0.00001	0.00001 ± 0.00001	40.000	0.0010 ± 0.0004	0.0007 ± 0.0002	1.429	0.00008 ± 0.00002	0.00014 ± 0.0001	0.571	0.0002 ± 0.00004	0.00004 ± 0.00002	5.000
ZEB1	0.0845 ± 0.0096	0.0886 ± 0.0056	0.954	0.0350 ± 0.0057	0.0343 ± 0.0034	1.020	0.0818 ± 0.0037	0.1628 ± 0.0196	0.502	0.0068 ± 0.0004	0.0655 ± 0.0094	0.104	0.0486 ± 0.0024	0.0552 ± 0.0083	0.880
CDH5	0.6792 ± 0.0132	3.0981 ± 0.3207	0.219	0.4247 ± 0.0985	0.5115 ± 0.0189	0.830	0.3888 ± 0.0087	0.3852 ± 0.0165	1.009	0.9632 ± 0.0871	9.4160 ± 2.8673	0.102	1.1429 ± 0.1359	2.1643 ± 0.0577	0.528
CDH2	0.0088 ± 0.0013	0.0103 ± 0.0015	0.854	0.0108 ± 0.0015	0.0028 ± 0.0009	3.857	0.0670 ± 0.0056	0.0001 ± 0.0002	670.000	0.0479 ± 0.0032	0.0146 ± 0.0039	3.281	0.1393 ± 0.0119	0.0079 ± 0.0003	17.633
NOS3	0.0450 ± 0.0008	0.1536 ± 0.0102	0.293	0.0066 ± 0.00011	0.0020 ± 0.0007	3.300	0.0015 ± 0.0004	0.0009 ± 0.0007	1.667	0.0057 ± 0.0005	0.2375 ± 0.0387	0.024	0.0262 ± 0.0026	0.0125 ± 0.0003	2.096

N/D—not defined (have not been measured).

The findings revealed at proteomic profiling were confirmed by fluorescent Western blotting for the proteins corresponding to some of the genes which expression has been measured at RT-qPCR, followed by total protein normalisation to confirm the equal protein loading across the bands. In keeping with the gene expression measurements, VCAM1, TWIST1, and KLF4 expression was higher in HITAECs as compared with HCAECs, whilst other transcription factors of endothelial-to-mesenchymal transition (Snail, Slug, and ZEB1), ICAM1, and eNOS showed minor if any expression differences (Figure 4A–G).

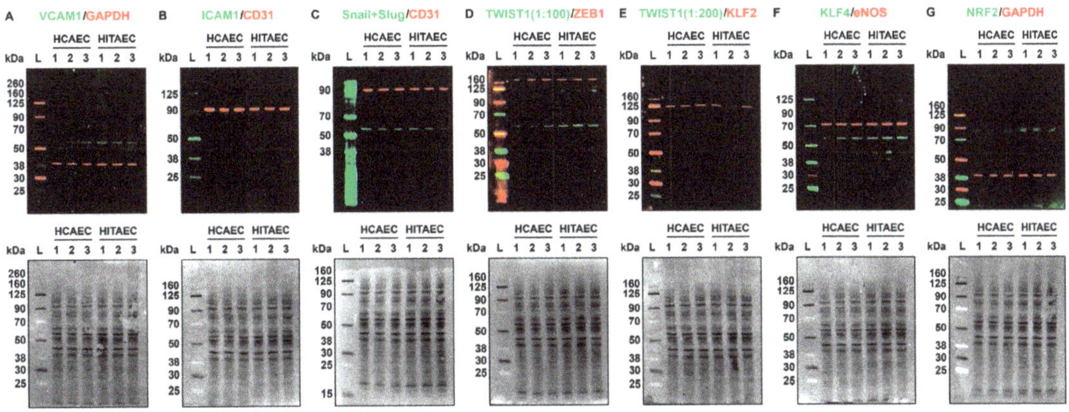

Figure 4. Fluorescent Western blotting for cell adhesion molecules (VCAM1 and ICAM1), transcription factors of endothelial-to-mesenchymal transition (Snail and Slug, TWIST1, and ZEB1), mechanosensitive transcription factors (KLF2, KLF4, and NRF2), endothelial nitric oxide synthase eNOS, and loading control (GAPDH and CD31) in human coronary artery endothelial cells (HCAECs) and human internal thoracic artery endothelial cells (HITAECs) cultured at static conditions. (**A**) VCAM1 (pro-inflammatory cell adhesion molecule, green)/GAPDH (loading control, red), fluorescent Western blot (**top**), and total protein staining confirming an equal protein loading (**bottom**); (**B**) ICAM1 (pro-inflammatory cell adhesion molecule, green)/CD31 (loading control, red), fluorescent Western blot (**top**), and total protein staining confirming an equal protein loading (**bottom**); (**C**) Snail and Slug (endothelial-to-mesenchymal transition transcription factor, green)/CD31 (loading control, red), fluorescent Western blot (**top**), and total protein staining confirming an equal protein loading (**bottom**); (**D**) TWIST1 (endothelial-to-mesenchymal transition transcription factor, green)/ZEB1 (another endothelial-to-mesenchymal transition transcription factor, red), fluorescent Western blot (**top**), and total protein staining confirming an equal protein loading (**bottom**); (**E**) TWIST1 (endothelial-to-mesenchymal transition transcription factor, green)/KLF2 (atheroprotective mechanosensitive transcription factor, red), fluorescent Western blot (**top**), and total protein staining confirming an equal protein loading (**bottom**); (**F**) KLF4 (atheroprotective mechanosensitive transcription factor, green)/eNOS (endothelial nitric oxide synthase, red), fluorescent Western blot (**top**), and total protein staining confirming an equal protein loading (**bottom**); (**G**) NRF2 (atheroprotective mechanosensitive transcription factor, green)/GAPDH (loading control, red), fluorescent Western blot (**top**), and total protein staining confirming an equal protein loading (**bottom**). Each band within the groups represent a protein lysate from one experiment (n = 3 experiments in total). Total protein normalisation was conducted by Fast Green FCF staining of the membranes after the fluorescent imaging to ensure the equal protein loading at all blots (in addition to loading controls such as GAPDH or CD31). Fluorescent ladder (L) and molecular weight signatures (kDa) are provided to the left of the HCAECs and HITAECs protein bands. Ratios of 1:100 and 1:200 are dilutions of the antibody against TWIST1, highlighted to show low expression of this protein in the quiescent ECs.

The results of selective gene expression measurements by RT-qPCR and protein measurements by Western blotting were concordant with those documented by whole transcriptomic sequencing and proteomic profiling, respectively. For instance, HITAECs were notable for molecular signatures of upregulated pro-inflammatory signaling (i.e., production of cytokines and chemokines, including interleukin-6) at the transcriptomic profiling (i.e., RNA-seq) and for increased expression of *CXCL8* and *CCL2* genes (encoding interleukin-8 and monocyte chemoattractant protein, respectively) at RT-qPCR, both at laminar flow and in static culture conditions. Further, HITAECs showed proteomic signatures of enhanced generation of nitrogen compounds and *NOS3* gene was evidently higher expressed at laminar flow. As HCAECs and HITAECs also exhibited minor differences in protein expression at Western blotting, we suggest that RT-qPCR and Western blotting results provide additional evidence for the molecular congruence between these EC lines.

As the concept of reciprocal and beneficial paracrine effects of HCAECs and HITAECs implies multiple interactions between their DEPs and DEGs, we carried out a functional enrichment analysis of protein–protein and gene–gene interaction networks using STRING database and Cytoscape software with the stringApp plugin. Bioinformatic analysis pipeline included: (1) filtration of DEPs and DEGs having $\geq$1 interaction (254 DEPs, 516 DEGs at laminar flow, and 466 DEGs under static conditions); (2) colour mapping in order to distinguish interacting DEPs and DEGs between HCAECs and HITAECs; (3) pathway enrichment analysis using GO, Reactome, UniProtKB, and KEGG terms; and (4) selection of such molecular terms relevant for arterial homeostasis.

Having employed this workflow, we found that interacting DEPs and DEGs in HCAECs and HITAECs were overrepresented in pathways (i.e., molecular terms) responsible for the maintenance of endothelial monolayer and basement membrane (various types of intercellular junctions as well as cell–cell and cell–matrix adhesion), as well as in angiogenesis, EC proliferation, elastic fiber formation, and nitric oxide synthesis pathways (Figures 5–7 and Supplementary Tables S34–S39). Most of the molecular terms were in concord between the proteomic and transcriptomic data, as well as between the transcriptomic data obtained under laminar flow and at static conditions. Hence, we found that the dataset of interacting DEPs and DEGs between HCAECs and HITAECs showed significant enrichment in arterial homeostasis pathways that suggests another argument towards beneficial interactions between these two EC lines.

To reinforce the study findings, we examined the data from 102 patients who underwent repeated coronary angiography 10 years after CABG surgery. Out of 311 bypasses, we documented 88 bypass dysfunctions (i.e., adverse outcomes), and the proportion of adverse outcomes was significantly higher when using SV grafts (54/160, 33.75%) as compared with utilising left or right ITA (34/151, 22.52%, $p = 0.038$, Supplementary Figure S4A). Hence, the relative contribution of SV graft dysfunction into the total adverse outcomes upon the CABG surgery was 61.36% (54 out of 88 adverse outcomes), in comparison with only 36.66% when using ITA conduits (34 out of 88 adverse outcomes, Supplementary Figure S4B). Among the causes of bypass dysfunctions, atherosclerosis and graft degeneration (triggered by endothelial dysfunction) were responsible for 42 out of 54 adverse outcomes (77.78%) in SV conduits but had been accountable only for 9 of 34 adverse outcomes (26.47%) in ITA grafts where competitive flow (a surgical complication) prevailed (23 of 34 adverse outcomes, 67.65%, Supplementary Figure S4B). Therefore, bioinformatic and molecular biology evidence for the synergy between HCAECs and HITAECs were concordant with the clinical observations showing the superiority of ITA conduits as compared with SV grafts.

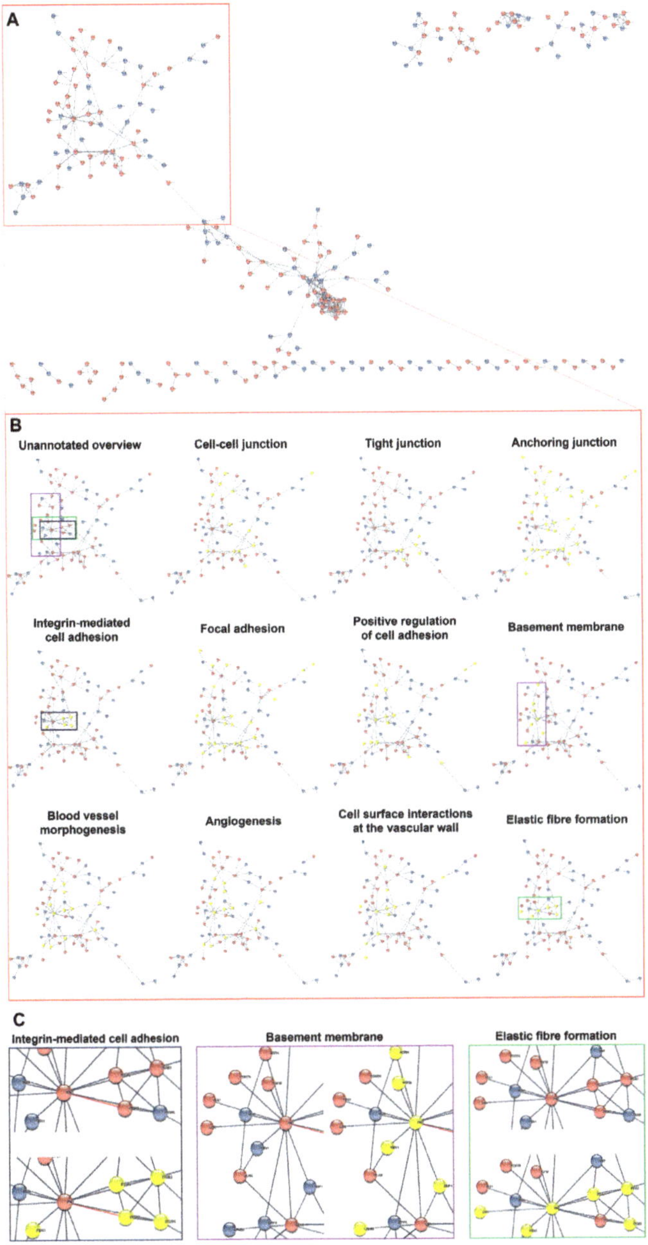

Figure 5. Bioinformatic analysis of protein–protein interactions between primary human coronary endothelial cells (HCAECs) and human internal thoracic artery endothelial cells (HITAECs). (**A**) Overview of protein–protein interactions between HCAECs (blue colour) and HITAECs (red colour); (**B**) annotation of the interacting proteins related to the specific molecular terms (yellow colour) in comparison with unannotated overview (the main cluster of interacting proteins is demarcated by red contour); and (**C**) annotations of clustered interacting proteins in selected molecular terms: integrin-mediated cell adhesion (demarcated by blue contour), basement membrane (demarcated by violet contour), and elastic fiber formation (demarcated by green contour).

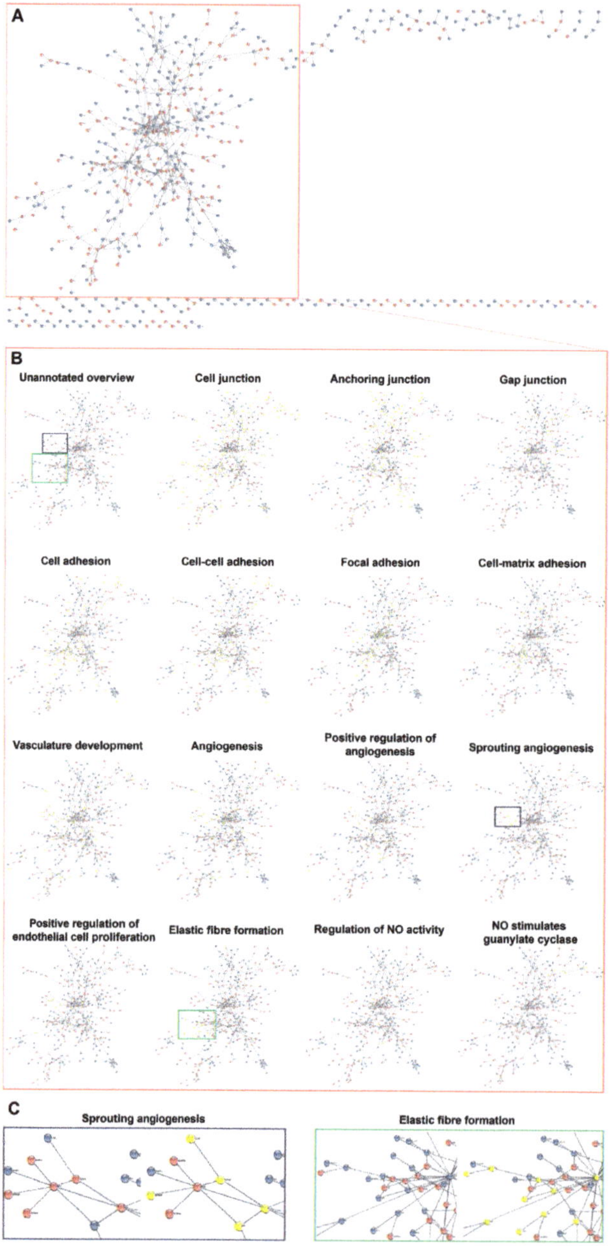

Figure 6. Bioinformatic analysis of gene–gene interactions between primary human coronary endothelial cells (HCAECs) and human internal thoracic artery endothelial cells (HITAECs) cultured under laminar flow. (**A**) Overview of gene–gene interactions between HCAECs (blue colour) and HITAECs (red colour) cultured under laminar flow; (**B**) annotation of the interacting genes related to the specific molecular terms (yellow colour) in comparison with unannotated overview (the main cluster of interacting genes is demarcated by red contour); and (**C**) annotations of clustered interacting genes in selected molecular terms: sprouting angiogenesis (demarcated by blue contour) and elastic fiber formation (demarcated by green contour).

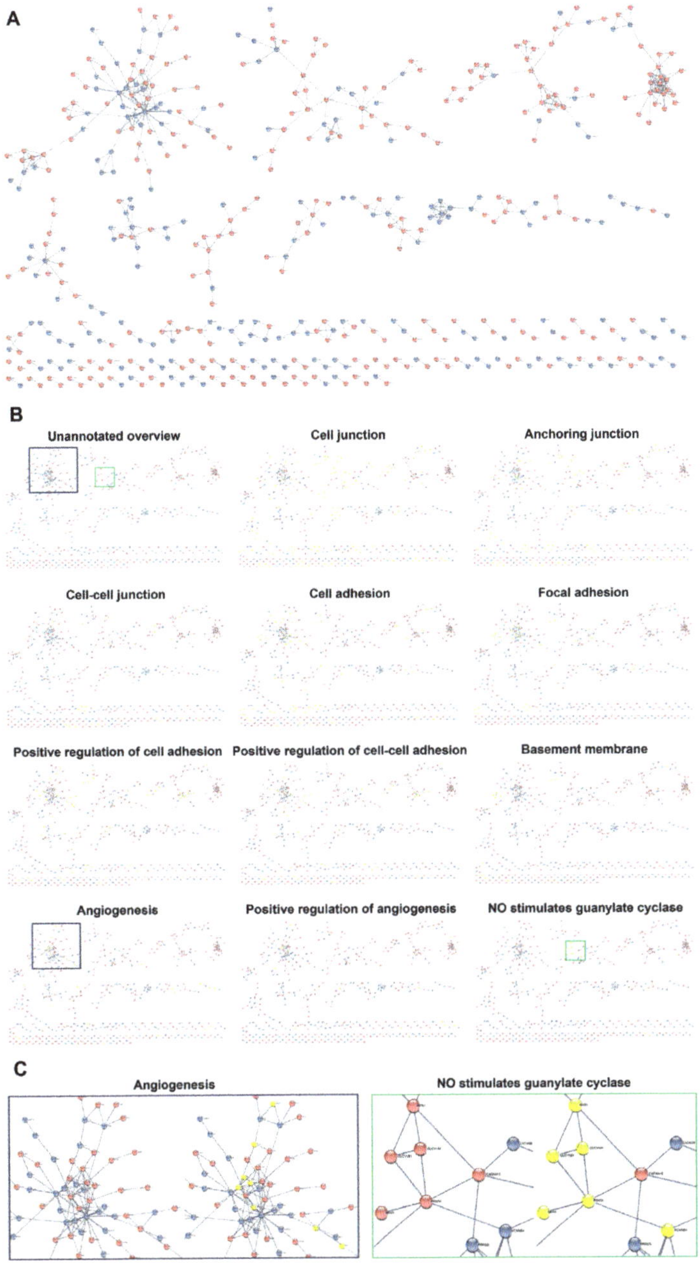

Figure 7. Bioinformatic analysis of gene–gene interactions between primary human coronary endothelial cells (HCAECs) and human internal thoracic artery endothelial cells (HITAECs) cultured at static conditions. (**A**) Overview of gene–gene interactions between HCAECs (blue colour) and HITAECs (red colour) cultured under laminar flow; (**B**) annotation of the interacting genes related to the specific molecular terms (yellow colour) in comparison with unannotated overview; and (**C**) annotations of clustered interacting genes in selected molecular terms: angiogenesis (demarcated by blue contour) and stimulation of guanylate cyclase by nitric oxide (demarcated by green contour).

3. Discussion

Although molecular heterogeneity between different EC lineages [10–15] and ECs in distinct organs of the human body is well established [6–9], its pathophysiological and clinical significance remain unclear. CABG surgery, which is a seminal technique to treat coronary artery disease, employs the construction of an artificial bypass between the coronary artery and aorta (if using SV) or between the coronary artery and ITA (in the case of single or bilateral ITA grafting) and therefore links the coronary artery with a venous or arterial conduit, bringing their ECs into close proximity [24–27]. MAG, a CABG variation which employs both ITAs or the left ITA and radial artery to build a bypass, has been associated with better survival, freedom from major adverse cardiovascular events, and quality of life in comparison with SAG which relies on using ITA and SV [33–44]. Earlier, we showed beneficial effects of co-culturing HCAECs and HITAECs (i.e., elevated nitric oxide synthase expression, downregulation of endothelial-to-mesenchymal transition transcription factors Snail and Slug, and release of pro-angiogenic molecules) in comparison with culturing HCAECs together with human SV ECs (HSaVEC) [91].

Hence, we suggested that synergistic interactions between the coronary and ITA endothelium are among the factors determining better clinical outcomes of MAG, in addition to (1) similar microanatomy, as the coronary artery, ITA, and radial artery are muscular arteries which tunica media is delineated with internal and external elastic laminae and contains multiple layers of VSMCs [60–69]; (2) anti-fibrotic, anti-atherogenic, and anti-proteolytic chemical composition depleted in collagen and enriched with decorin in combination with curbed protease activity in arteries [70–73]; (3) contractile phenotype of arterial VSMCs [60,74–83]; (4) favourable secretory profile of arterial ECs, which release increased levels of vasodilators (such as nitric oxide) and pro-angiogenic molecules [84–94]; (5) resistance of arterial cell populations to oxidative stress, an imperative consequence of inflammation [92–94]; and (6) better vasoreactivity [95–99] and anti-thrombotic profile [100,101] of arterial ECs and VSMCs. As ECs play a key role in maintaining physiological vasodilation in response to blood pressure, have angiocrine function in terms of released extracellular vesicles and soluble factors, and ensure resistance of blood vessels to thrombosis [1–5], reciprocal and beneficial interactions between HCAECs and HITAECs might be of pathophysiological significance but largely depend on their heterogeneity. In this study, we aimed to perform an unbiased analysis of major proteins and global gene expression in HCAECs and HITAECs lysates by means of UHPLC-MS/MS and RNA sequencing, respectively. Rather than relying on single specific markers, we have analysed bioinformatic categories (i.e., molecular terms) encompassing the entire set of genes or proteins which are engaged in various biological processes (including biochemical pathways), share certain molecular functions, or are located in distinct cellular or extracellular compartments. Pathway enrichment analysis of molecular terms through Gene Ontology, UniProtKB Keywords, Reactome, and Kyoto Encyclopedia of Genes and Genomes (KEGG) databases included calculation of observed-verses-expected number of DEGs or DEPs in bioinformatic categories related to the structure and assembly of the endothelial monolayer (EC-ECM and EC-BM adhesion, organisation of intercellular junctions, cytoskeletal rearrangements, and synthesis and folding of ECM components) and to endothelial function (ubiquitination and autophagy, intracellular transport and extracellular secretion, bioenergetic processes, DNA repair, transcription, and translation).

We found that both HCAECs and HITAECs showed the molecular signatures of extracellular matrix (ECM) production, basement membrane (BM) synthesis, cell–cell and cell–ECM interactions, and extracellular vesicle (EV) release. Formation of BM, collagen biosynthesis and folding, and organisation of cell–cell contacts were particularly pronounced in HCAECs, whilst molecular signatures of pro-inflammatory signaling, protein and nitrogen generation, and ribosome biogenesis were overrepresented in HITAECs. Though transcriptome analysis showed notable heterogeneity between HCAECs and HITAECs, no specific markers of either EC type have been found at the protein level. As the molecular categories which were upregulated in HCAECs and HITAECs were coherent, we suggested synergistic interactions between these ECs, in agreement with our previous findings [91]. In accord to this hypothesis, the bioinformatic analysis of the molecular interactions revealed that arterial homeostasis pathways are significantly enriched in the dataset of DEPs and DEGs between HCAECs and HITAECs. Collectively, these findings provide a molecular rationale for extended use of ITA grafts and particularly for the ROMA trial, which is now conducted to evaluate the clinical arguments for prioritising MAG over SAG and to provide a definitive answer whether total arterial revascularisation and bilateral ITA grafting are beneficial at least for certain patient cohorts.

Bioinformatic analysis of proteomic and transcriptomic data obtained from three sequential experiments revealed 244 DEPs and from 729 to 1014 DEGs upregulated in HCAECs, 287 DEPs and from 849 to 926 DEGs upregulated in HITAECs, and 2794 proteins as well as from 17,789 to 19,228 genes which have not been differentially expressed between HCAECs and HITAECs (if applying a logarithmical fold change ≥ 1 and FDR-corrected p value ≤ 0.05). Moreover, the HCAEC/HITAEC interactome (i.e., the DEPs and DEGs having $\geq$1 interaction) included 254 DEPs, 516 DEGs at laminar flow, and 466 DEGs under static conditions. Among the molecular terms differentially expressed in both HCAECs and HITAECs were those accountable for the biosynthesis and folding of the ECM and BM components (e.g., collagen), adhesion of ECs to the ECM and BM, and formation of intercellular junctions. Previous studies of arterial wall composition have shown that type I, type III, type IV, type V, and type VI collagen, elastin, fibronectin, vitronectin, chondroitin sulfate, dermatan sulfate, decorin, versican, and biglycan are the major components of medial and adventitial ECM (although medial ECM is enriched and adventitial ECM is deficient in elastin), whilst the BM consists of type IV, type XV, and type XVIII collagen, laminin, nidogen, perlecan, agrin, and fibronectin [102–106]. Adhesion of ECs to the ECM and BM is largely mediated by integrins, whereas junctions between the ECs are formed by claudins and occludin (tight junctions constructing the intercellular barrier near the luminal surface), VE-cadherin (adherens junctions located mostly at the lateral surfaces joining adjacent ECs within the monolayer), and connexins (gap junctions passing ions and small molecules through the intercellular channels) [107–110]. Assembly of endothelial monolayer and proper regulation of endothelial integrity, geometry, and permeability ensure original specification, physiological elongation, and favourable molecular profile of arterial ECs at high shear stress [111–113]. In addition, chemical composition of cell membrane, which acts as a scaffold for the formation of intercellular junctions, also regulates endothelial response to high shear stress which is typical for arteries [114]. Therefore, similarity of molecular terms related to the ECM, BM, and formation of intercellular junctions in HCAECs and HITAECs suggested the structural congruence of HCAECs and HITAECs in the context of artificial coronary bypass. Intriguingly, glycosaminoglycans of the BM such as chondroitin sulfate, heparan sulfate, or dermatan sulfate also compose the glycocalyx, a meshwork of membrane-bound proteoglycans and glycoproteins lining the luminal surface of the ECs, and upregulation of these molecules in both HCAECs and HITAECs is fruitful to maintain endothelial physiology [115–118].

Further, HCAECs and HITAECs overexpressed numerous functional molecular terms including synthesis of mitochondrial ribosomes, mitochondrial transcription and translation, energy generation in mitochondria, Ca^{2+}-dependent signaling, secretion of extracellular vesicles, DNA metabolism and repair, RNA processing, ubiquitination, and autophagy. Such upregulation patterns suggested rapid metabolism to support the biosynthesis of ECM and BM components indicated above, similar to the scenario occurring in tissue-engineered vascular grafts during the replacement of biodegradable polymers with newly formed vascular tissue [119,120]. Another reason for active energy consumption is the need to support and regulate endothelial barrier semi-permeability during the vasoreactivity and regulation of blood pressure. This task requires large amounts of ATP to rearrange the intercellular junctions and maintain intracellular Ca^{2+} metabolism, which is also indispensable for the enzymatic digestion and biosynthesis of nitric oxide and prostacyclin, the potent vasodilators [121–124]. With regards to nucleotide metabolism, DNA repair defects have been associated with age-related and premature endothelial dysfunction which develops as reduced nitric oxide release and chronic low-grade inflammation [125–131]. The same has been reported for decreased ubiquitination and impaired autophagy, as removal of dysfunctional organelles, supramolecular complexes, and molecules also becomes compromised with age [132–134], and ubiquitination participates in regulating rearrangements of intercellular junctions and integrity of the endothelial barrier [135,136]. Notably, both HCAECs and HITAECs were characterised by an upregulated export of extracellular vesicles which serve as shuttles for juxtacrine and paracrine protein transfer and mediate protective effects on heart [137] and blood vessels [138,139], having been proposed as potential therapeutic agent to treat myocardial ischemia [140–142].

Importantly, the dataset of interacting DEPs and DEGs between HCAECs and HITAECs was enriched with molecular terms related to arterial homeostasis such as those related to cell–cell and cell–matrix junctions or their positive regulation, basement membrane assembly, angiogenesis (in particular sprouting angiogenesis) and its positive regulation, proliferation and migration of ECs (as these processes are indispensable for angiogenesis), nitric oxide biosynthesis, and formation of elastic fibers. Along with coherent structural and functional molecular terms enriched in HCAECs and HITAECs proteome/transcriptome, such an in silico interactome profile suggests the synergistic impact of HCAECs and HITAECs into the functioning of the continuous endothelial monolayer within the coronary bypass in the CABG surgery context.

Although we confirmed the substantial molecular heterogeneity of HCAECs and HITAECs (244 and 287 DEPs, respectively), we did not find any definitive protein marker (having a logarithmical fold change > 5 and relevant for endothelial biology) specific for either of the mentioned ECs, and multiple molecular terms were concurrently upregulated in both of these cell lines. This suggested that differences in biochemical pathways do not affect their paracrine interactions to a major extent and pointed to their functional congruence in the context of artificial anastomosis. Likewise, the absence of specific protein markers of distinct EC lineages in adventitial vasa vasorum within the SV of patients advised for CABG surgery has been previously reported by our group [143,144]. Although the time of EC culture under laminar flow and at static conditions have not coincided and therefore these experiments could not be compared head-to-head, the culture of ECs at laminar flow is preferrable to recapitulate the physiological conditions. The comparison of transcriptomic and proteomic data demonstrated that number of DEGs (from 729 to 1014) exceeds the number of DEPs (from 244 to 287) 3- to 5-fold if applying the same logarithmical fold change ($\geq$2), which is probably because of post-transcriptional and translational regulation and higher coverage of transcriptomic analysis. The study limitations included the inability to compare the proteomic data at laminar flow and under static conditions as the amount of total protein extracted from ECs cultured in flow chambers was insufficient to perform an adequate UHPLC-MS/MS analysis.

To conclude, we showed that the molecular profile of HCAECs and HITAECs has common upregulated molecular terms which are related to the structure of the endothelial monolayer and describe numerous aspects of EC physiology, whilst the HCAEC/HITAEC interactome is enriched with arterial homeostasis pathways. Taken together, these findings provide the arguments confirming molecular congruence of the coronary artery and ITA in the context of bypass surgery that contributes to better outcomes of MAG in comparison with SAG. Although molecular heterogeneity between HCAECs and HITAECs is undisputed and is quantified by up to $\approx$300 DEPs and $\approx$1000 DEGs, neither of these EC lines showed any distinctive protein markers.

4. Materials and Methods

4.1. Cell Culture

For the experiments, we used commercially available primary HCAECs (300K-05a, Cell Applications, San Diego, CA, USA) and HITAECs (308K-05a, Cell Applications, San Diego, CA, USA) which have been cryopreserved at the 2nd passage. Cell culture was performed as in our previous studies [91,145–147]. Briefly, we used MesoEndo Growth Medium (212-500, Cell Applications, San Diego, CA, USA), trypsin/ethylenediaminetetraacetic acid kit (090K, Cell Applications, San Diego, CA, USA), and T-75 flasks (90076, Techno Plastic Products, Trasadingen, Switzerland) for subculturing both types of ECs. Passaging was carried out at 80–90% confluence. After 3 passages (i.e., at the 5th passage in total), HCAECs and HITAECs were seeded into flow channel slides (80126, Ibidi, Gräfelfing, Germany) or in fresh T-75 (90076, Techno Plastic Products, Trasadingen, Switzerland) for culturing cells under flow or under static conditions, respectively. In flow culture studies, HCAECs and HITAECs were seeded into flow channel slides (80126, Ibidi, Gräfelfing, Germany) at 90% confluence (≈350,000 cells per slide), left for 16 h for proper adhesion, and then cultured under laminar flow (15 dyn/cm^2) using the respective perfusion set of 50 cm length, 1.6 mm internal diameter, and 10 mL reservoirs (Yellow/Green, 10964, Ibidi, Gräfelfing, Germany) in the flow culture system (Ibidi Pump System Quad, Ibidi, Gräfelfing, Germany) for 48 h. In static conditions, HCAECs and HITAECs were also incubated for 48 h after reaching >95% confluence (i.e., after an endothelial monolayer was established). Standard cell culture conditions (37 °C, 95% air: 5% CO_2 atmosphere, high humidity, and sterile conditions) were continuously maintained (MCO-18AIC, Sanyo, Tokyo, Japan).

4.2. *Whole-Transcriptome Analysis*

Whole-transcriptome analysis was conducted employing RNA sequencing, which was carried out in SB RAS Genomics Core Facility (Institute of Chemical Biology and Fundamental Medicine of the Siberian Branch of the Russian Academy of Sciences, Novosibirsk). Upon the withdrawal of culture medium and washing in ice-cold phosphate buffered saline (PBS, pH 7.4, 10010023, Thermo Fisher Scientific, Waltham, MA, USA), cells (one T-75 flask (equal to ≈ 3,000,000 cells), or 4 flow channel slides (equal to ≈ 400,000 cells), n = 3 flasks or 3 four-slide batches of flow channel slides per cell line) were lysed with TRIzol (15596018, Thermo Fisher Scientific, Waltham, MA, USA) with the following total RNA isolation (Purelink RNA Micro Scale Kit, 12183016, Thermo Fisher Scientific, Waltham, MA, USA) and DNAse treatment (DNASE70, Sigma-Aldrich, Saint Louis, MO, USA) according to the manufacturer's protocols. The RNA integrity index (RIN) was assessed using an RNA 6000 Pico Kit (5067-1513, Agilent Technologies, Santa Clara, CA, USA) and Bioanalyzer 2100 (Agilent Technologies, Santa Clara, CA, USA). RNA quantification was carried out using NanoDrop 2000 (Thermo Fisher Scientific, Waltham, MA, USA) and Qubit 4 (Thermo Fisher Scientific, Waltham, MA, USA).

For the 1 μg of isolated RNA, we performed rRNA depletion (RiboCop rRNA Depletion Kit V1.2, 037.96, Lexogen, Wien, Austria) followed by DNA library preparation (MGIEasy RNA Directional Library Prep Set, MGI Tech, Shenzhen, China) and quality control (High Sensitivity DNA Kit, 5067-4626, Agilent Technologies, Santa Clara, CA, USA). DNA libraries were then quantified by qPCR (CFX96 Touch, Bio-Rad, Hercules, CA, USA), pooled in equimolar amounts, and sequenced (MGIseq-2000, MGI Tech, Shenzhen, China) using a DNBSEQ-G400RS High-throughput Sequencing Set (FCL PE100, 1000016950, MGI Tech, Shenzhen, China).

Read mapping to the human genome (hg38) was conducted using STAR v2.7.6a [148]. Gene expression (exon coverage) was evaluated by HTSeq-count v0.12.4 [149] using Ensembl annotation (v.38.93). To identify DEGs, we used DESeq2 package (https://bioconductor.org/packages/release/bioc/html/DESeq2.html (accessed on 25 August 2023)) [150]. DEGs were defined as those with a logarithmical fold change ≥ 1 and false discovery rate (FDR)-corrected p value ≤ 0.05. Bioinformatic analysis was performed using Gene Ontology [151,152], UniProtKB Keywords [153], Reactome [154,155], and Kyoto Encyclopedia of Genes and Genomes (KEGG) [156,157] databases. The RNA sequencing data have been deposited in Sequence Read Archive (accession number: PRJNA891895), "https://www.ncbi.nlm.nih.gov/bioproject/PRJNA891895/" (accessed on 25 August 2023).

4.3. Proteomic Profiling

Proteomic profiling was performed by means of UHPLC-MS/MS with ion mobility in the Centre for Molecular and Cell Technologies (Saint Petersburg State University Research Park). Upon the withdrawal of culture medium and washing in ice-cold phosphate buffered saline (PBS, pH 7.4, 10010023, Thermo Fisher Scientific, Waltham, MA, USA), HCAECs and HITAECs (one T-75 flask, equal to ≈ 3,000,000 cells, $n = 3$ flasks) were lysed with a radioimmunoprecipitation assay (RIPA) buffer (89901, Thermo Fisher Scientific, Waltham, MA, USA) supplied with a Halt protease and phosphatase inhibitor cocktail (78444, Thermo Fisher Scientific, Waltham, MA, USA) according to the manufacturer's protocol and centrifuged at 14,000× *g* (Microfuge 20R, Beckman Coulter, Brea, CA, USA) for 15 min. Protein quantification was conducted using a BCA Protein Assay Kit (23227, Thermo Fisher Scientific, Waltham, MA, USA) and Multiskan Sky microplate spectrophotometer (Thermo Fisher Scientific, Waltham, MA, USA) in accordance with the manufacturer's protocol.

To prepare the samples for the tryptic digestion, we first removed the RIPA buffer by 1-h acetone precipitation (650501, Sigma-Aldrich, Saint Louis, MO, USA) at −20 °C and centrifugation at 13,000× *g* for 15 min at 4 °C (Microfuge 20R, Beckman Coulter, Brea, CA, USA). Then, the protein pellet was resuspended in 250 µL acetone for 15 min at −20 °C and centrifugation was repeated. After removal of the supernatant and evaporating the residual acetone for 5–10 min, the protein pellet was resuspended in 8 mol/L urea (U5128, Sigma-Aldrich, Saint Louis, MO, USA) in 50 mmol/L ammonium bicarbonate (09830, Sigma-Aldrich, Saint Louis, MO, USA), incubated for 20 min on ice (at 4 °C), ultrasonicated in a water bath (Sapphire, Moscow, Russia), and incubated for another 10 min on ice (at 4 °C). The protein concentration was measured by a Qubit 4 fluorometer (Q33238, Thermo Fisher Scientific, Waltham, MA, USA) with a QuDye Protein Quantification Kit (25102, Lumiprobe, Cockeysville, MD, USA) according to the manufacturer's protocol. Protein samples (15 µg) were then incubated in 5 mmol/L dithiothreitol (D0632, Sigma-Aldrich, Saint Louis, MO, USA) for 1 h at 37 °C with the subsequent incubation in 15 mmol/L iodoacetamide for 30 min in the dark at room temperature (I1149, Sigma-Aldrich, Saint Louis, MO, USA). Next, the samples were diluted with 7 volumes of 50 mmol/L ammonium bicarbonate and incubated for 16 h at 37 °C with 300 ng of trypsin (1:50 trypsin:protein ratio; VA9000, Promega, Madison, WI, USA). The peptides were then desalted with stage tips (Tips-RPS-M.T2.200.96, Affinisep, Le Houlme, France) according to the manufacturer's protocol using methanol (1880092500, Sigma-Aldrich, Saint Louis, MO, USA), acetonitrile (1000291000, Sigma-Aldrich, Saint Louis, MO, USA), and 0.1% formic acid (33015, Sigma-Aldrich, Saint Louis, MO, USA). Desalted peptides were dried in a centrifuge concentrator (Concentrator plus, Eppendorf, Hamburg, Germany) for 3 h and finally dissolved in water for chromatography (1153334000, Sigma-Aldrich, Saint Louis, MO, USA) supplied with 0.1% formic acid (33015, Sigma-Aldrich, Saint Louis, MO, USA) for the further shotgun proteomics analysis.

Approximately 500 ng of peptides per sample were used for shotgun proteomics analysis by UHPLC-MS/MS with ion mobility in a trapped ion mobility spectrometry time-of-flight (TimsToF) Pro mass spectrometer with a nanoElute UHPLC system (Bruker, Billerica, MA, USA). UHPLC was performed in the two-column separation mode with an Acclaim PepMap 5 mm Trap Cartridge (Thermo Fisher Scientific) and a Bruker Fifteen separation column (C18 ReproSil AQ, 150 mm × 0.75 mm, 1.9 µm, 120 A; Bruker, Billerica, MA, USA) in a gradient mode with 400 nL/min flow rate and 40 °C. Phase A was water/0.1% formic acid (33015, Sigma-Aldrich, Saint Louis, MO, USA) and phase B was acetonitrile/0.1% formic acid (1000291000, Sigma-Aldrich, Saint Louis, MO, USA; 33015, Sigma-Aldrich, Saint Louis, MO, USA). The gradient was from 2% to 30% phase B for 42 min, then to 95% phase B for 6 min with subsequent washing with 95% phase B for 6 min. Before each sample, trap and separation columns were equilibrated with 10 and 4 column volumes, respectively.

CaptiveSpray ion source was used for electrospray ionization with 1600 V of capillary voltage, 3 L/min N_2 flow, and 180 °C source temperature. The mass spectrometry acquisition was performed in data-dependent acquisition parallel accumulation serial fragmentation (DDA-PASEF) mode with 0.5 s cycle in positive polarity with the fragmentation of ions with at least two charges in an m/z range from 100 to 1700 and ion mobility range from 0.85 to 1.30 1/K0. Protein identification was performed in PEAKS Studio Xpro software (a license granted to St. Petersburg State University; Bioinformatics Solutions, Waterloo, ON, Canada) "https://www.bioinfor.com/peaks-software/" (accessed on 25 August 2023) using the human protein SwissProt database "https://www.uniprot.org/" (accessed on 20 July 2022; organism: Human [9606]; uploaded on 2 March 2021; 20,394 sequences) and protein contaminants database CRAP (version of 4 March 2019). The search parameters were as follows: parent mass error tolerance 10 ppm and fragment mass error tolerance 0.05 ppm, protein and peptide FDR <1% and 0.1%, respectively, two possible missed cleavage sites, and proteins with $\geq$2 unique peptides. Cysteine carbamidomethylation was set as fixed modification. Methionine oxidation, N-terminal acetylation, and asparagine and glutamine deamidation were set as variable modifications.

Then, label-free quantification by peak area under the curve was used for further analysis in R (version 3.6.1; R Core Team, 2019). The biological groups were qualitatively compared by the "VennDiagram" package "https://cran.r-project.org/web/packages/VennDiagram/index.html" (accessed on 25 August 2023) [158]. Then, proteins with missing values in >2 replicates were removed, and the rest of the missing values were imputed by the k-nearest neighbours algorithm. Multivariate data analysis for quantitative protein expression data was performed by non-metric multidimensional scaling using the "Vegan" package "https://cran.r-project.org/web/packages/vegan/index.html" (accessed on 25 August 2023) [159] and by clusterisation of samples by sparse partial least squares discriminant analysis in the "MixOmics" package "https://bioconductor.org/packages/release/bioc/html/mixOmics.html" (accessed on 25 August 2023) [160]. Differentially expressed proteins were identified through the moderated *t*-test by the "limma" package "https://bioconductor.org/packages/release/bioc/html/limma.html" (accessed on 25 August 2023) [161] and were defined as those with a logarithmical fold change $\geq$1 and FDR-corrected p value $\leq$ 0.05. Pathway enrichment analysis of differentially expressed proteins was performed using Gene Ontology [151,152], UniProtKB Keywords [153], Reactome [154,155], and Kyoto Encyclopedia of Genes and Genomes (KEGG) [156,157] databases. The "ggplot2" "https://cran.r-project.org/web/packages/ggplot2/index.html" (accessed on 25 August 2023) [162] and "EnhancedVolcano" "https://bioconductor.org/packages/release/bioc/html/EnhancedVolcano.html" (accessed on 25 August 2023) [163] packages were used for visualisation. The mass spectrometry proteomics data have been deposited to the ProteomeXchange Consortium via the PRIDE [164] partner repository with the dataset identifier PXD037861.

4.4. Bioinformatic Analysis of the HCAEC/HITAEC Interactome

To analyse the profile of interacting DEPs and DEGs in HCAECs and HITAECs, we applied the Cytoscape software (version 3.10.1, Cytoscape Consortium, USA) [165] with a stringApp utilising the following workflow: (1) filtration of DEPs and DEGs having $\geq$1 interaction; (2) colour mapping in order to distinguish interacting DEPs and DEGs between HCAECs and HITAECs; (3) pathway enrichment analysis using GO, Reactome, UniProtKB, and KEGG terms; and (4) selection of such molecular terms relevant for arterial homeostasis.

4.5. RT-qPCR Analysis

Upon the RNA extraction for whole-transcriptome analysis, we performed reverse transcription using a High-Capacity cDNA Reverse Transcription Kit (4368814, Thermo Fisher Scientific, Waltham, MA, USA) and then measured the gene expression level by RT-qPCR. The same RNA aliquots have been used to allocate RNA for RNA-seq and RT-qPCR in order to ensure the correct verification of whole-transcriptome analysis. RT-qPCR was conducted using customised primers (500 nmol/L each, Evrogen, Moscow, Russia, Supplementary Table S40), cDNA (20 ng), and PowerUp SYBR Green Master Mix (A25778,

Thermo Fisher Scientific, Waltham, MA, USA) according to the manufacturer's protocol for Tm $\geq$ 60 °C (fast cycling mode). Technical replicates (n = 3 per each sample) were performed in all qPCR experiments. Quantification of the mRNA levels was performed by calculation of ΔCt and by using the $2^{-\Delta\Delta Ct}$ method. Relative transcript levels were expressed as a value relative to the average of three housekeeping genes (*GAPDH*, *ACTB*, and *B2M*) and to the HCAECs group ($2^{-\Delta\Delta Ct}$).

4.6. Western Blotting

Equal amounts of the same protein lysates that were selected for proteomic profiling (10 µg per sample) were prepared for fluorescent Western blotting as previously described [120]. A Chameleon Duo Pre-Stained Protein Ladder (928–60000, LI-COR Biosciences, Lincoln, NE, USA) was loaded as a molecular weight marker. The proteins were separated, and the protein transfer was performed using nitrocellulose transfer stacks as previously described [120]. Nitrocellulose membranes were then incubated in protein-free Block'n'Boost! solution (K-028, Molecular Wings, Kemerovo, Russia) for 1 h to prevent non-specific binding.

The blots were probed with (1) rabbit antibodies to VCAM1 (1:250 dilution, SL0920R, Sunlong Biotech, Hangzhou, China) and mouse antibodies to GAPDH (1:1000, SLM33033M, Sunlong Biotech, Hangzhou, China); (2) rabbit antibodies to ICAM1 (1:250, SL0608R, Sunlong Biotech, Hangzhou, China) and mouse antibodies to CD31 (1:2000, ab9498, Abcam, Cambridge, UK); (3) rabbit antibodies to Snail and Slug (1:250, ab180714, Abcam, Cambridge, UK) and mouse antibodies to CD31 (1:2000, ab9498, Abcam, Cambridge, UK); (4) rabbit antibodies to ZEB1 (70512, Cell Signaling Technology, Danvers, MA, USA) and mouse antibodies to TWIST1 (1:100, sc-81417, Santa Cruz Biotechnology, Dallas, TX, USA); (5) rabbit antibodies to KLF2 (1:200, SL2772R, Sunlong Biotech, Hangzhou, China) and mouse antibodies to TWIST1 (1:200, sc-81417, Santa Cruz Biotechnology, Dallas, TX, USA); (6) rabbit antibodies to KLF4 (1:500, ab215036, Abcam, Cambridge, UK) and mouse antibodies to eNOS (1:500, SLM33176M, Sunlong Biotech, Hangzhou, China); and (7) rabbit antibodies to NRF2 (1:200, ab62352, Abcam, Cambridge, UK) and mouse antibodies to GAPDH (1:1000, SLM33033M, Sunlong Biotech, Hangzhou, China). IRDye 680RD-conjugated goat anti-mouse (926-68070, LI-COR Biosciences, Lincoln, NE, USA) and IRDye 800CW-conjugated goat anti-rabbit (926-32211, LI-COR Biosciences, Lincoln, NE, USA) or IRDye 680RD-conjugated goat anti-rabbit (926-68071, LI-COR Biosciences, Lincoln, NE, USA) and IRDye 800CW-conjugated goat anti-mouse (926-32210, LI-COR Biosciences, Lincoln, NE, USA) IgG secondary antibodies were used at a 1:1000 dilution.

Incubation with the antibodies and fluorescent detection was performed using an Odyssey XF imaging system (LI-COR Biosciences, Lincoln, NE, USA) at a 700 nm channel (685 nm excitation and 730 nm emission). Total protein normalisation was conducted after the fluorescent detection using 0.1% Fast Green FCF (F8130, Solarbio Life Sciences, Beijing, China) as previously described [120]. The total protein visualisation was performed using an Odyssey XF imaging system (LI-COR Biosciences, Lincoln, NE, USA) in a 600 nm channel (520 nm excitation and 600 nm emission).

4.7. Analysis of Bypass Dysfunctions after CABG Surgery at 10 Years of Follow-Up

To analyse the long-term efficiency of SV verses ITA grafts applied for creating a bypass during CABG surgery, we collected the data from 102 case histories of patients who underwent CABG and conducted a repeated coronary angiography (GE Healthcare Innova 3100 Cardiac Angiography System, General Electric Healthcare, Chicago, IL, USA) at 10 years of follow-up. The study was conducted according to the latest revision of the Declaration of Helsinki (2013), and the study protocol was approved by the Local Ethical Committee of the Research Institute for Complex Issues of Cardiovascular Diseases (Kemerovo, Russia, protocol code 021/2023, date of approval: 2 February 2023). Written informed consent has been provided by all study participants after receiving a full explanation of the study's purposes. In total, we analysed 311 bypasses between (1) the SV and right coronary artery, obtuse marginal artery, or diagonal branches of the left anterior descending artery; (2) the left ITA and left anterior descending artery, obtuse marginal artery, or diagonal branches of the left anterior descending artery; and (3) the right ITA and right coronary artery, obtuse marginal artery, or left anterior descending artery. Adverse outcomes included development of atherosclerosis in the coronary artery, competitive flow, and graft degeneration at 10 years of follow-up. Favourable outcomes included freedom from adverse outcomes at 10 years of follow-up. Comparison of the proportions was carried out using a Pearson's chi-squared test with Yates's correction for continuity.

5. Conclusions

Bioinformatic analysis of RNA sequencing and proteomic profiling data showed that the molecular heterogeneity of HCAECs and HITAECs does not contradict their functional congruence. HCAECs and HITAECs had similar upregulated molecular terms related to their structure (adhesion to ECM and BM, biosynthesis and folding of ECM and BM, and assembly of intercellular junctions) and function (biogenesis of mitochondrial ribosomes, mitochondrial transcription and translation, energy generation in mitochondria, Ca^{2+}-dependent signaling, secretion of extracellular vesicles, DNA metabolism and repair, and RNA processing and autophagy), and no specific protein markers have been revealed for either of the mentioned EC lines. This can be considered as a molecular basis of their synergistic effects which have been revealed earlier in a co-culture model. The coherence of HCAECs and HITAECs molecular profiles might also better explain the mid- and long-term outcomes of MAG, a CABG surgery modality including the use of >1 artery to create a bypass.

Supplementary Materials: The following supporting information can be downloaded at: https://www.mdpi.com/article/10.3390/ijms241915032/s1.

Author Contributions: Conceptualization, A.F. and A.K.; data curation, A.F., A.L., M.K. and A.K.; formal analysis, A.F., A.L., M.K., B.Z., A.T., D.S., V.M., A.S., E.G., Y.M. and A.K.; funding acquisition, A.K.; investigation, A.F., A.L., M.K., B.Z., A.T., D.S., V.M., A.S., E.G., Y.M. and A.K.; methodology, A.F., A.L., M.K., B.Z., A.T., D.S., V.M., A.S., E.G., Y.M. and A.K.; project administration, A.K.; resources, A.L., M.K. and A.K.; software, A.L., M.K. and A.K.; supervision, A.F. and A.K.; validation, A.F., A.L., M.K. and A.K.; visualisation, A.L., M.K. and A.K.; writing—original draft, A.F., A.L., M.K. and A.K.; writing—review and editing, A.K. All authors have read and agreed to the published version of the manuscript.

Funding: This study was supported by the Ministry of Science and Higher Education of the Russian Federation (National Project Science and Universities) within the Complex Program of Basic Research under the Siberian Branch of the Russian Academy of Sciences within the Basic Research Topic of the Research Institute for Complex Issues of Cardiovascular Diseases No. 0419-2021-0001 "Novel anti-atherosclerotic therapies and machine learning solutions for automated diagnosis and prognostication of cardiovascular disease." The APC was funded by the Ministry of Science and Higher Education of the Russian Federation.

Institutional Review Board Statement: This study was conducted according to the Good Clinical Practice guidelines and the latest revision of the Declaration of Helsinki (2013), and the study protocol was approved by the Local Ethical Committee of the Research Institute for Complex Issues of Cardiovascular Diseases (Kemerovo, Russia, protocol code 021/2023, approved on 2 February 2023).

Informed Consent Statement: Written informed consent was provided by all study participants after receiving a full explanation of the study's purposes.

Data Availability Statement: The datasets used and analysed during the current study are available from the corresponding author upon reasonable request.

Conflicts of Interest: The authors declare no conflict of interest. The funders had no role in the design of the study; in the collection, analyses, or interpretation of data; in the writing of the manuscript; or in the decision to publish the results.

References

1. Rafii, S.; Butler, J.M.; Ding, B.S. Angiocrine Functions of Organ-Specific Endothelial Cells. *Nature* **2016**, *529*, 316–325. [CrossRef]
2. Pasquier, J.; Ghiabi, P.; Chouchane, L.; Razzouk, K.; Rafii, S.; Rafii, A. Angiocrine Endothelium: From Physiology to Cancer. *J. Transl. Med.* **2020**, *18*, 52. [CrossRef] [PubMed]
3. Gomez-Salinero, J.M.; Itkin, T.; Rafii, S. Developmental Angiocrine Diversification of Endothelial Cells for Organotypic Regeneration. *Dev. Cell* **2021**, *56*, 3042–3051. [CrossRef] [PubMed]
4. Kutikhin, A.G.; Shishkova, D.K.; Velikanova, E.A.; Sinitsky, M.Y.; Sinitskaya, A.V.; Markova, V.E. Endothelial Dysfunction in the Context of Blood-Brain Barrier Modeling. *J. Evol. Biochem. Physiol.* **2022**, *58*, 781–806. [CrossRef] [PubMed]
5. Bishop, D.; Schwarz, Q.; Wiszniak, S. Endothelial-Derived Angiocrine Factors as Instructors of Embryonic Development. *Front. Cell Dev. Biol.* **2023**, *11*, 1172114. [CrossRef]
6. Feng, W.; Chen, L.; Nguyen, P.K.; Wu, S.M.; Li, G. Single Cell Analysis of Endothelial Cells Identified Organ-Specific Molecular Signatures and Heart-Specific Cell Populations and Molecular Features. *Front. Cardiovasc. Med.* **2019**, *6*, 165. [CrossRef]
7. Paik, D.T.; Tian, L.; Williams, I.M.; Rhee, S.; Zhang, H.; Liu, C.; Mishra, R.; Wu, S.M.; Red-Horse, K.; Wu, J.C. Single-Cell RNA Sequencing Unveils Unique Transcriptomic Signatures of Organ-Specific Endothelial Cells. *Circulation* **2020**, *142*, 1848–1862. [CrossRef]
8. Stone, O.A.; Zhou, B.; Red-Horse, K.; Stainier, D.Y.R. Endothelial Ontogeny and the Establishment of Vascular Heterogeneity. *Bioessays* **2021**, *43*, e2100036. [CrossRef]
9. Jambusaria, A.; Hong, Z.; Zhang, L.; Srivastava, S.; Jana, A.; Toth, P.T.; Dai, Y.; Malik, A.B.; Rehman, J. Endothelial Heterogeneity across Distinct Vascular Beds during Homeostasis and Inflammation. *Elife* **2020**, *9*, e51413. [CrossRef]
10. Dejana, E.; Hirschi, K.K.; Simons, M. The Molecular Basis of Endothelial Cell Plasticity. *Nat. Commun.* **2017**, *8*, 14361. [CrossRef]
11. Jakab, M.; Augustin, H.G. Understanding Angiodiversity: Insights from Single Cell Biology. *Development* **2020**, *147*, dev146621. [CrossRef] [PubMed]
12. Greenspan, L.J.; Weinstein, B.M. To Be or Not to Be: Endothelial Cell Plasticity in Development, Repair, and Disease. *Angiogenesis* **2021**, *24*, 251–269. [CrossRef]
13. Naiche, L.A.; Villa, S.R.; Kitajewski, J.K. Endothelial Cell Fate Determination: A Top Notch Job in Vascular Decision-Making. *Cold Spring Harb. Perspect. Med.* **2022**, *12*, a041183. [CrossRef]
14. Becker, L.M.; Chen, S.H.; Rodor, J.; de Rooij, L.P.M.H.; Baker, A.H.; Carmeliet, P. Deciphering Endothelial Heterogeneity in Health and Disease at Single-Cell Resolution: Progress and Perspectives. *Cardiovasc. Res.* **2023**, *119*, 6–27. [CrossRef]
15. Trimm, E.; Red-Horse, K. Vascular Endothelial Cell Development and Diversity. *Nat. Rev. Cardiol.* **2023**, *20*, 197–210. [CrossRef] [PubMed]
16. Norrmén, C.; Tammela, T.; Petrova, T.V.; Alitalo, K. Biological Basis of Therapeutic Lymphangiogenesis. *Circulation* **2011**, *123*, 1335–1351. [CrossRef]
17. Campbell, K.T.; Silva, E.A. Biomaterial-Based Strategies for Engineering New Lymphatic Vasculature. *Adv. Healthc. Mater.* **2020**, *9*, e2000895. [CrossRef] [PubMed]
18. Shimizu, Y.; Che, Y.; Murohara, T. Therapeutic Lymphangiogenesis Is a Promising Strategy for Secondary Lymphedema. *Int. J. Mol. Sci.* **2023**, *24*, 7774. [CrossRef]
19. Elliott, M.B.; Ginn, B.; Fukunishi, T.; Bedja, D.; Suresh, A.; Chen, T.; Inoue, T.; Dietz, H.C.; Santhanam, L.; Mao, H.Q.; et al. Regenerative and Durable Small-Diameter Graft as an Arterial Conduit. *Proc. Natl. Acad. Sci. USA* **2019**, *116*, 12710–12719. [CrossRef]
20. Kutikhin, A.G.; Tupikin, A.E.; Matveeva, V.G.; Shishkova, D.K.; Antonova, L.V.; Kabilov, M.R.; Velikanova, E.A. Human Peripheral Blood-Derived Endothelial Colony-Forming Cells Are Highly Similar to Mature Vascular Endothelial Cells yet Demonstrate a Transitional Transcriptomic Signature. *Cells* **2020**, *9*, 876. [CrossRef]
21. Seiffert, N.; Tang, P.; Keshi, E.; Reutzel-Selke, A.; Moosburner, S.; Everwien, H.; Wulsten, D.; Napierala, H.; Pratschke, J.; Sauer, I.M.; et al. In Vitro Recellularization of Decellularized Bovine Carotid Arteries Using Human Endothelial Colony Forming Cells. *J. Biol. Eng.* **2021**, *15*, 15. [CrossRef]
22. Velikanova, E.A.; Sinitsky, M.Y.; Sinitskaya, A.V.; Matveeva, V.G.; Khanova, M.Y.; Antonova, L.V. Evaluation of the Feasibility of Endothelial Colony-Forming Cells to Develop Tissue-Engineered Vascular Grafts Based on the Gene Expression Profile Analysis. *Sovrem. Tekhnol. Med.* **2022**, *14*, 15–19. [CrossRef] [PubMed]
23. Kraus, X.; van de Flierdt, E.; Renzelmann, J.; Thoms, S.; Witt, M.; Scheper, T.; Blume, C. Peripheral Blood Derived Endothelial Colony Forming Cells as Suitable Cell Source for Pre-Endothelialization of Arterial Vascular Grafts under Dynamic Flow Conditions. *Microvasc. Res.* **2022**, *143*, 104402. [CrossRef] [PubMed]
24. Melly, L.; Torregrossa, G.; Lee, T.; Jansens, J.L.; Puskas, J.D. Fifty Years of Coronary Artery Bypass Grafting. *J. Thorac. Dis.* **2018**, *10*, 1960–1967. [CrossRef] [PubMed]
25. Squiers, J.J.; Mack, M.J. Coronary Artery Bypass Grafting-Fifty Years of Quality Initiatives Since Favaloro. *Ann. Cardiothorac. Surg.* **2018**, *7*, 516–520. [CrossRef] [PubMed]
26. Beerkens, F.J.; Claessen, B.E.; Mahan, M.; Gaudino, M.F.L.; Tam, D.Y.; Henriques, J.P.S.; Mehran, R.; Dangas, G.D. Contemporary Coronary Artery Bypass Graft Surgery and Subsequent Percutaneous Revascularization. *Nat. Rev. Cardiol.* **2022**, *19*, 195–208. [CrossRef]
27. Welt, F.G.P. CABG versus PCI End of the Debate? *N. Engl. J. Med.* **2022**, *386*, 185–187. [CrossRef]

28. Serruys, P.W.; Morice, M.C.; Kappetein, A.P.; Colombo, A.; Holmes, D.R.; Mack, M.J.; Ståhle, E.; Feldman, T.E.; van den Brand, M.; Bass, E.J.; et al. Percutaneous Coronary Intervention versus Coronary-Artery Bypass Grafting for Severe Coronary Artery Disease. *N. Engl. J. Med.* **2009**, *360*, 961–972. [CrossRef]
29. Mohr, F.W.; Morice, M.C.; Kappetein, A.P.; Feldman, T.E.; Ståhle, E.; Colombo, A.; Mack, M.J.; Holmes, D.R.; Morel, M.A.; Van Dyck, N.; et al. Coronary Artery Bypass Graft Surgery versus Percutaneous Coronary Intervention in Patients with Three-Vessel Disease and Left Main Coronary Disease: 5-Year Follow-Up of the Randomised, Clinical SYNTAX Trial. *Lancet* **2013**, *381*, 629–638. [CrossRef]
30. Head, S.J.; Milojevic, M.; Daemen, J.; Ahn, J.M.; Boersma, E.; Christiansen, E.H.; Domanski, M.J.; Farkouh, M.E.; Flather, M.; Fuster, V.; et al. Mortality after Coronary Artery Bypass Grafting versus Percutaneous Coronary Intervention with Stenting for Coronary Artery Disease: A Pooled Analysis of Individual Patient Data. *Lancet* **2018**, *391*, 939–948. [CrossRef]
31. Thuijs, D.J.F.M.; Kappetein, A.P.; Serruys, P.W.; Mohr, F.W.; Morice, M.C.; Mack, M.J.; Holmes, D.R., Jr.; Curzen, N.; Davierwala, P.; Noack, T.; et al. Percutaneous coronary intervention versus coronary artery bypass grafting in patients with three-vessel or left main coronary artery disease: 10-year follow-up of the multicentre randomised controlled SYNTAX trial. *Lancet* **2019**, *394*, 1325–1334. [CrossRef] [PubMed]
32. Gaudino, M.; Hameed, I.; Farkouh, M.E.; Rahouma, M.; Naik, A.; Robinson, N.B.; Ruan, Y.; Demetres, M.; Biondi-Zoccai, G.; Angiolillo, D.J.; et al. Overall and Cause-Specific Mortality in Randomized Clinical Trials Comparing Percutaneous Interventions With Coronary Bypass Surgery: A Meta-analysis. *JAMA Intern. Med.* **2020**, *180*, 1638–1646. [CrossRef] [PubMed]
33. Taggart, D.P.; Altman, D.G.; Flather, M.; Gerry, S.; Gray, A.; Lees, B.; Benedetto, U.; ART (Arterial Revascularization Trial) Investigators. Associations Between Adding a Radial Artery Graft to Single and Bilateral Internal Thoracic Artery Grafts and Outcomes: Insights From the Arterial Revascularization Trial. *Circulation* **2017**, *136*, 454–463. [CrossRef] [PubMed]
34. Rocha, R.V.; Tam, D.Y.; Karkhanis, R.; Nedadur, R.; Fang, J.; Tu, J.V.; Gaudino, M.; Royse, A.; Fremes, S.E. Multiple Arterial Grafting Is Associated With Better Outcomes for Coronary Artery Bypass Grafting Patients. *Circulation* **2018**, *138*, 2081–2090. [CrossRef] [PubMed]
35. Gaudino, M.; Rahouma, M.; Abouarab, A.; Tam, D.Y.; Di Franco, A.; Leonard, J.; Benedetto, U.; Iannaccone, M.; D'Ascenzo, F.; Biondi-Zoccai, G.; et al. Meta-analysis Comparing Outcomes of Drug Eluting Stents Versus Single and Multiarterial Coronary Artery Bypass Grafting. *Am. J. Cardiol.* **2018**, *122*, 2018–2025. [CrossRef] [PubMed]
36. Samadashvili, Z.; Sundt, T.M., 3rd; Wechsler, A.; Chikwe, J.; Adams, D.H.; Smith, C.R.; Jordan, D.; Girardi, L.; Lahey, S.J.; Gold, J.P.; et al. Multiple Versus Single Arterial Coronary Bypass Graft Surgery for Multivessel Disease. *J. Am. Coll. Cardiol.* **2019**, *74*, 1275–1285. [CrossRef]
37. Gaudino, M.; Lorusso, R.; Rahouma, M.; Abouarab, A.; Tam, D.Y.; Spadaccio, C.; Saint-Hilary, G.; Leonard, J.; Iannaccone, M.; D'Ascenzo, F.; et al. Radial Artery Versus Right Internal Thoracic Artery Versus Saphenous Vein as the Second Conduit for Coronary Artery Bypass Surgery: A Network Meta-Analysis of Clinical Outcomes. *J. Am. Heart Assoc.* **2019**, *8*, e010839. [CrossRef]
38. Taggart, D.P.; Audisio, K.; Gerry, S.; Robinson, N.B.; Rahouma, M.; Soletti, G.J.; Cancelli, G.; Benedetto, U.; Lees, B.; Gray, A.; et al. Effect of Total Arterial Grafting in the Arterial Revascularization Trial. *J. Thorac. Cardiovasc. Surg.* **2022**, *163*, 1002–1009.e6. [CrossRef]
39. Saraiva, F.A.; Leite-Moreira, J.P.; Barros, A.S.; Lourenço, A.P.; Benedetto, U.; Leite-Moreira, A.F. Multiple versus Single Arterial Grafting in Coronary Artery Bypass Grafting: A Meta-Analysis of Randomized Controlled Trials and Propensity Score Studies. *Int. J. Cardiol.* **2020**, *320*, 55–63. [CrossRef]
40. Gaudino, M.; Di Franco, A.; Flather, M.; Gerry, S.; Bagiella, E.; Gray, A.; Pearcey, L.; Saw, T.H.; Lees, B.; Benedetto, U.; et al. Association of Age with 10-Year Outcomes After Coronary Surgery in the Arterial Revascularization Trial. *J. Am. Coll. Cardiol.* **2021**, *77*, 18–26. [CrossRef]
41. Saraiva, F.A.; Moreira, R.; Cerqueira, R.J.; Mancio, J.; Barros, A.S.; Lourenço, A.P.; Leite-Moreira, A.F. Multiple versus single arterial grafting in the elderly: A meta-analysis of randomized controlled trials and propensity score studies. *J. Cardiovasc. Surg.* **2022**, *63*, 169–178. [CrossRef] [PubMed]
42. Taggart, D.P.; Audisio, K.; Gerry, S.; Robinson, N.B.; Rahouma, M.; Soletti, G.J.; Cancelli, G.; Benedetto, U.; Lees, B.; Gray, A.; et al. Single versus multiple arterial grafting in diabetic patients at 10 years: The Arterial Revascularization Trial. *Eur. Heart J.* **2022**, *43*, 4644–4652. [CrossRef] [PubMed]
43. Thuijs, D.J.F.M.; Davierwala, P.; Milojevic, M.; Deo, S.V.; Noack, T.; Kappetein, A.P.; Serruys, P.W.; Mohr, F.W.; Morice, M.C.; Mack, M.J.; et al. Long-term survival after coronary bypass surgery with multiple versus single arterial grafts. *Eur. J. Cardiothorac. Surg.* **2022**, *61*, 925–933. [CrossRef]
44. Davierwala, P.M.; Gao, C.; Thuijs, D.J.F.M.; Wang, R.; Hara, H.; Ono, M.; Noack, T.; Garg, S.; O'leary, N.; Milojevic, M.; et al. Single or multiple arterial bypass graft surgery vs. percutaneous coronary intervention in patients with three-vessel or left main coronary artery disease. *Eur. Heart J.* **2022**, *43*, 1334–1344. [CrossRef]
45. Taggart, D.P.; Altman, D.G.; Gray, A.M.; Lees, B.; Gerry, S.; Benedetto, U.; Flather, M.; ART Investigators. Randomized Trial of Bilateral versus Single Internal-Thoracic-Artery Grafts. *N. Engl. J. Med.* **2016**, *375*, 2540–2549. [CrossRef] [PubMed]
46. Rubino, A.S.; Gatti, G.; Reichart, D.; Tauriainen, T.; De Feo, M.; Onorati, F.; Pappalardo, A.; Chocron, S.; Gulbins, H.; Dalén, M.; et al. Early Outcome of Bilateral Versus Single Internal Mammary Artery Grafting in the Elderly. *Ann. Thorac. Surg.* **2018**, *105*, 1717–1723. [CrossRef] [PubMed]

47. Iribarne, A.; Schmoker, J.D.; Malenka, D.J.; Leavitt, B.J.; McCullough, J.N.; Weldner, P.W.; DeSimone, J.P.; Westbrook, B.M.; Quinn, R.D.; Klemperer, J.D.; et al. Does Use of Bilateral Internal Mammary Artery Grafting Reduce Long-Term Risk of Repeat Coronary Revascularization? A Multicenter Analysis. *Circulation* **2017**, *136*, 1676–1685. [CrossRef]
48. Buttar, S.N.; Yan, T.D.; Taggart, D.P.; Tian, D.H. Long-term and short-term outcomes of using bilateral internal mammary artery grafting versus left internal mammary artery grafting: A meta-analysis. *Heart* **2017**, *103*, 1419–1426. [CrossRef]
49. Little, M.; Gray, A.M.; Altman, D.G.; Benedetto, U.; Flather, M.; Gerry, S.; Lees, B.; Murphy, J.; Gaudino, M.; Taggart, D.P.; et al. Cost-effectiveness of bilateral vs. single internal thoracic artery grafts at 10 years. *Eur. Heart J. Qual. Care Clin. Outcomes* **2022**, *8*, 324–332. [CrossRef]
50. Taggart, D.P.; Benedetto, U.; Gerry, S.; Altman, D.G.; Gray, A.M.; Lees, B.; Gaudino, M.; Zamvar, V.; Bochenek, A.; Buxton, B.; et al. Bilateral versus Single Internal-Thoracic-Artery Grafts at 10 Years. *N. Engl. J. Med.* **2019**, *380*, 437–446. [CrossRef]
51. Pevni, D.; Nesher, N.; Kramer, A.; Paz, Y.; Farkash, A.; Ben-Gal, Y. Does bilateral versus single thoracic artery grafting provide survival benefit in female patients? *Interact. Cardiovasc. Thorac. Surg.* **2019**, *28*, 860–867. [CrossRef] [PubMed]
52. Gaudino, M.; Alexander, J.H.; Bakaeen, F.G.; Ballman, K.; Barili, F.; Calafiore, A.M.; Davierwala, P.; Goldman, S.; Kappetein, P.; Lorusso, R.; et al. Randomized comparison of the clinical outcome of single versus multiple arterial grafts: The ROMA trial-rationale and study protocol. *Eur. J. Cardiothorac. Surg.* **2017**, *52*, 1031–1040. [CrossRef] [PubMed]
53. Gaudino, M.F.L.; Taggart, D.P.; Fremes, S.E. The ROMA trial: Why it is needed. *Curr. Opin. Cardiol.* **2018**, *33*, 622–626. [CrossRef] [PubMed]
54. Gaudino, M.; Bakaeen, F.G.; Benedetto, U.; Di Franco, A.; Fremes, S.; Glineur, D.; Girardi, L.N.; Grau, J.; Puskas, J.D.; Ruel, M.; et al. Arterial Grafts for Coronary Bypass: A Critical Review After the Publication of ART and RADIAL. *Circulation* **2019**, *140*, 1273–1284. [CrossRef] [PubMed]
55. Gaudino, M.; Audisio, K.; Rahouma, M.; Chadow, D.; Cancelli, G.; Soletti, G.J.; Gray, A.; Lees, B.; Gerry, S.; Benedetto, U.; et al. Comparison of Long-term Clinical Outcomes of Skeletonized vs Pedicled Internal Thoracic Artery Harvesting Techniques in the Arterial Revascularization Trial. *JAMA Cardiol.* **2021**, *6*, 1380–1386. [CrossRef]
56. Kusu-Orkar, T.E.; Kermali, M.; Masharani, K.; Noshirwani, A.; MacCarthy-Ofosu, B.; Oguamanam, N.; Bin Saeid, J.; Muir, A.D.; Harky, A. Skeletonized or Pedicled Harvesting of Left Internal Mammary Artery: A Systematic Review and Meta-analysis. *Semin. Thorac. Cardiovasc. Surg.* **2021**, *33*, 10–18. [CrossRef]
57. Iddawela, S.; Mellor, S.L.; Zahra, S.A.; Khare, Y.; Harky, A. Pedicled or skeletonized bilateral internal mammary artery harvesting a meta-analysis and trial sequential analysis. *Expert Rev. Cardiovasc. Ther.* **2021**, *19*, 647–654. [CrossRef]
58. Dreifaldt, M.; Samano, N.; Geijer, H.; Lidén, M.; Bodin, L.; Souza, D. Pedicled versus skeletonized internal thoracic artery grafts: A randomized trial. *Asian Cardiovasc. Thorac. Ann.* **2021**, *29*, 490–497. [CrossRef]
59. Sá, M.P.; Cavalcanti, P.E.; de Andrade Costa Santos, H.J.; Soares, A.F.; Albuquerque Miranda, R.G.; Araújo, M.L.; Lima, R.C. Skeletonized versus pedicled bilateral internal mammary artery grafting: Outcomes and concerns analyzed through a meta-analytical approach. *Int. J. Surg.* **2015**, *16*, 146–152. [CrossRef]
60. Otsuka, F.; Yahagi, K.; Sakakura, K.; Virmani, R. Why is the mammary artery so special and what protects it from atherosclerosis? *Ann. Cardiothorac. Surg.* **2013**, *2*, 519–526. [CrossRef]
61. Martínez-González, B.; Reyes-Hernández, C.G.; Quiroga-Garza, A.; Rodríguez-Rodríguez, V.E.; Esparza-Hernández, C.N.; Elizondo-Omaña, R.E.; Guzmán-López, S. Conduits Used in Coronary Artery Bypass Grafting: A Review of Morphological Studies. *Ann. Thorac. Cardiovasc. Surg.* **2017**, *23*, 55–65. [CrossRef] [PubMed]
62. Gharibeh, L.; Ferrari, G.; Ouimet, M.; Grau, J.B. Conduits' Biology Regulates the Outcomes of Coronary Artery Bypass Grafting. *JACC Basic Transl. Sci.* **2021**, *6*, 388–396. [CrossRef] [PubMed]
63. Shadrin, I.Y.; Holmes, D.R.; Behfar, A. Left Internal Mammary Artery as an Endocrine Organ: Insights Into Graft Biology and Long-term Impact Following Coronary Artery Bypass Grafting. *Mayo Clin. Proc.* **2023**, *98*, 150–162. [CrossRef] [PubMed]
64. Canver, C.C.; Ricotta, J.J.; Bhayana, J.N.; Fiedler, R.C.; Mentzer, R.M., Jr. Use of duplex imaging to assess suitability of the internal mammary artery for coronary artery surgery. *J. Vasc. Surg.* **1991**, *13*, 294–300. [CrossRef]
65. Dodge, J.T., Jr.; Brown, B.G.; Bolson, E.L.; Dodge, H.T. Lumen diameter of normal human coronary arteries. Influence of age, sex, anatomic variation, and left ventricular hypertrophy or dilation. *Circulation* **1992**, *86*, 232–246. [CrossRef]
66. Waller, B.F.; Orr, C.M.; Slack, J.D.; Pinkerton, C.A.; Van Tassel, J.; Peters, T. Anatomy, histology, and pathology of coronary arteries: A review relevant to new interventional and imaging techniques—Part I. *Clin. Cardiol.* **1992**, *15*, 451–457. [CrossRef]
67. Canham, P.B.; Finlay, H.M.; Boughner, D.R. Contrasting structure of the saphenous vein and internal mammary artery used as coronary bypass vessels. *Cardiovasc. Res.* **1997**, *34*, 557–567. [CrossRef]
68. Jung, Y.; Ahn, B.H.; Kim, G.S.; Jeong, I.S.; Lee, K.S.; Song, S.Y.; Na, K.J.; Oh, S.G. Change in luminal diameter of the left internal thoracic artery anastomosed to the totally occluded left anterior descending coronary artery. *J. Cardiothorac. Surg.* **2016**, *11*, 157. [CrossRef]
69. Gopal, D.; Singh, N.G.; Jagadeesh, A.M.; Ture, A.; Thimmarayappa, A. Comparison of left internal mammary artery diameter before and after left stellate ganglion block. *Ann. Card Anaesth.* **2013**, *16*, 238–242. [CrossRef]
70. Ylä-Herttuala, S.; Sumuvuori, H.; Karkola, K.; Möttönen, M.; Nikkari, T. Glycosaminoglycans in normal and atherosclerotic human coronary arteries. *Lab Invest.* **1986**, *54*, 402–407.
71. Sisto, T.; Ylä-Herttuala, S.; Luoma, J.; Riekkinen, H.; Nikkari, T. Biochemical composition of human internal mammary artery and saphenous vein. *J. Vasc. Surg.* **1990**, *11*, 418–422. [CrossRef] [PubMed]

72. Merrilees, M.J.; Beaumont, B.; Scott, L.J. Comparison of deposits of versican, biglycan and decorin in saphenous vein and internal thoracic, radial and coronary arteries: Correlation to patency. *Coron. Artery Dis.* **2001**, *12*, 7–16. [CrossRef]
73. Anstadt, M.P.; Franga, D.L.; Portik-Dobos, V.; Pennathur, A.; Bannan, M.; Mawulawde, K.; Ergul, A. Native matrix metalloproteinase characteristics may influence early stenosis of venous versus arterial coronary artery bypass grafting conduits. *Chest* **2004**, *125*, 1853–1858. [CrossRef] [PubMed]
74. Predel, H.G.; Yang, Z.; von Segesser, L.; Turina, M.; Bühler, F.R.; Lüscher, T.F. Implications of pulsatile stretch on growth of saphenous vein and mammary artery smooth muscle. *Lancet* **1992**, *340*, 878–879. [CrossRef] [PubMed]
75. Yang, Z.; Oemar, B.S.; Carrel, T.; Kipfer, B.; Julmy, F.; Lüscher, T.F. Different proliferative properties of smooth muscle cells of human arterial and venous bypass vessels: Role of PDGF receptors, mitogen-activated protein kinase, and cyclin-dependent kinase inhibitors. *Circulation* **1998**, *97*, 181–187. [CrossRef]
76. Del Rizzo, D.F.; Yurkova, N.; Moon, M.C.; Litchie, B.; Zahradka, P. Platelet-derived growth factor-induced expression of c-fos in human vascular smooth muscle cells: Implications for long-term graft patency. *Ann. Thorac. Surg.* **2002**, *74*, 90–95. [CrossRef] [PubMed]
77. Friedl, R.; Li, J.; Schumacher, B.; Hanke, H.; Waltenberger, J.; Hannekum, A.; Stracke, S. Intimal hyperplasia and expression of transforming growth factor-beta1 in saphenous veins and internal mammary arteries before coronary artery surgery. *Ann. Thorac. Surg.* **2004**, *78*, 1312–1318. [CrossRef]
78. Hata, J.A.; Petrofski, J.A.; Schroder, J.N.; Williams, M.L.; Timberlake, S.H.; Pippen, A.; Corwin, M.T.; Solan, A.K.; Jakoi, A.; Gehrig, T.R.; et al. Modulation of phosphatidylinositol 3-kinase signaling reduces intimal hyperplasia in aortocoronary saphenous vein grafts. *J. Thorac. Cardiovasc. Surg.* **2005**, *129*, 1405–1413. [CrossRef]
79. Frischknecht, K.; Greutert, H.; Weisshaupt, C.; Kaspar, M.; Yang, Z.; Luscher, T.F.; Carrel, T.P.; Tanner, F.C. Different vascular smooth muscle cell apoptosis in the human internal mammary artery and the saphenous vein. Implications for bypass graft disease. *J. Vasc. Res.* **2006**, *43*, 338–346. [CrossRef]
80. Mekontso-Dessap, A.; Kirsch, M.; Guignambert, C.; Zadigue, P.; Adnot, S.; Loisance, D.; Eddahibi, S. Vascular-wall remodeling of 3 human bypass vessels: Organ culture and smooth muscle cell properties. *J. Thorac. Cardiovasc. Surg.* **2006**, *131*, 651–658. [CrossRef]
81. Turner, N.A.; Ho, S.; Warburton, P.; O'Regan, D.J.; Porter, K.E. Smooth muscle cells cultured from human saphenous vein exhibit increased proliferation, invasion, and mitogen-activated protein kinase activation in vitro compared with paired internal mammary artery cells. *J. Vasc. Surg.* **2007**, *45*, 1022–1028. [CrossRef] [PubMed]
82. Mitra, A.K.; Jia, G.; Gangahar, D.M.; Agrawal, D.K. Temporal PTEN inactivation causes proliferation of saphenous vein smooth muscle cells of human CABG conduits. *J. Cell. Mol. Med.* **2009**, *13*, 177–187. [CrossRef] [PubMed]
83. Zhu, T.X.; Lan, B.; Meng, L.Y.; Yang, Y.L.; Li, R.X.; Li, E.M.; Zheng, S.Y.; Xu, L.Y. ECM-related gene expression profile in vascular smooth muscle cells from human saphenous vein and internal thoracic artery. *J. Cardiothorac. Surg.* **2013**, *8*, 155. [CrossRef] [PubMed]
84. Yang, Z.H.; Diederich, D.; Schneider, K.; Siebenmann, R.; Stulz, P.; von Segesser, L.; Turina, M.; Bühler, F.R.; Lüscher, T.F. Endothelium-derived relaxing factor and protection against contractions induced by histamine and serotonin in the human internal mammary artery and in the saphenous vein. *Circulation* **1989**, *80*, 1041–1048. [CrossRef]
85. Yang, Z.H.; von Segesser, L.; Bauer, E.; Stulz, P.; Turina, M.; Lüscher, T.F. Different activation of the endothelial L-arginine and cyclooxygenase pathway in the human internal mammary artery and saphenous vein. *Circ. Res.* **1991**, *68*, 52–60. [CrossRef]
86. Tadjkarimi, S.; O'Neil, G.S.; Luu, T.N.; Allen, S.P.; Schyns, C.J.; Chester, A.H.; Yacoub, M.H. Comparison of cyclic GMP in human internal mammary artery and saphenous vein: Implications for coronary artery bypass graft patency. *Cardiovasc. Res.* **1992**, *26*, 297–300. [CrossRef]
87. Thorin-Trescases, N.; Hamilton, C.A.; Reid, J.L.; McPherson, K.L.; Jardine, E.; Berg, G.; Bohr, D.; Dominiczak, A.F. Inducible L-arginine/nitric oxide pathway in human internal mammary artery and saphenous vein. *Am. J. Physiol.* **1995**, *268*, H1122–H1132. [CrossRef]
88. Liu, Z.G.; Ge, Z.D.; He, G.W. Difference in endothelium-derived hyperpolarizing factor-mediated hyperpolarization and nitric oxide release between human internal mammary artery and saphenous vein. *Circulation* **2000**, *102*, III296–III301. [CrossRef]
89. Broeders, M.A.; Doevendans, P.A.; Maessen, J.G.; van Gorsel, E.; Egbrink, M.G.; Daemen, M.J.; Tangelder, G.J.; Reneman, R.S.; van der Zee, R. The human internal thoracic artery releases more nitric oxide in response to vascular endothelial growth factor than the human saphenous vein. *J. Thorac. Cardiovasc. Surg.* **2001**, *122*, 305–309. [CrossRef]
90. Gaudino, M.; Toesca, A.; Maggiano, N.; Pragliola, C.; Possati, G. Localization of nitric oxide synthase type III in the internal thoracic and radial arteries and the great saphenous vein: A comparative immunohistochemical study. *J. Thorac. Cardiovasc. Surg.* **2003**, *125*, 1510–1515. [CrossRef]
91. Shishkova, D.; Markova, V.; Sinitsky, M.; Tsepokina, A.; Frolov, A.; Zagorodnikov, N.; Bogdanov, L.; Kutikhin, A. Co-Culture of Primary Human Coronary Artery and Internal Thoracic Artery Endothelial Cells Results in Mutually Beneficial Paracrine Interactions. *Int. J. Mol. Sci.* **2020**, *21*, 8032. [CrossRef]
92. Schmalfuss, C.M.; Chen, L.Y.; Bott, J.N.; Staples, E.D.; Mehta, J.L. Superoxide Anion Generation, Superoxide Dismutase Activity, and Nitric Oxide Release in Human Internal Mammary Artery and Saphenous Vein Segments. *J. Cardiovasc. Pharmacol. Ther.* **1999**, *4*, 249–257. [CrossRef] [PubMed]

93. Shapira, O.M.; Xu, A.; Aldea, G.S.; Vita, J.A.; Shemin, R.J.; Keaney, J.F., Jr. Enhanced nitric oxide-mediated vascular relaxation in radial artery compared with internal mammary artery or saphenous vein. *Circulation* **1999**, *100*, II322–II327. [CrossRef] [PubMed]
94. Mangoush, O.; Athanasiou, T.; Nakamura, K.; Johnson, P.; Smoienski, R.; Sarathchandra, P.; Oury, T.; Chester, A.H.; Amrani, M. Anti-oxidant properties of the internal thoracic artery and the radial artery. *Heart Lung Circ.* **2008**, *17*, 40–47. [CrossRef] [PubMed]
95. Uydeş-Doğan, B.S.; Nebigil, M.; Aslamaci, S.; Onuk, E.; Kanzik, I.; Akar, F. The comparison of vascular reactivities of arterial and venous grafts to vasodilators: Management of graft spasm. *Int. J. Cardiol.* **1996**, *53*, 137–145. [CrossRef]
96. Hammerer-Lercher, A.; Fersterer, J.; Holzmann, S.; Bonatti, J.; Ruttmann, E.; Hoefer, D.; Mair, J.; Puschendorf, B. Direct comparison of relaxation and cGMP production in human coronary bypass grafts in response to stimulation with natriuretic peptides and a nitric oxide donor. *Clin. Sci.* **2006**, *111*, 225–231. [CrossRef]
97. Mirkhani, H.; Shafa, M.; Khazraei, H. Comparison of the effects of levosimendan and papaverine on human internal mammary artery and saphenous vein. *Cardiovasc. Drugs Ther.* **2009**, *23*, 355–359. [CrossRef]
98. Nguyen, H.G.; Korach, A.; Collura, C.; Eskenazi, B.R.; Vita, J.A.; Shapira, O.M. Differential effects of natriuretic peptides on arterial and venous coronary artery bypass conduits. *Ann. Thorac. Surg.* **2009**, *87*, 748–756. [CrossRef]
99. Nishioka, H.; Kitamura, S.; Kameda, Y.; Taniguchi, S.; Kawata, T.; Mizuguchi, K. Difference in acetylcholine-induced nitric oxide release of arterial and venous grafts in patients after coronary bypass operations. *J. Thorac. Cardiovasc. Surg.* **1998**, *116*, 454–459. [CrossRef]
100. Augustin, H.G.; Koh, G.Y. Organotypic vasculature: From descriptive heterogeneity to functional pathophysiology. *Science* **2017**, *357*, eaal2379. [CrossRef]
101. Payeli, S.K.; Latini, R.; Gebhard, C.; Patrignani, A.; Wagner, U.; Lüscher, T.F.; Tanner, F.C. Prothrombotic gene expression profile in vascular smooth muscle cells of human saphenous vein, but not internal mammary artery. *Arterioscler. Thromb. Vasc. Biol.* **2008**, *28*, 705–710. [CrossRef] [PubMed]
102. Xu, J.; Shi, G.P. Vascular wall extracellular matrix proteins and vascular diseases. *Biochim. Biophys. Acta* **2014**, *1842*, 2106–2119. [CrossRef] [PubMed]
103. Del Monte-Nieto, G.; Fischer, J.W.; Gorski, D.J.; Harvey, R.P.; Kovacic, J.C. Basic Biology of Extracellular Matrix in the Cardiovascular System, Part 1/4: JACC Focus Seminar. *J. Am. Coll. Cardiol.* **2020**, *75*, 2169–2188. [CrossRef] [PubMed]
104. Barallobre-Barreiro, J.; Loeys, B.; Mayr, M.; Rienks, M.; Verstraeten, A.; Kovacic, J.C. Extracellular Matrix in Vascular Disease, Part 2/4: JACC Focus Seminar. *J. Am. Coll. Cardiol.* **2020**, *75*, 2189–2203. [CrossRef] [PubMed]
105. Cai, Z.; Gong, Z.; Li, Z.; Li, L.; Kong, W. Vascular Extracellular Matrix Remodeling and Hypertension. *Antioxid. Redox Signal.* **2021**, *34*, 765–783. [CrossRef]
106. Mammoto, A.; Matus, K.; Mammoto, T. Extracellular Matrix in Aging Aorta. *Front. Cell Dev. Biol.* **2022**, *10*, 822561. [CrossRef]
107. Komarova, Y.A.; Kruse, K.; Mehta, D.; Malik, A.B. Protein Interactions at Endothelial Junctions and Signaling Mechanisms Regulating Endothelial Permeability. *Circ. Res.* **2017**, *120*, 179–206. [CrossRef]
108. Wettschureck, N.; Strilic, B.; Offermanns, S. Passing the Vascular Barrier: Endothelial Signaling Processes Controlling Extravasation. *Physiol. Rev.* **2019**, *99*, 1467–1525. [CrossRef]
109. Duong, C.N.; Vestweber, D. Mechanisms Ensuring Endothelial Junction Integrity Beyond VE-Cadherin. *Front. Physiol.* **2020**, *11*, 519. [CrossRef]
110. Claesson-Welsh, L.; Dejana, E.; McDonald, D.M. Permeability of the Endothelial Barrier: Identifying and Reconciling Controversies. *Trends Mol. Med.* **2021**, *27*, 314–331. [CrossRef]
111. Arora, S.; Yim, E.K.F.; Toh, Y.C. Environmental Specification of Pluripotent Stem Cell Derived Endothelial Cells Toward Arterial and Venous Subtypes. *Front. Bioeng. Biotechnol.* **2019**, *7*, 143. [CrossRef] [PubMed]
112. Gifre-Renom, L.; Daems, M.; Luttun, A.; Jones, E.A.V. Organ-Specific Endothelial Cell Differentiation and Impact of Microenvironmental Cues on Endothelial Heterogeneity. *Int. J. Mol. Sci.* **2022**, *23*, 1477. [CrossRef] [PubMed]
113. Di Russo, J.; Luik, A.L.; Yousif, L.; Budny, S.; Oberleithner, H.; Hofschröer, V.; Klingauf, J.; van Bavel, E.; Bakker, E.N.; Hellstrand, P.; et al. Endothelial basement membrane laminin 511 is essential for shear stress response. *EMBO J.* **2017**, *36*, 183–201. [CrossRef]
114. Yamamoto, K.; Nogimori, Y.; Imamura, H.; Ando, J. Shear stress activates mitochondrial oxidative phosphorylation by reducing plasma membrane cholesterol in vascular endothelial cells. *Proc. Natl. Acad. Sci. USA* **2020**, *117*, 33660–33667. [CrossRef] [PubMed]
115. Moore, K.H.; Murphy, H.A.; George, E.M. The glycocalyx: A central regulator of vascular function. *Am. J. Physiol. Regul. Integr. Comp. Physiol.* **2021**, *320*, R508–R518. [CrossRef] [PubMed]
116. Suzuki, A.; Tomita, H.; Okada, H. Form follows function: The endothelial glycocalyx. *Transl. Res.* **2022**, *247*, 158–167. [CrossRef]
117. Villalba, N.; Baby, S.; Yuan, S.Y. The Endothelial Glycocalyx as a Double-Edged Sword in Microvascular Homeostasis and Pathogenesis. *Front. Cell Dev. Biol.* **2021**, *9*, 711003. [CrossRef]
118. Hu, Z.; Cano, I.; D'Amore, P.A. Update on the Role of the Endothelial Glycocalyx in Angiogenesis and Vascular Inflammation. *Front. Cell Dev. Biol.* **2021**, *9*, 734276. [CrossRef]
119. Antonova, L.; Kutikhin, A.; Sevostianova, V.; Lobov, A.; Repkin, E.; Krivkina, E.; Velikanova, E.; Mironov, A.; Mukhamadiyarov, R.; Senokosova, E.; et al. Controlled and Synchronised Vascular Regeneration upon the Implantation of Iloprost- and Cationic Amphiphilic Drugs-Conjugated Tissue-Engineered Vascular Grafts into the Ovine Carotid Artery: A Proteomics-Empowered Study. *Polymers* **2022**, *14*, 5149. [CrossRef]

120. Antonova, L.V.; Sevostianova, V.V.; Silnikov, V.N.; Krivkina, E.O.; Velikanova, E.A.; Mironov, A.V.; Shabaev, A.R.; Senokosova, E.A.; Khanova, M.Y.; Glushkova, T.V.; et al. Comparison of the Patency and Regenerative Potential of Biodegradable Vascular Prostheses of Different Polymer Compositions in an Ovine Model. *Int. J. Mol. Sci.* **2023**, *24*, 8540. [CrossRef]
121. Eelen, G.; de Zeeuw, P.; Treps, L.; Harjes, U.; Wong, B.W.; Carmeliet, P. Endothelial Cell Metabolism. *Physiol. Rev.* **2018**, *98*, 3–58. [CrossRef]
122. Li, X.; Sun, X.; Carmeliet, P. Hallmarks of Endothelial Cell Metabolism in Health and Disease. *Cell Metab.* **2019**, *30*, 414–433. [CrossRef] [PubMed]
123. Li, X.; Kumar, A.; Carmeliet, P. Metabolic Pathways Fueling the Endothelial Cell Drive. *Annu. Rev. Physiol.* **2019**, *81*, 483–503. [CrossRef] [PubMed]
124. Peng, H.; Wang, X.; Du, J.; Cui, Q.; Huang, Y.; Jin, H. Metabolic Reprogramming of Vascular Endothelial Cells: Basic Research and Clinical Applications. *Front. Cell Dev. Biol.* **2021**, *9*, 626047. [CrossRef] [PubMed]
125. Donato, A.J.; Machin, D.R.; Lesniewski, L.A. Mechanisms of Dysfunction in the Aging Vasculature and Role in Age-Related Disease. *Circ. Res.* **2018**, *123*, 825–848. [CrossRef] [PubMed]
126. Ungvari, Z.; Tarantini, S.; Kiss, T.; Wren, J.D.; Giles, C.B.; Griffin, C.T.; Murfee, W.L.; Pacher, P.; Csiszar, A. Endothelial dysfunction and angiogenesis impairment in the ageing vasculature. *Nat. Rev. Cardiol.* **2018**, *15*, 555–565. [CrossRef]
127. Ungvari, Z.; Tarantini, S.; Sorond, F.; Merkely, B.; Csiszar, A. Mechanisms of Vascular Aging, A Geroscience Perspective: JACC Focus Seminar. *J. Am. Coll. Cardiol.* **2020**, *75*, 931–941. [CrossRef]
128. Sinitsky, M.Y.; Kutikhin, A.G.; Tsepokina, A.V.; Shishkova, D.K.; Asanov, M.A.; Yuzhalin, A.E.; Minina, V.I.; Ponasenko, A.V. Mitomycin C induced genotoxic stress in endothelial cells is associated with differential expression of proinflammatory cytokines. *Mutat. Res. Genet. Toxicol. Environ. Mutagen.* **2020**, *858–860*, 503252. [CrossRef]
129. Sinitsky, M.; Sinitskaya, A.; Shishkova, D.; Tupikin, A.; Asanov, M.; Khutornaya, M.; Kabilov, M.; Ponasenko, A. Identification of Key Genes and Pathways in Genotoxic Stress Induced Endothelial Dysfunction: Results of Whole Transcriptome Sequencing. *Biomedicines* **2022**, *10*, 2067. [CrossRef]
130. Sinitsky, M.; Asanov, M.; Sinitskaya, A.; Shishkova, D.; Khutornaya, M.; Minina, V.; Ponasenko, A. Atorvastatin Can Modulate DNA Damage Repair in Endothelial Cells Exposed to Mitomycin C. *Int. J. Mol. Sci.* **2023**, *24*, 6783. [CrossRef]
131. Bautista-Niño, P.K.; Portilla-Fernandez, E.; Rubio-Beltrán, E.; van der Linden, J.J.; de Vries, R.; van Veghel, R.; de Boer, M.; Durik, M.; Ridwan, Y.; Brandt, R.; et al. Local endothelial DNA repair deficiency causes aging-resembling endothelial-specific dysfunction. *Clin. Sci.* **2020**, *134*, 727–746. [CrossRef] [PubMed]
132. Mameli, E.; Martello, A.; Caporali, A. Autophagy at the interface of endothelial cell homeostasis and vascular disease. *FEBS J.* **2022**, *289*, 2976–2991. [CrossRef] [PubMed]
133. Pacinella, G.; Ciaccio, A.M.; Tuttolomondo, A. Endothelial Dysfunction and Chronic Inflammation: The Cornerstones of Vascular Alterations in Age-Related Diseases. *Int. J. Mol. Sci.* **2022**, *23*, 15722. [CrossRef] [PubMed]
134. Marzoog, B.A. Endothelial cell autophagy in the context of disease development. *Anat. Cell Biol.* **2023**, *56*, 16–24. [CrossRef] [PubMed]
135. Cai, J.; Culley, M.K.; Zhao, Y.; Zhao, J. The role of ubiquitination and deubiquitination in the regulation of cell junctions. *Protein Cell* **2018**, *9*, 754–769. [CrossRef]
136. Totland, M.Z.; Rasmussen, N.L.; Knudsen, L.M.; Leithe, E. Regulation of gap junction intercellular communication by connexin ubiquitination: Physiological and pathophysiological implications. *Cell Mol. Life Sci.* **2020**, *77*, 573–591. [CrossRef] [PubMed]
137. Yadid, M.; Lind, J.U.; Ardoña, H.A.M.; Sheehy, S.P.; Dickinson, L.E.; Eweje, F.; Bastings, M.M.C.; Pope, B.; O'Connor, B.B.; Straubhaar, J.R.; et al. Endothelial extracellular vesicles contain protective proteins and rescue ischemia-reperfusion injury in a human heart-on-chip. *Sci. Transl. Med.* **2020**, *12*, eaax8005. [CrossRef]
138. Li, T.; Wang, B.; Ding, H.; Chen, S.; Cheng, W.; Li, Y.; Wu, X.; Wang, L.; Jiang, Y.; Lu, Z.; et al. Effect of Extracellular Vesicles From Multiple Cells on Vascular Smooth Muscle Cells in Atherosclerosis. *Front. Pharmacol.* **2022**, *13*, 857331. [CrossRef]
139. He, Y.; Li, Q.; Feng, F.; Gao, R.; Li, H.; Chu, Y.; Li, S.; Wang, Y.; Mao, R.; Ji, Z.; et al. Extracellular vesicles produced by human-induced pluripotent stem cell-derived endothelial cells can prevent arterial stenosis in mice via autophagy regulation. *Front. Cardiovasc. Med.* **2022**, *9*, 922790. [CrossRef]
140. Abel, F.; Murke, F.; Gaida, M.; Garnier, N.; Ochsenfarth, C.; Theiss, C.; Thielmann, M.; Kleinbongard, P.; Giebel, B.; Peters, J.; et al. Extracellular vesicles isolated from patients undergoing remote ischemic preconditioning decrease hypoxia-evoked apoptosis of cardiomyoblasts after isoflurane but not propofol exposure. *PLoS ONE* **2020**, *15*, e0228948. [CrossRef]
141. Desgres, M.; Lima Correa, B.; Petrusca, L.; Autret, G.; Pezzana, C.; Marigny, C.; Guillas, C.; Bellamy, V.; Vilar, J.; Perier, M.C.; et al. Therapeutic potential of extracellular vesicles derived from cardiac progenitor cells in rodent models of chemotherapy-induced cardiomyopathy. *Front. Cardiovasc. Med.* **2023**, *10*, 1206279. [CrossRef]
142. Alfi, E.; Thairi, C.; Femminò, S.; Alloatti, G.; Moccia, F.; Brizzi, M.F.; Pagliaro, P.; Penna, C. Extracellular vesicles (EVs) in ischemic conditioning and angiogenesis: Focus on endothelial derived EVs. *Vascul. Pharmacol.* **2021**, *140*, 106873. [CrossRef]
143. Markova, V.; Bogdanov, L.; Velikanova, E.; Kanonykina, A.; Frolov, A.; Shishkova, D.; Lazebnaya, A.; Kutikhin, A. Endothelial Cell Markers Are Inferior to Vascular Smooth Muscle Cells Markers in Staining Vasa Vasorum and Are Non-Specific for Distinct Endothelial Cell Lineages in Clinical Samples. *Int. J. Mol. Sci.* **2023**, *24*, 1959. [CrossRef] [PubMed]

144. Bogdanov, L.A.; Velikanova, E.A.; Kanonykina, A.Y.; Frolov, A.V.; Shishkova, D.K.; Lazebnaya, A.I.; Kutikhin, A.G. Vascular smooth muscle cell contractile proteins as universal markers of vessels of microcirculatory bed. *Compl. Iss. Cardiovasc. Dis.* **2022**, *11*, 162–176. [CrossRef]
145. Shishkova, D.; Lobov, A.; Zainullina, B.; Matveeva, V.; Markova, V.; Sinitskaya, A.; Velikanova, E.; Sinitsky, M.; Kanonykina, A.; Dyleva, Y.; et al. Calciprotein Particles Cause Physiologically Significant Pro-Inflammatory Response in Endothelial Cells and Systemic Circulation. *Int. J. Mol. Sci.* **2022**, *23*, 14941. [CrossRef]
146. Shishkova, D.; Velikanova, E.; Bogdanov, L.; Sinitsky, M.; Kostyunin, A.; Tsepokina, A.; Gruzdeva, O.; Mironov, A.; Mukhamadiyarov, R.; Glushkova, T.; et al. Calciprotein Particles Link Disturbed Mineral Homeostasis with Cardiovascular Disease by Causing Endothelial Dysfunction and Vascular Inflammation. *Int. J. Mol. Sci.* **2021**, *22*, 12458. [CrossRef] [PubMed]
147. Shishkova, D.; Markova, V.; Sinitsky, M.; Tsepokina, A.; Velikanova, E.; Bogdanov, L.; Glushkova, T.; Kutikhin, A. Calciprotein Particles Cause Endothelial Dysfunction under Flow. *Int. J. Mol. Sci.* **2020**, *21*, 8802. [CrossRef] [PubMed]
148. Dobin, A.; Davis, C.A.; Schlesinger, F.; Drenkow, J.; Zaleski, C.; Jha, S.; Batut, P.; Chaisson, M.; Gingeras, T.R. STAR: Ultrafast universal RNA-seq aligner. *Bioinformatics* **2013**, *29*, 15–21. [CrossRef]
149. Anders, S.; Pyl, P.T.; Huber, W. HTSeq—A Python framework to work with high-throughput sequencing data. *Bioinformatics* **2015**, *31*, 166–169. [CrossRef]
150. Love, M.I.; Huber, W.; Anders, S. Moderated estimation of fold change and dispersion for RNA-seq data with DESeq2. *Genome Biol.* **2014**, *15*, 550. [CrossRef]
151. Ashburner, M.; Ball, C.A.; Blake, J.A.; Botstein, D.; Butler, H.; Cherry, J.M.; Davis, A.P.; Dolinski, K.; Dwight, S.S.; Eppig, J.T.; et al. Gene ontology: Tool for the unification of biology. The Gene Ontology Consortium. *Nat. Genet.* **2000**, *25*, 25–29. [CrossRef] [PubMed]
152. Gene Ontology Consortium. The Gene Ontology resource: Enriching a GOld mine. *Nucleic Acids Res.* **2021**, *49*, D325–D334. [CrossRef]
153. UniProt Consortium. UniProt: The universal protein knowledgebase in 2021. *Nucleic Acids Res.* **2021**, *49*, D480–D489. [CrossRef] [PubMed]
154. Gillespie, M.; Jassal, B.; Stephan, R.; Milacic, M.; Rothfels, K.; Senff-Ribeiro, A.; Griss, J.; Sevilla, C.; Matthews, L.; Gong, C.; et al. The reactome pathway knowledgebase 2022. *Nucleic Acids Res.* **2022**, *50*, D687–D692. [CrossRef] [PubMed]
155. Griss, J.; Viteri, G.; Sidiropoulos, K.; Nguyen, V.; Fabregat, A.; Hermjakob, H. ReactomeGSA Efficient Multi-Omics Comparative Pathway Analysis. *Mol. Cell. Proteomics* **2020**, *19*, 2115–2125. [CrossRef]
156. Kanehisa, M.; Goto, S. KEGG: Kyoto encyclopedia of genes and genomes. *Nucleic Acids Res.* **2000**, *28*, 27–30. [CrossRef] [PubMed]
157. Kanehisa, M.; Furumichi, M.; Sato, Y.; Ishiguro-Watanabe, M.; Tanabe, M. KEGG: Integrating viruses and cellular organisms. *Nucleic Acids Res.* **2021**, *49*, D545–D551. [CrossRef]
158. Chen, H.; Boutros, P.C. VennDiagram: A package for the generation of highly-customizable Venn and Euler diagrams in R. *BMC Bioinform.* **2011**, *12*, 35. [CrossRef]
159. Dixon, P. VEGAN, A Package of R Functions for Community Ecology. *J. Veget. Sci.* **2003**, *14*, 927–930. [CrossRef]
160. Rohart, F.; Gautier, B.; Singh, A.; Lê Cao, K.A. mixOmics: An R package for 'omics feature selection and multiple data integration. *PLoS Comput. Biol.* **2017**, *13*, e1005752. [CrossRef]
161. Ritchie, M.E.; Phipson, B.; Wu, D.; Hu, Y.; Law, C.W.; Shi, W.; Smyth, G.K. limma powers differential expression analyses for RNA-sequencing and microarray studies. *Nucleic Acids Res.* **2015**, *43*, e47. [CrossRef] [PubMed]
162. Wickham, H. *ggplot2: Elegant Graphics for Data Analysis*; Springer: New York, NY, USA, 2016.
163. Blighe, K.; Rana, S.; Lewis, M. *EnhancedVolcano: Publication-Ready Volcano Plots with Enhanced Colouring and Labeling*, R package version 1.14.0; R Core Team: Vienna, Austria, 2022.
164. Perez-Riverol, Y.; Bai, J.; Bandla, C.; García-Seisdedos, D.; Hewapathirana, S.; Kamatchinathan, S.; Kundu, D.J.; Prakash, A.; Frericks-Zipper, A.; Eisenacher, M.; et al. The PRIDE database resources in 2022: A hub for mass spectrometry-based proteomics evidences. *Nucleic Acids Res.* **2022**, *50*, D543–D552. [CrossRef] [PubMed]
165. Shannon, P.; Markiel, A.; Ozier, O.; Baliga, N.S.; Wang, J.T.; Ramage, D.; Amin, N.; Schwikowski, B.; Ideker, T. Cytoscape: A software environment for integrated models of biomolecular interaction networks. *Genome Res.* **2003**, *13*, 2498–2504. [CrossRef] [PubMed]

International Journal of
Molecular Sciences

MDPI

Article

Osteoprotegerin Is Essential for the Development of Endothelial Dysfunction Induced by Angiotensin II in Mice

Mieczysław Dutka [1,*], Wojciech Garczorz [2], Agnieszka Kosowska [2], Elzbieta Buczek [3], Piotr Godek [4], Wojciech Wojakowski [4] and Tomasz Francuz [2]

[1] Department of Biochemistry and Molecular Biology, Faculty of Health Sciences, University of Bielsko-Biala, 43-309 Bielsko-Biala, Poland

[2] Department of Biochemistry, Faculty of Medical Sciences in Katowice, Medical University of Silesia, 40-055 Katowice, Poland; wojtekg@sum.edu.pl (W.G.); akosowska@sum.edu.pl (A.K.); tfrancuz@sum.edu.pl (T.F.)

[3] Jagiellonian Centre for Experimental Therapeutics (JCET), Jagiellonian University, 30-348 Krakow, Poland; elzbieta.buczek@jcet.eu

[4] Department of Cardiology and Structural Heart Disease, Faculty of Medical Sciences in Katowice, Medical University of Silesia, 40-055 Katowice, Poland; piotrgodek77@gmail.com (P.G.); wwojakowski@sum.edu.pl (W.W.)

* Correspondence: mdutka@ubb.edu.pl

Abstract: Opinions on the effects of osteoprotegerin (OPG) have evolved over the years from a protein protecting the vasculature from calcification to a cardiovascular risk factor contributing to inflammation within the vascular wall. Nowadays, the link between OPG and angiotensin II (Ang II) appears to be particularly important. In this study, the endothelial function was investigated in OPG-knockout mice (B6.129.S4-OPG, OPG^-) and wild-type (C57BL/6J, OPG^+) mice under basic conditions and after Ang II exposure by assessing the endothelium-dependent diastolic response of aortic rings to acetylcholine in vitro. A further aim of the study was to compare the effect of Ang II on the expression of cytokines in the aortic wall of both groups of mice. Our study shows that rings from OPG^- mice had their normal endothelial function preserved after incubation with Ang II, whereas those from OPG^+ mice showed significant endothelial dysfunction. We conclude that the absence of OPG, although associated with a pro-inflammatory cytokine profile in the vascular wall, simultaneously protects against Ang II-induced increases in pro-inflammatory cytokines in the murine vascular wall. Our study also demonstrates that the absence of OPG can result in a decrease in the concentration of pro-inflammatory cytokines in the vascular wall after Ang II exposure. The presence of OPG is therefore crucial for the development of Ang II-induced inflammation in the vascular wall and for the development of Ang II-induced endothelial dysfunction.

Keywords: osteoprotegerin; endothelium; endothelial dysfunction; angiotensin II; cytokines; inflammation

1. Introduction

Osteoprotegerin (OPG) is a glycoprotein that belongs to the tumour necrosis factor superfamily (TNFSF). This superfamily currently comprises more than 20 different ligands and more than 30 related receptors [1]. OPG belongs to the group of soluble receptors and exists mainly in a free form, not bound to the cell membrane [1–3]. OPG is best known as a regulator of bone remodelling under physiological conditions and in various clinical situations. The effect of OPG on bone metabolism is mediated by its function as a decoy receptor, which blocks the interaction between the receptor activator of nuclear factor kappa B (RANK) and its ligand (RANKL) [3–6]. Sites of OPG production include various organs such as kidneys, intestines, stomach and bones, as well as matrix cells, megakaryocytes, immune cells such as B lymphocytes or dendritic cells, vascular endothelial cells (ECs) and vascular smooth muscle cells (VSMCs) [5,7].

A growing body of research confirms that OPG may also be involved in cardiovascular disease processes or may be a prognostic indicator of cardiovascular diseases [6,8]. Initial observations in mice with a knockout of the OPG gene showed that, in addition to increased osteoporosis, there was also increased calcification of the aortic wall and renal arteries in these OPG-deficient animals [7,9–11].

These first observations formed the basis for viewing OPG as a factor protecting the vasculature from calcification. The similarities between the regulation of osteoclastogenesis in bone and this calcification of the vascular wall and the involvement of the RANK-RANKL-OPG signalling axis in this regulation seemed to support such a hypothesis.

However, subsequent clinical observations have yielded opposite results. High OPG concentrations have been found to be associated with increased cardiovascular risk in patients with coronary artery disease (CAD) [3,5,7,12–14]. These high OPG concentrations have also been confirmed as a predictor of a higher incidence of hospitalisation for exacerbation of heart failure (HF) with reduced ejection fraction of ischaemic aetiology [5]. Significant changes in plasma OPG concentrations have also been observed in patients with unstable angina (UA) and in patients with acute myocardial infarction (AMI) [13,15–18]. Studies have also confirmed that high plasma OPG levels are a strong predictor of cardiovascular death in patients with myocardial infarction, both STEMI (ST-segment elevation myocardial infarction) and NSTEMI (non-ST-segment elevation myocardial infarction) [15,19].

Higher concentrations of OPG have also been found in patients with retinopathy and diabetic neuropathy and in patients with arterial hypertension [5,8]. Therefore, an increased concentration of OPG is regarded as a marker of vascular pathologies associated with diabetes and arterial hypertension, as well as an indicator of endothelial dysfunction and high cardiovascular risk [5,8,12,20]. This has also been confirmed in hypertensive paediatric patients [21]. High plasma OPG concentrations are an indicator of the risk of development of chronic kidney disease (CKD) in patients with arterial hypertension [22]. The detailed mechanisms linking OPG with the regulation of blood pressure are unknown. However, some polymorphisms of the OPG gene, such as rs2073618, have been reported to be associated with the development of hypertension and with a higher cardiovascular risk in patients with type-2 diabetes [23].

The mechanisms of action of OPG that may explain its pathogenic role in arterial wall damage and atherosclerotic plaque development remain unclear. Among other things, OPG is thought to contribute to inflammation within the vascular wall and to enhance leukocyte adhesion to the vascular endothelium [6,24,25]. The importance of angiotensin II (Ang II), platelet-derived growth factor (PDGF), and basic fibroblast growth factor (bFGF) in stimulating OPG expression in VSMCs and contributing to the development of atherosclerotic lesions has been raised [8].

The link between OPG and Ang II, which plays an important role in the development of age-related adverse changes in the phenotype of VSMCs and ECs and in the pathogenesis of atherosclerosis, is of particular relevance [4]. Ang II acts directly on the vascular endothelium, leading to its dysfunction, the development of inflammation, and the progression of atherosclerosis [26]. Reciprocal stimulatory interactions between OPG and Ang II have been demonstrated [3,27–29]. Ang II has been shown to increase OPG expression in human and murine vascular walls. OPG has also been shown to increase the expression of the AT1 receptor for Ang II in these cells [3,30]. This is one of the postulated mechanisms by which OPG may promote endothelial dysfunction and the development of atherosclerotic lesions.

Taking into account the links between OPG and Ang II described above and the discrepancies between the results of studies in OPG-knockout mice (suggesting a vascular-protective effect of OPG) and of later preclinical and clinical studies (suggesting an adverse cardiovascular effect of OPG), the aims of our study were established. The first aim of our study was to assess the endothelial function in OPG-knockout mice (OPG^-) and mice with normal OPG production (OPG^+). This was achieved by measuring and comparing the acetylocholine-induced endothelium-dependent relaxation response of aortas from OPG^-

mice and those from OPG$^+$ mice, both under basic conditions and after Ang II exposure. A further aim of the study was to assess the effect of Ang II on the expression of individual cytokines in the aortic wall of both these groups of mice. The cytokine profile in the aortic wall of OPG$^-$ and OPG$^+$ mice was compared. It should be emphasised that the studied mice differed only in the knockout of the OPG gene and in the ability to produce OPG, as the OPG$^-$ mice were derived from C57BL/6J wild-type mice (OPG$^+$).

2. Results

2.1. Nitric Oxide-Dependent Endothelial Function in the Isolated Murine Aorta

The endothelial NO-dependent relaxation induced by acetylcholine (Ach) and the endothelium-independent response to sodium nitroprusside (SNP) were tested. In wild-type mice, a significant impairment in the NO-dependent response to ACh was found in the aortic rings incubated for 24 h with Ang II (1 μM) when compared to the control rings (Figure 1A). In contrast, the use of this Ang II-induced endothelial dysfunction model in OPG$^-$ mice showed an effect which has not been previously described in the literature. These rings, despite 24 h of incubation with 1 μM of Ang II, retained normal endothelial function and had a normal relaxation response to acetylcholine. As expected, the aortic rings from OPG$^+$ mice, incubated for 24 h with Ang II (1 μM), showed a significant impairment in NO-dependent response to ACh when compared to OPG$^-$ mice. A comparison of the control rings (not exposed to any agent) from the OPG$^-$ and the OPG$^+$ mice showed no statistically significant difference in the endothelium-dependent relaxation response to acetylcholine (Figure 1A). There were no differences found in the responses to SNP between all experimental groups (Figure 1B).

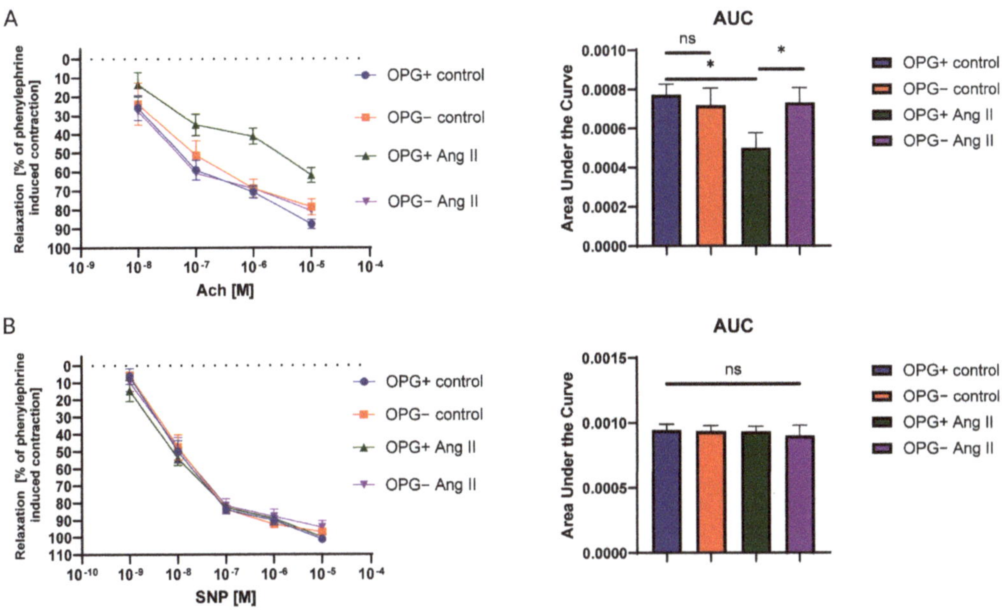

Figure 1. Acetylcholine-induced endothelium-dependent relaxation of aortic rings from wild-type mice (OPG$^+$) and OPG-knockout mice (OPG$^-$) under basic conditions (control) and after incubation with angiotensin II (Ang II) (**A**). For comparison, sodium nitroprusside-induced endothelium-independent relaxation of aortic rings from OPG$^+$ and OPG$^-$ mice under basic conditions (control) and after incubation with Ang II is presented (**B**). Mean values ± SEM are shown. n = 9 per group. * $p < 0.05$. Unpaired Student *t*-test.

2.2. Analysis of Cytokine Panel

Murine aortic rings isolated from wild-type and OPG-knockout mice were evaluated. Protein levels of BCA-1/CXCL 13, I-309/CCL1, Eotaxin-2/CCL24, Fractalkine/CX3CL1, IL-1B, I-TAC/CXCL11, MIP-1b/CCL2, and IL-10 were analysed via multiplex bead-based (Luminex) assays. The average results from eight murine rings are presented in Figure 2. An increase in pro-inflammatory cytokines was observed in OPG$^-$ mice when compared to the OPG$^+$ mice. The concentrations of the following pro-inflammatory cytokines increased: Eotaxin-2/CCL24 by 52.0%, BCA-1/CXCL 13 by 25.7%, Fractalkine/CX3CL1 by 26.6%, I-309/CCL1 by 51.0%, IL-1B by 34.4%, I-TAC/CXCL11 by 39.4%, and MCP-1/CCL2 by 18.7%. The anti-inflammatory IL-10 concentration in OPG$^-$-knockout mice increased by 48.4% (Figure 2).

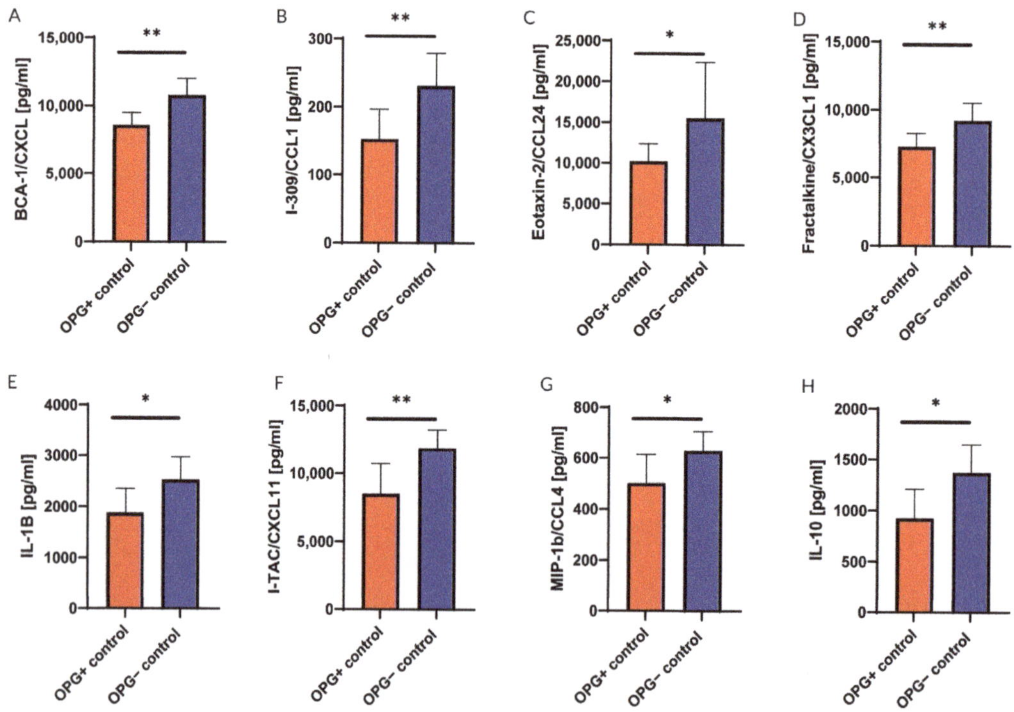

Figure 2. Cytokine concentrations in aortic rings isolated from wild-type mice (OPG$^+$) and OPG-knockout mice (OPG$^-$). Protein levels of BCA-1/CXCL 13 (**A**), I-309/CCL1 (**B**), Eotaxin-2/CCL24 (**C**), Fractalkine/CX3CL1 (**D**), IL-1B (**E**), I-TAC/CXCL11 (**F**), MIP-1b/CCL2 (**G**) and IL-10 (**H**) were analysed by multiplex. Mean values ± SEM are shown. n = 8 per group. * $p < 0.05$, ** $p < 0.01$. OPG$^-$ vs. OPG$^+$ under basic conditions (control group). Unpaired Student t-test (**A**,**B**,**D–H**) and Mann–Whitney test (**C**).

When aortic rings from OPG$^+$ and OPG$^-$ mice were incubated with 1 μM of Ang II for 24 h and compared with aortic rings incubated in culture medium alone (control), it was found that IL-6 levels in the aortic wall homogenates from OPG$^+$ mice increased significantly (77%) after incubation with Ang II. This effect was not observed in the aortic wall of OPG$^-$ mice where IL-6 levels remained unchanged despite incubation with Ang II (Figure 3).

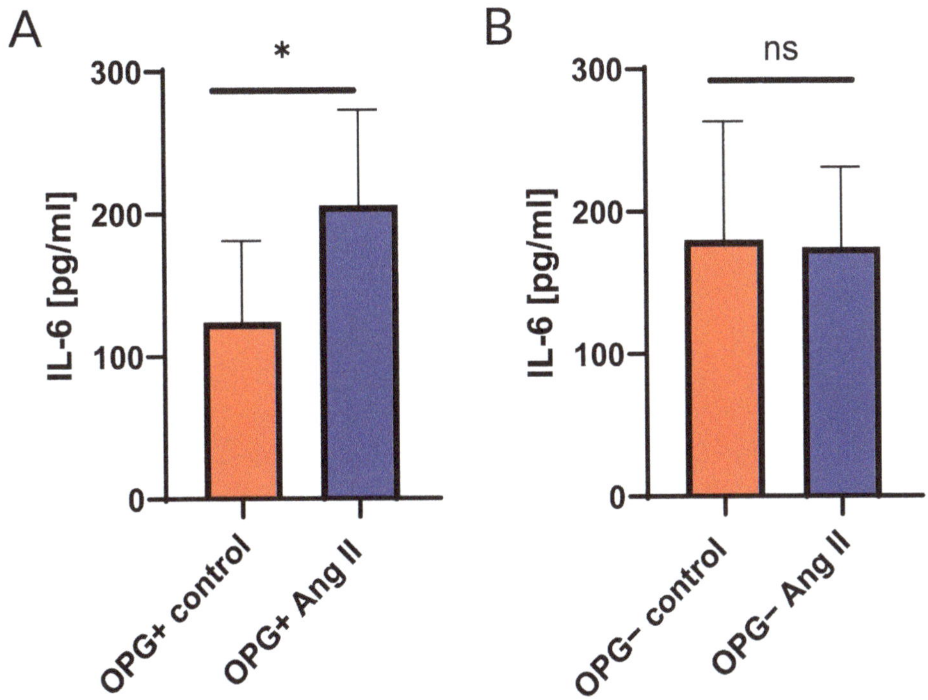

Figure 3. Cytokine concentrations in aortic rings isolated from wild-type mice (OPG^+) (**A**) and OPG-knockout mice (OPG^-) (**B**) under basic conditions (control) and after incubation with angiotensin II (Ang II). Protein levels of IL-6 were analysed using multiplex assay. Mean values $\pm$ SEM are shown. n = 8 per group. * $p < 0.05$. Mann–Whitney test.

Furthermore, OPG^- mice showed significantly lower levels of the tested cytokines in aortic ring homogenates incubated with Ang II compared to the control group. No such effect was observed in OPG^+ mice. In the aortic wall of OPG^- mice, the concentrations of the following cytokines decreased upon incubation with Ang II: BCA-1/CXCL 13 by 21.7%, I-309/CCL1 by 29.4%, IL-4 by 17.6%, I-TAC/CXCL11 by 22.8%, and IP-10/CXCL 10 by 21.7% (Figure 4).

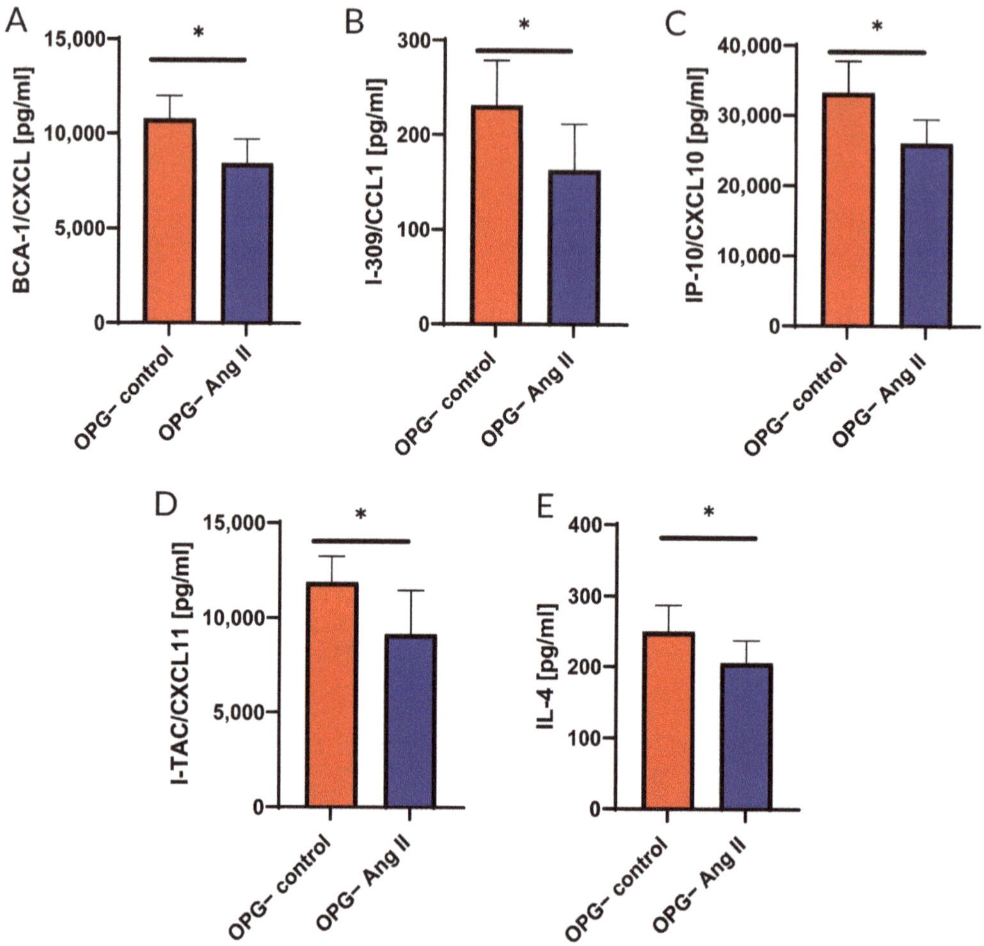

Figure 4. Cytokine concentrations in aortic rings isolated from OPG-knockout mice (OPG$^-$) under basic conditions (control) and after incubation with angiotensin II (Ang II). Protein levels of BCA-1/CXCL 13 (**A**), I-309/CCL1 (**B**), IP-10/CXCL 10 (**C**), I-TAC/CXCL11 (**D**), and IL-4 (**E**) were analysed using multiplex assay. Mean values ± SEM are shown. n = 8 per group. * $p < 0.05$. Unpaired Student *t*-test.

3. Discussion

3.1. Endothelial Function

Given the data indicating the involvement of OPG in endothelial dysfunction and the development of atherosclerotic cardiovascular diseases, the endothelial function was investigated by assessing the endothelium-dependent relaxation response of aortic rings from OPG$^+$ and OPG$^-$ mice. Due to the reported association between OPG and Ang II, this assessment was performed both under basic conditions and after exposure to Ang II (Figure 1). A comparison of control rings (not exposed to any agent) from OPG$^-$ and OPG$^+$ mice showed no statistically significant difference in terms of the endothelium-dependent relaxation response to acetylcholine. However, when exposed to Ang II, aortic rings from OPG$^-$ mice differed from those from OPG$^+$ mice in that they retained normal endothelial function and normal relaxation response to acetylcholine despite 24 h of incubation with Ang II.

In contrast, aortic rings from OPG^{+} mice showed a significant impairment of the endothelium-dependent relaxation response to acetylcholine after 24 h of incubation with Ang II compared to control rings incubated in the culture medium alone. Such a response is typically observed in a model of Ang II-induced endothelial dysfunction [31]. To our knowledge, this study is the first to show that knockout of the OPG gene protects against Ang II-induced endothelial dysfunction. This suggests a link between the endothelial dysfunction-inducing effects of Ang II and OPG. The OPG^{-} mice used in this experiment are from the same strain as the wild-type (OPG^{+}) mice studied. The only difference is that they are unable to produce OPG because the gene for OPG has been knocked out. The presence of OPG is therefore a key factor in the ability of Ang II to induce endothelial dysfunction.

3.2. Cytokine Profile

In view of the results obtained in this functional study indicating that OPG is involved in the induction of endothelial dysfunction by Ang II and the well-known link between Ang II action on the vascular wall and inflammation [26], the cytokine profile in the vascular wall of the OPG^{+} and OPG^{-} mice was also assessed. Analysis of cytokines showed that the aortic wall of OPG-knockout mice exhibited a pro-inflammatory profile. The levels of various proteins, including BCA-1/CXCL13, Eotaxin-2/CCL24, Fractalkine/CX3CL1, I-309/CCL1, IL-1B, I-TAC/CXCL11, and MCP-1/CCL2, were significantly increased in the aortic wall of OPG-knockout mice when compared to wild-type mice. These proteins play critical roles in the complex landscape of cardiovascular diseases (CVDs). Each of these proteins contributes to different aspects of the inflammatory and immune responses associated with cardiovascular pathophysiology [32–34].

The pro-inflammatory cytokine profile in the aortic wall of OPG^{-} mice found in this study could explain the first observations made by Bucay et al. and Mizuno et al. in mice with a knockout gene for OPG [9,10]. At the time, it was noted that these mice not only had increased osteoporosis and a higher incidence of bone fractures but also had increased calcification of the aortic wall and renal arteries [7,9–11]. These early observations provided the basis for considering OPG as a vascular protective factor against calcification, and the similarities between the regulation of osteoclastogenesis in bones and this calcification of the vascular wall and the involvement of the RANK-RANKL-OPG signalling axis in this regulation seemed to support such a hypothesis. However, this was not confirmed by subsequent studies in humans. These studies showed, among other things, that older women with severe osteoporosis have high OPG levels and that these levels are higher the more advanced the osteoporosis [7,35,36]. In addition, high OPG levels in these women correlated strongly and positively with cardiovascular mortality [7,37,38]. Other studies have shown that high OPG concentrations in patients with CAD correlate strongly and positively with the severity of CAD and cardiovascular mortality [3,7,39–41]. It has also been confirmed that an increase in OPG levels during acute coronary syndromes is an indicator of the risk of adverse cardiovascular events and poor prognosis [16,17]. This was initially thought to be a protective mechanism, with the belief that OPG levels increase in response to harmful agents and that high OPG levels may have a protective effect or at least be a marker of the potency of the damaging effects of other factors. However, subsequent studies have provided ample evidence of the direct adverse effects of OPG on the blood vessel wall, including increased leukocyte adhesion to the endothelial surface, activation of the renin–angiotensin–system (RAS), pro-inflammatory and pro-fibrotic effects, and the induction of endothelial dysfunction at early stages of atherogenesis [42]. The known mechanisms of OPG action on vascular wall cells now allow a better understanding of the clinical observations, indicating a strong association between high OPG concentrations, the presence and course of CVDs, and the development of HF and cardiovascular mortality. It is now believed that, although, at the initial stage, the increase in OPG concentrations may be a response of the vascular wall to various damaging agents, at a later stage, the persistence of high OPG concentrations results in the activation of mechanisms of adverse OPG action that ultimately contribute to vascular damage and atherogenesis [42].

In our study, we also found that incubation of the aortic wall of OPG^+ mice with Ang II resulted in a significant increase in IL-6 levels (a 77% increase) in the aortic wall under the influence of Ang II. In OPG^- mice, this increase in IL-6 was absent in response to Ang II (Figure 3). This indicates a differential response of the vascular wall to Ang II depending on the availability of OPG. This differential response was also observed for other cytokines. Indeed, it was found that in OPG^- mice, incubation of aortic rings with Ang II was associated with lower concentrations of the cytokines tested compared to the control group. This was not observed in OPG^+ mice. The decrease in cytokine levels after incubation with Ang II involved proteins such as BCA-1/CXCL13, I-309/CCL1, IL-4, I-TAC/CXCL11, and IP-10/CXCL10 (Figure 4). Thus, when there was a lack of OPG, there was no Ang II-mediated increase in IL-6 levels, and there was an Ang II-mediated decrease in levels of the aforementioned cytokines. This indicates the importance of the link between OPG and Ang II, which plays a major role in the pathogenesis of atherosclerosis [4]. Previous studies have confirmed that Ang II acts directly on the vascular endothelium, leading to endothelial dysfunction, the development of inflammation, and the progression of atherosclerosis [26]. Reciprocal stimulatory interactions between OPG and Ang II have been demonstrated [3,27–29]. Ang II has been shown to increase OPG expression in human and murine vascular cells. OPG has also been shown to increase the expression of the AT1 receptor for Ang II in these cells [3,30]. This is one of the postulated mechanisms by which OPG may promote endothelial dysfunction and the development of atherosclerotic lesions. This may explain the results of our functional myograph studies in which, despite the incubation of the aortic rings with Ang II, a normal endothelium-dependent response to acetylcholine was observed in the absence of OPG in the OPG^- mice. The results obtained in both parts of the experiments suggest that the presence of OPG in the model of induction of endothelial dysfunction is crucial for eliciting the inflammatory effect of Ang II.

3.3. *Mechanisms of Action of OPG in Vascular Wall*

There are three ways in which OPG exerts its biological effect on the cells of the vascular walls. Firstly, by attaching itself through a specific domain to its ligand RANKL, OPG prevents RANKL from joining its receptor, RANK. Secondly, OPG triggers cell-surface signalling by direct action on the cells. It achieves this through a heparin-binding domain, which is able to bind to heparan sulphate proteoglycans, which can be found on the surface of cells. Such action has been confirmed in bones as well as in cells of the vascular wall and immune system [3,6,25,43]. Thirdly, OPG diminishes or eliminates the effects of TRAIL. It does this by attaching itself to its ligand TRAIL, thereby preventing TRAIL binding to its receptors [6].

RAS is crucial in the development of adverse changes, which occur with age, in the VSMCs and ECs phenotype, as well as the pathogenesis of atherosclerosis [4]. Direct action on the vascular endothelium by the main mediator of RAS, which is Ang II, causes dysfunction, further inflammation, and the development of atherosclerosis. Heightened expression of vascular endothelial growth factors (VEGFs), VEGF-A and VEGF-B, caused by the activation of the angiotensin II type 1 (AT1) receptor, enhance inflammation and remodelling in blood vessels by triggering pro-inflammatory mechanisms and pathological angiogenesis. These VEGF actions are intensified by OPG [26]. Both atheroma-derived cells harvested during endarterectomy and ECs from human dermal microvasculature were tested under cell culture conditions and cultivated with and without irbesartan, which is the blocker of the AT1 receptor [44]. In these cells, a reduction in the concentration levels of IL-6, interleukin-8 (IL-8), and OPG has been confirmed with the use of irbesartan. Furthermore, the blockade of the AT1 receptor in these cells caused a decrease in extracellular signal-regulated kinase-1 and -2 (ERK1 and ERK2) expression as well as a reduction in their phosphorylation, which is usually activated by RANKL when it is bound to RANK. Similarly, there was also a reduction in RANKL-induced ERK1 and ERK2 phosphorylation in a study with mice using losartan—another blocker of AT1 [45]. This would suggest that, at the level of ERK1/2 phosphorylation regulation, there is a convergent action of RANKL and Ang II. OPG can also directly activate ERK1/2 phosphorylation, which is linked to pathological angiogenesis [4,44,45].

Furthermore, it has been confirmed that mutual stimulating interactions exist between OPG and RAS [3,27–29]. Ang II increases OPG expression in vascular wall cells in both humans and mice, while irbesartan reduces the OPG expression in these cells by blocking the AT1 receptor. In the same way that Ang II has a dose-dependent effect in enhancing OPG expression in vascular wall cells, OPG has a dose-dependent effect in enhancing the expression of the AT1 receptor [3,30].

Ang II causes an increase in the expression of VEGF, which results in an over-expression of RANK in ECs and intensifies the angiogenic response of these cells to RANKL. A possible additional RANKL action, which occurs via the PI3-kinase/Akt signalling pathway, is to maintain EC integrity and induce a pro-survival effect on ECs [4]. This effect is inhibited when OPG binds with RANKL, thereby impeding its link with RANK and the activation of the PI3-kinase/Akt signalling pathway. When PI3-kinase is inhibited, the pro-survival effect of RANKL in relation to ECs is blocked [46]. Ang II enhances the expression of VEGF, which suppresses the PI3-kinase/Akt signalling pathway [47].

3.4. Conclusions, Potential Clinical Implications, and Future Perspectives

Based on our results, we may conclude that the OPG gene knockout protects against Ang II-induced endothelial dysfunction in mice. The absence of OPG, although associated with a pro-inflammatory cytokine profile in the vascular wall, simultaneously protects against Ang II-induced increases in pro-inflammatory cytokine concentrations in the murine vascular wall. As shown in our study, the absence of OPG can even lead to a decrease in the concentration of pro-inflammatory cytokines in the vascular wall exposed to Ang II. The presence of OPG is therefore crucial for the development of Ang II-induced inflammation in the vascular wall and for the development of Ang II-induced endothelial dysfunction. OPG may therefore be a potential therapeutic target in cardiovascular diseases with significant activation of the RAS and consequently high concentrations of Ang II inducing inflammation in the vascular wall and endothelial dysfunction.

There are several areas of particular interest, one of which is the interaction between OPG and TRAIL, which suppresses the mesenchymal stem cell (MSC) migratory activity caused by TRAIL. This suppressive activity of OPG on MSC migration has been demonstrated in vitro. This is of particular interest because there is, among other things, an increase in MSCs migrating from the bone marrow to the infarcted area of the myocardium during the AMI. It is currently believed that these cells help to regenerate the heart muscle and protect the left ventricle from unfavourable post-infarction remodelling [19]. This TRAIL activity related to MSC, together with the anti-inflammatory and anti-atherosclerotic effects of TRAIL, means that the regulation of its activity by tumour necrosis factor -alpha (TNF-α) and OPG continues to arouse interest. It is possible that the increase in OPG concentrations, which reduces the positive effects of TRAIL on MSCs and on the vascular system, may have important pathogenic implications for AMI [19]. The prospect of disabling this OPG action is an exciting concept in treating CVDs in the future.

Research is also underway to determine the possibility of diminishing the effects of OPG on TRAIL, where it acts on the vascular cell walls. Of particular interest are the studies which demonstrate that TRAIL stimulates endothelial nitric oxide synthase (eNOS) and increases the production of nitric oxide (NO) in ECs [48]. The results, to date, have been encouraging, as the search continues to eliminate the unwanted effects of OPG and enhance the effect of TRAIL in the vascular system. Whether this can be achieved or, indeed, whether it will prove to be beneficial is still unknown, but bearing in mind the mechanisms of action of OPG and TRAIL in the cardiovascular system, it does appear to be a potential therapeutic target in CVDs.

Furthermore, it is thought that OPG is a chemotactic factor in the infiltration of inflammatory cells into the vascular wall, which occurs in the initial stages of atherosclerotic lesions [4,25,49–53]. Pro-inflammatory cytokines, such as IL-6 and interleukin-1ß (IL-1ß), are sourced from activated inflammatory cells. The ability of OPG, firstly, to interact with these cytokines and, secondly, to enhance adhesion molecule expression in ECs now forms the rationale for the search for new strategies in the treatment of CVDs, with the cytokines and their receptors as potential therapeutic targets.

This knowledge concerning the mechanisms of action of OPG on the vascular wall has led to a better understanding of the clinical observations, which demonstrate a strong relationship between CVDs and high OPG concentrations. These mechanisms of action are also now considered extremely important for the pathogenesis of CVDs and for future CVD therapies. Researchers are currently investigating what the best methods may be for neutralising the effects of OPG on the cells in the CV system and whether these methods will provide clinical benefits. There is no doubt, however, that, due to these mechanisms of action on the CV system, the signal axis with a central role of OPG is a potential therapeutic target in CVDs.

For the next step in our study, we plan to carry out in vivo research to assess the differences in responses to Ang II in OPG^+ and OPG^- mice. This will be performed based on a murine model of endothelial dysfunction induced by long-term intraperitoneal administration of Ang II with an osmotic pump. This experimental model [54] will allow us not only to assess the endothelial function but also to compare vascular remodelling, hypertension, oxidative stress and damage to various organs, as well as cytokine and adhesion molecule expression in OPG^+ and OPG^- mice exposed to Ang II.

3.5. *Limitation of the Study*

The main limitation of this study is the use of the mouse model. Due to the complex regulation of OPG in the human body, a mouse model with the knockout of the OPG gene may not fully correlate to human physiology. Moreover, although Ang II is widely used in experiments as an inductor of endothelial dysfunction, it does not fully reflect the complexity of such dysfunction.

4. Materials and Methods

Thoracic aortic segments from male wild-type mice (C57BL/6J, OPG^+) and from OPG-knockout mice (B6.129.S4-OPG, OPG^-), which were directly derived from C57BL/6J mice, were used for the experiment. The animals were purchased from The Jackson Laboratory, Farmington, CT, USA. All mice were kept under specific pathogen-free conditions (SPF) and fed a standard laboratory diet and water ad libitum. All experimental procedures used in this study were carried out in accordance with the Guidelines for the Care and Treatment of Animals of the European Communities and the Guide for the Care and Use of Laboratory Animals published by the US National Institutes of Health (NIH publication number 85-23, revised 1996). The mice were anaesthetised with ketamine/xylazine (100/10 mg/kg body weight). Each thoracic aorta was quickly removed and placed in Krebs-Heinseleit (KH) buffer with the following composition (mM): NaCl 118.0, $CaCl_2$ 2.52, $MgSO_4$ 1.16, $NaHCO_3$ 24.88, KH_2PO_4 1.18, KCl 4.7, glucose 10.0, pyruvic acid 2.0, EDTA 0.5. Aortas were carefully dissected from the surrounding tissues and cut into rings (2 mm long). Aortic rings were randomly divided into experimental groups (control, Ang II) and incubated for 24 h in medium (MEM, 0.1% FBS) only (control group) or with Ang II (1 μM) (Ang II group), at 37 °C (CellCulture CO_2 incubator, ESCO), as previously described by other authors [31]. After 24 h of incubation, the aortic rings were directly transferred to the organ bath for functional studies using a set of myographs. In another part of the experiment, after the same 24 h of incubation, the aortic rings were frozen in PathScan Lysis Buffer (Cell Signaling Technology, Danvers, MA, USA) at −80 °C for subsequent biochemical analyses (Figure 5).

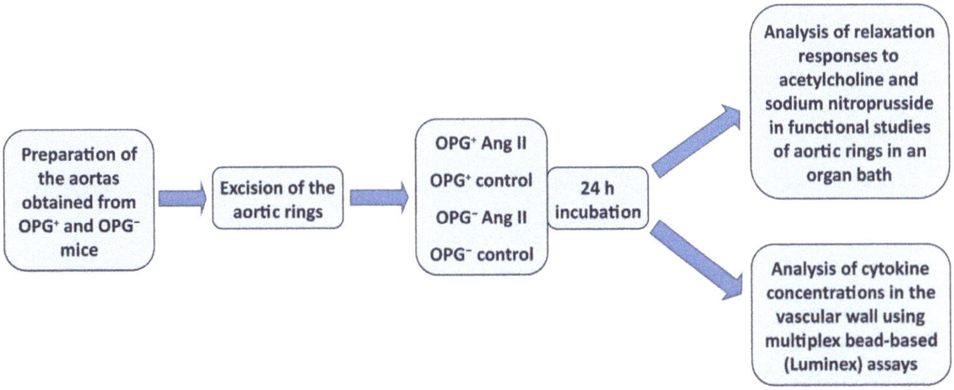

Figure 5. Research diagram.

4.1. Evaluation of Nitric Oxide-Dependent Endothelial Function in the Isolated Murine Aorta

After the 24 h of incubation described above, the aortic rings were mounted on two pins in the organ chambers of the wire myograph (620 M, Danish Myo Technology, Hinnerup, Denmark), filled with 5 mL of KH buffer, and gassed with carbogen (95% O_2, 5% CO_2) at 37 °C. After assembly, the aortic rings were equilibrated for 30 min without stretching. The resting tension of the rings was then gradually increased to 10 mN. After the equilibration period, aortic viability was assessed by contractile responses to potassium chloride (30 and 60 mM of KCl), and maximal contraction to phenylephrine (Phe; 3 μM) was evoked. NO-dependent endothelial function was assessed by the relaxation response to cumulative concentrations of acetylcholine (ACh; 0.01–10 μM) in vessels pre-contracted with phenylephrine (Phe; 0.1–1 μM). Endothelium-independent relaxation was determined using cumulative concentrations of sodium nitroprusside (SNP; 0.001–10 μM). All tissue responses were recorded using a data-acquisition system and recording software (Power Lab, LabChart 3.01, AD Instruments, Bella Vista NSW, Australia). The relaxation response was expressed as a percentage of the pre-contraction induced by phenylephrine.

4.2. Fluorescent Bead-Based Luminex Cytokine Assay

The murine aortic rings, which had been previously frozen at −80 °C, were thawed and homogenised on ice in PathScan Lysis Buffer (Cell Signaling Technology, Danvers, MA, USA) using TissueRuptor (Qiagen, Germantown, MD, USA). The solution was then centrifuged (10 min. at 10,000× *g* 4 °C), and the total protein in the supernatant was evaluated using the BCA method (MERCK KGaA, Darmstadt, Germany). The protein concentration was normalised, and an equal amount of total protein was used in the Luminex assay. Cytokine concentrations were measured using multiplex bead-based (Luminex) assays on a Bio-Plex 200 Suspension Array System according to the manufacturer's instructions. Bio-Plex Pro Mouse Assays (Bio-Rad Laboratories, Watford, UK) were used. Data were acquired on a validated and calibrated Bio-Plex 200 system (Bio-Rad Laboratories, Watford, UK) and analysed using Bio-Plex Manager 6.0 software (Bio-Rad Laboratories, Watford, UK) with a detection target of 50 beads per region, high RP1 target for CAL2 calibration, and recommended doublet discriminator (DD) gates of 5000–25,000 for Bio-Plex. The median fluorescence intensity (MFI) was measured. The concentration of each cytokine was calculated from the standard curve using Bio-Plex software 6.0 (Bio-Rad Laboratories, Watford, UK).

4.3. Statistical Analysis

Data were analysed by Prism 9.5.0 software (GraphPad, CA, USA). Results are presented as the mean ± SEM. The normality of the results was analysed using the Shapiro–Wilk test. To calculate statistical significance, an Unpaired Student's *t*-test or Mann–Whitney test was used.

Author Contributions: Conceptualisation, M.D. and W.W.; Methodology, M.D., E.B. and W.G.; Software, M.D.; Formal Analysis, T.F.; Investigation, M.D., E.B. and W.G.; Resources, A.K. and P.G.; Data Curation, M.D.; Writing—Original Draft Preparation, M.D.; Writing—Review and Editing, M.D., W.G., A.K., T.F., P.G. and E.B.; Supervision, W.W. and T.F.; Project Administration, W.W. and T.F.; Funding Acquisition, W.W. and T.F. All authors have read and agreed to the published version of the manuscript.

Funding: This article was supported by a grant from Narodowe Centrum Nauki (National Centre of Science) in Poland. Grant Number: 2016/21/B/NZ5/01902.

Institutional Review Board Statement: Ethical review and approval were waived for this study, as the law in Poland does not require the approval of the Local Ethics Committee when animal tissues are taken from euthanised animals which have not been subjected to any experimental procedures. Therefore, in this type of study, the Local Ethics Committee is not involved (according to the Polish Law—"The protection of animals used for scientific and educational purposes" dated 15 January 2015, chapter 1, article 2.1. point 6, Statute Book 26.02.2015, Position 266). The study was performed in vitro on animal tissues provided by the Department for Experimental Medicine, Medical University of Silesia, ul. Medyków 4, 40-752 Katowice, Poland, and taken from euthanised animals.

Informed Consent Statement: Not applicable.

Data Availability Statement: The data that support the findings of this study are available from the corresponding author upon reasonable request.

Conflicts of Interest: The authors declare no conflicts of interest.

References

1. Ueland, T.; Yndestad, A.; Dahl, C.P.; Gullestad, L.; Aukrust, P. TNF Revisited: Osteoprotegerin and TNF—Related Molecules in Heart Failure. *Curr. Heart Fail. Rep.* **2012**, *9*, 92–100. [CrossRef] [PubMed]
2. Korzon-Burakowska, A.; Burakowski, S. Oś osteoprotegeryna/RANKL/RANK—Rola w powikłaniach cukrzycy oraz w chorobie wieńcowej. *Diabetol. Prakt.* **2007**, *8*, 161–164.
3. Bernardi, S.; Bossi, F.; Toffoli, B.; Fabris, B. Roles and Clinical Applications of OPG and TRAIL as Biomarkers in Cardiovascular Disease. *Biomed. Res. Int.* **2016**, *2016*, 1752854. [CrossRef] [PubMed]
4. Rochette, L.; Meloux, A.; Rigal, E.; Zeller, M.; Cottin, Y.; Cottin, Y.; Vergely, C. The Role of Osteoprotegerin and Its Ligands in Vascular Function. *Int. J. Mol. Sci.* **2019**, *20*, 705. [CrossRef] [PubMed]
5. Montagnana, M.; Lippi, G.; Danese, E.; Guidi, G.C. The role of osteoprotegerin in cardiovascular disease. *Ann. Med.* **2013**, *45*, 254–264. [CrossRef] [PubMed]
6. Celebi Torabfam, G.; Porsuk, M.H. The Role of the Receptor Activator of Nuclear Factor Kappa-B Ligand/Osteoprotegerin Ratio in Vascular Diseases: A Therapeutic Approach. *Angiology* **2024**, *2024*, 00033197231226275. [CrossRef] [PubMed]
7. Corallini, F.; Rimondi, E.; Secchiero, P. TRAIL and osteoprotegerin: A role in endothelial physiopathology? *Front. Biosci.* **2008**, *13*, 135–147. [CrossRef] [PubMed]
8. Stępień, E. Osteoprotegerin as a possible novel predictor of cardiovascular dysfunction. *Kardiochirurgia I Torakochirurgia Pol.* **2012**, *9*, 82–85.
9. Bucay, N.; Sarosi, I.; Dunstan, C.R.; Morony, S.; Tarpley, J.; Capparelli, C.; Scully, S.; Tan, H.L.; Xu, W.; Lacey, D.L.; et al. Osteoprotegerin-deficient mice develop early onset osteoporosis and arterial calcification. *Genes Dev.* **1998**, *12*, 1260–1268. [CrossRef]
10. Mizuno, A.; Amizuka, N.; Irie, K.; Murakami, A.; Fujise, N.; Kanno, T.; Sato, Y.; Nakagawa, N.; Yasuda, H.; Mochizuki, S.; et al. Severe osteoporosis in mice lacking osteoclastogenesis inhibitory factor/osteoprotegerin. *Biochem. Biophys. Res. Comm.* **1998**, *247*, 610–615. [CrossRef]
11. Hofbauer, L.C.; Schoppet, M. Clinical implications of the osteoprotegerin/RANKL/RANK system for bone and vascular disease. *JAMA* **2004**, *292*, 490–495. [CrossRef] [PubMed]
12. Bjerre, M. Osteoprotegerin (OPG) as a biomarker for diabetic cardiovascular complications. *SpringerPlus* **2013**, *2*, 658. [CrossRef] [PubMed]

13. Özkalaycı, F.; Gülmez, Ö.; Uğur-Altun, B.; Pandi-Perumal, S.R.; Altun, A. The Role of Osteoprotegerin as a Cardioprotective versus Reactive Inflammatory Marker: The Chicken or the Egg Paradox. *Balkan Med. J.* **2018**, *35*, 225–232. [CrossRef] [PubMed]
14. Shin, J.Y.; Shin, J.G.; Chung, C.H. Elevated Serum Osteoprotegerin Levels Are Associated with Vascular Endothelial Dysfunction in Type 2 Diabetes. *Diabetes Care* **2006**, *9*, 1664–1666. [CrossRef] [PubMed]
15. Secchiero, P.; Corallini, F.; Beltrami, A.; Ceconi, C.; Bonasia, V.; Di Chiara, A.; Ferrari, R.; Zauli, G. An imbalanced OPG/TRAIL ratio is associated to severe acute myocardial infarction. *Atherosclerosis* **2010**, *210*, 274–277. [CrossRef] [PubMed]
16. Bjerre, M.; Munk, K.; Sloth, A.D.; Nielsen, S.T.; Flyvbjerg, A.; Bøtker, H.E. High osteoprotegerin leves predict MACCE in STEMI patients, but are not assotiated with myocardial salvage. *Scand. Cardiovasc. J.* **2014**, *48*, 209–215. [CrossRef]
17. Pedersen, S.; Mogelvang, R.; Bjerre, M.; Frystyk, J.; Flyvbjerg, A.; Galatius, S.; Sørensen, T.B.; Iversen, A.; Hvelplund, A.; Jensen, J.S. Osteoprotegerin predicts long-term outcam in patients with ST-segment elevation myocardial infarction treated with primary percutaneous coronary intervention. *Cardiology* **2012**, *123*, 31–38. [CrossRef] [PubMed]
18. Erkol, A.; Oduncu, V.; Pala, S.; Kizilirmak, F.; Kilicgedik, A.; Yılmaz, F.; Güler, A.; Karabay, C.Y.; Kırma, C. Plasma osteoprotegerin level on admission is associated with no-reflow phenomenon after primary angioplasty and subsequent left ventricular remodeling in patients with acute ST-segment elevation myocardial infarction. *Atherosclerosis* **2012**, *221*, 254–259. [CrossRef] [PubMed]
19. Corallini, F.; Secchiero, P.; Beltrami, A.P.; Cesselli, D.; Puppato, E.; Ferrari, R.; Beltrami, C.A.; Zauli, G. TNF–alfa modulates the migratory response of mesenchymal stem cells to TRAIL. *Cell. Mol. Life Sci.* **2010**, *67*, 1307–1314. [CrossRef] [PubMed]
20. Kamimura, D.; Suzuki, T.; Furniss, A.L.; Griswold, M.E.; Kullo, I.J.; Lindsey, M.L.; Winniford, M.D.; Butler, K.R.; Mosley, T.H.; Hall, M.E. Elevated serum osteoprotegerin is associated with increased left ventricular mass index and myocardial stiffness. *J. Cardiovasc. Med.* **2017**, *18*, 954–961. [CrossRef]
21. Skrzypczyk, P.; Stelmaszczyk-Emmel, A.; Szyszka, M.; Ofiara, A.; Pańczyk-Tomaszewska, M. Circulating calcification inhibitors are associated with arterial damage in pediatric patients with primary hypertension. *Pediatr. Nephrol.* **2021**, *36*, 2371–2382. [CrossRef] [PubMed]
22. Bernardi, S.; Toffoli, B.; Bossi, F.; Candido, R.; Stenner, E.; Carretta, R.; Barbone, F.; Fabris, B. Circulating osteoprotegerin is associated with chronic kidney disease in hypertensive patients. *BMC Nephrol.* **2017**, *18*, 219. [CrossRef] [PubMed]
23. Sailaja, A.N.; Nanda, N.; Suryanarayana, B.S.; Pal, G.K. Association of rs2073618 polymorphism and osteoprotegerin levels with hypertension and cardiovascular risks in patients with type 2 diabetes mellitus. *Sci. Rep.* **2023**, *13*, 17451. [CrossRef]
24. Collin-Osdoby, P.; Rothe, L.; Anderson, F.; Nelson, M.; Maloney, W.; Osdoby, P. Receptor Activator of NF-kB and Osteoprotegerin Expression by Human Microvascular Endothelial Cells, Regulation by Inflammatory Cytokines, and Role in Human Osteoclastogenesis. *J. Biol. Chem.* **2001**, *276*, 20659–20672. [CrossRef] [PubMed]
25. Zauli, G.; Corallini, F.; Bossi, F.; Fischetti, F.; Durigutto, P.; Celeghini, C.; Tedesco, F.; Secchiero, P. Osteoprotegerin increases leukocyte adhesion to endothelial cells both in vitro and in vivo. *Blood* **2007**, *110*, 536–543. [CrossRef] [PubMed]
26. Malyankar, U.M.; Scatena, M.; Suchland, K.L.; Yun, T.J.; Clark, E.A.; Giachelli, C.M. Osteoprotegerin is an alpha vbeta 3-induced, NF-kappa B-dependent survival factor for endothelial cells. *J. Biol. Chem.* **2000**, *275*, 20959–20962. [CrossRef] [PubMed]
27. Toffoli, B.; Pickering, R.J.; Tsorotes, D.; Wang, B.; Bernardi, S.; Kantharidis, P.; Fabris, B.; Zauli, G.; Secchiero, P.; Thomas, M.C. Osteoprotegerin promotes vascular fibrosis via a TGF-β1 autocrine loop. *Atherosclerosis* **2011**, *218*, 61–68. [CrossRef] [PubMed]
28. Zhang, J.; Fu, M.; Myles, D.; Zhu, X.; Du, J.; Cao, X.; Chen, Y.E. PDGF induces osteoprotegerin expression in vascular smooth muscle cells by multiple signal pathways. *FEBS Lett.* **2002**, *521*, 180–184. [CrossRef] [PubMed]
29. Moran, C.S.; McCann, M.; Karan, M.; Norman, P.; Ketheesan, N.; Golledge, J. Association of osteoprotegerin with human abdominal aortic aneurysm progression. *Circulation* **2005**, *111*, 3119–3125. [CrossRef] [PubMed]
30. Moran, C.S.; Cullen, B.; Campbell, J.H.; Golledge, J. Interaction between angiotensin II, osteoprotegerin, and peroxisome proliferator-activated receptor-γ in abdominal aortic aneurysm. *J. Vasc. Res.* **2009**, *46*, 209–217. [CrossRef]
31. Mateuszuk, Ł.; Campagna, R.; Kutryb-Zając, B.; Kuś, K.; Słominska, E.M.; Smolenski, R.T.; Chlopicki, S. Reversal of endothelial dysfunction by nicotinamide mononucleotide via extracellular conversion to nicotinamide riboside. *Biochem. Pharmacol.* **2020**, *178*, 114019. [CrossRef] [PubMed]
32. van der Vorst, E.P.C.; Daissormont, I.; Aslani, M.; Seijkens, T.; Wijnands, E.; Lutgens, E.; Duchene, J.; Santovito, D.; Döring, Y.; Halvorsen, B.; et al. Interruption of the CXCL13/CXCR5 Chemokine Axis Enhances Plasma IgM Levels and Attenuates Atherosclerosis Development. *Thromb. Haemost.* **2020**, *120*, 344–347. [CrossRef] [PubMed]
33. Luo, S.; Zhu, R.; Yu, T.; Fan, H.; Hu, Y.; Mohanta, S.K.; Hu, D. Chronic Inflammation: A Common Promoter in Tertiary Lymphoid Organ Neogenesis. *Front. Immunol.* **2019**, *10*, 2938. [CrossRef]
34. Wang, Z.; Xu, H.; Chen, M.; Lu, Y.; Zheng, L.; Ma, L. CCL24/CCR3 axis plays a central role in angiotensin II-induced heart failure by stimulating M2 macrophage polarization and fibroblast activation. *Cell Biol. Toxicol.* **2023**, *39*, 1413–1431. [CrossRef] [PubMed]
35. Boukhris, R.; Becker, K.L. Calcification of the aorta and osteoporosis. A roentgenographic study. *JAMA* **1972**, *219*, 1307–1311. [CrossRef] [PubMed]
36. Kado, D.M.; Browner, W.S.; Blackwell, T.; Gore, R.; Cummings, R.S. Rate of bone loss is associated with mortality in older women: A prospective study. *J. Bone Miner. Res.* **2000**, *15*, 1974–1980. [CrossRef] [PubMed]
37. Yano, K.; Tsuda, E.; Washida, N.; Kobayashi, F.; Goto, M.; Harada, A.; Ikeda, K.; Higashio, K.; Yamada, Y. Immunological characterization of circulating osteoprotegerin/osteoclasto-genesis inhibitory factor: Increased serum concentrations in postmenopausal women with osteoporosis. *J. Bone Miner. Res.* **1999**, *14*, 518–527. [CrossRef] [PubMed]

38. Price, P.A.; June, H.H.; Buckley, J.R.; Williamson, M.K. Osteoprotegerin inhibits artery calcification induced by warfarin and by vitamin D. *Arterioscler. Thromb. Vasc. Biol.* **2001**, *21*, 1610–1616. [CrossRef] [PubMed]
39. Browner, W.S.; Lui, L.Y.; Cummings, S.R. Associations of serum osteoprotegerin levels with diabetes, stroke, bone density, fractures, and mortality in elderly women. *J. Clin. Endocrinol. Metab.* **2001**, *86*, 631–637. [CrossRef] [PubMed]
40. Jono, S.; Ikari, Y.; Shioi, A.; Mori, K.; Miki, T.; Hara, K.; Nishizawa, Y. Serum osteoprotegerin levels are associated with the presence and severity of coronary artery disease. *Circulation* **2002**, *106*, 1192–1194. [CrossRef]
41. Knudsen, S.T.; Foss, C.H.; Poulsen, P.L.; Andersen, N.H.; Mogensen, C.E.; Rasmussen, L.M. Increased plasma concentrations of osteoprotegerin in type 2 diabetic patients with microvascular complications. *Eur. J. Endocrinol.* **2003**, *149*, 39–42. [CrossRef]
42. Dutka, M.; Bobiński, R.; Wojakowski, W.; Francuz, T.; Pająk, C.; Zimmer, K. Osteoprotegerin and RANKL-RANK-OPG-TRAIL signalling axis in heart failure and other cardiovascular diseases. *Heart Fail. Rev.* **2022**, *27*, 1395–1411. [CrossRef]
43. Wright, H.L.; McCarthy, H.S.; Middleton, J.; Marshall, M.J. RANK, RANKL and osteoprotegerin in bone biology and disease. *Curr. Rev. Musculoskelet. Med.* **2009**, *2*, 56–64. [CrossRef]
44. Clancy, P.; Koblar, S.A.; Golledge, J. Angiotensin receptor 1 blockade reduces secretion of inflammation associated cytokines from cultured human carotid atheroma and vascular cells in association with reduced extracellular signal regulated kinase expression and activation. *Atherosclerosis* **2014**, *236*, 108–115. [CrossRef]
45. Chen, S.; Grover, M.; Sibai, T.; Black, J.; Rianon, N.; Rajagopal, A.; Munivez, E.; Bertin, T.; Dawson, B.; Chen, Y.; et al. Losartan increases bone mass and accelerates chondrocyte hypertrophy in developing skeleton. *Mol. Genet. Metab.* **2015**, *115*, 53–60. [CrossRef]
46. Min, J.K.; Kim, Y.M.; Kim, Y.M.; Kim, E.C.; Gho, Y.S.; Kang, I.J.; Lee, S.Y.; Kong, Y.Y.; Kwon, Y.G. Vascular endothelial growth factor up-regulates expression of receptor activator of NF-kappa B (RANK) in endothelial cells. Concomitant increase of angiogenic responses to RANK ligand. *J. Biol. Chem.* **2003**, *278*, 39548–39557. [CrossRef]
47. Potente, M.; Carmeliet, P. The Link between Angiogenesis and Endothelial Metabolism. *Annu. Rev. Physiol.* **2017**, *79*, 43–66. [CrossRef]
48. Di Pietro, R.; Mariggiò, M.A.; Guarnieri, S.; Sancilio, S.; Giardinelli, A.; Di Silvestre, S.; Consoli, A.; Zauli, G.; Pandolfi, A. Tumor necrosis factor-related apoptosis-inducing ligand (TRAIL) regulates endothelial nitric oxide synthase (eNOS) activity and its localization within the human vein endothelial cells (HUVEC) in culture. *J. Cell. Biochem.* **2006**, *97*, 782–794. [CrossRef]
49. Bernardi, S.; Fabris, B.; Thomas, M.; Toffoli, B.; Tikellis, C.; Candido, R.; Catena, C.; Mulatero, P.; Barbone, F.; Radillo, O.; et al. Osteoprotegerin increases in metabolic syndrome and promotes adipose tissue proinflammatory changes. *Mol. Cell. Endocrinol.* **2014**, *394*, 13–20. [CrossRef]
50. Mangan, S.H.; Van Campenhout, A.; Rush, C.; Golledge, J. Osteoprotegerin upregulates endothelial cell adhesion molecule response to tumor necrosis factor-alpha associated with induction of angiopoietin-2. *Cardiovasc. Res.* **2007**, *76*, 494–505. [CrossRef] [PubMed]
51. Bennett, B.J.; Scatena, M.; Kirk, E.A.; Rattazzi, M.; Varon, R.M.; Averill, M.; Schwartz, S.M.; Giachelli, C.M.; Rosenfeld, M.E. Osteoprotegerin inactivation accelerates advanced atherosclerotic lesion progression and calcification in older ApoE−/− mice. *Arterioscler. Thromb. Vasc. Biol.* **2006**, *26*, 2117–2124. [CrossRef] [PubMed]
52. Kobayashi, Y. The regulatory role of nitric oxide in proinflammatory cytokine expression during the induction and resolution of inflammation. *J. Leukoc. Biol.* **2010**, *88*, 1157–1162. [CrossRef]
53. Quercioli, A.; Mach, F.; Bertolotto, M.; Lenglet, S.; Vuilleumier, N.; Galan, K.; Pagano, S.; Braunersreuther, V.; Pelli, G.; Pistoia, V.; et al. Receptor activator of NF-κB ligand (RANKL) increases the release of neutrophil products associated with coronary vulnerability. *Thromb. Haemost.* **2012**, *107*, 124–139. [CrossRef] [PubMed]
54. Trejo-Moreno, C.; Jiménez-Ferrer, E.; Castro-Martínez, G.; Méndez-Martínez, M.; Santana, M.A.; Arrellín-Rosas, G.; Pedraza-Chaverri, J.; Medina-Campos, O.N.; Hernández-Téllez, B.; Ramírez-Pliego, O.; et al. Characterization of a murine model of endothelial dysfunction induced by chronic intraperitoneal administration of angiotensin II. *Sci. Rep.* **2021**, *11*, 21193. [CrossRef] [PubMed]

International Journal of
Molecular Sciences

MDPI

Article

Wall Shear Stress (WSS) Analysis in Atherosclerosis in Partial Ligated Apolipoprotein E Knockout Mouse Model through Computational Fluid Dynamics (CFD)

Minju Cho [1,†], Joon Seup Hwang [1,†], Kyeong Ryeol Kim [1] and Jun Ki Kim [1,2,*]

1 Department of Convergence Medicine, Brain Korea 21 Project, College of Medicine, University of Ulsan, Seoul 05505, Republic of Korea
2 Biomedical Engineering Research Center, Asan Institute for Life Science, Asan Medical Center, Seoul 05505, Republic of Korea
* Correspondence: kim@amc.seoul.kr; Tel.: +82-2-3010-8619
† These authors contributed equally to this work.

Abstract: Atherosclerosis involves an inflammatory response due to plaque formation within the arteries, which can lead to ischemic stroke and heart disease. It is one of the leading causes of death worldwide, with various contributing factors such as hyperlipidemia, hypertension, obesity, diabetes, and smoking. Wall shear stress (WSS) is also known as a contributing factor of the formation of atherosclerotic plaques. Since the causes of atherosclerosis cannot be attributed to a single factor, clearly understanding the mechanisms and causes of its occurrence is crucial for preventing the disease and developing effective treatment strategies. To better understand atherosclerosis and define the correlation between various contributing factors, computational fluid dynamics (CFD) analysis is primarily used. CFD simulates WSS, the frictional force caused by blood flow on the vessel wall with various hemodynamic changes. Using apolipoprotein E knockout (ApoE-KO) mice subjected to partial ligation and a high-fat diet at 1-week, 2-week, and 4-week intervals as an atherosclerosis model, CFD analysis was conducted along with the reconstruction of carotid artery blood flow via magnetic resonance imaging (MRI) and compared to the inflammatory factors and pathological staining. In this experiment, a comparative analysis of the effects of high WSS and low WSS was conducted by comparing the standard deviation of time-averaged wall shear stress (TAWSS) at each point within the vessel wall. As a novel approach, the standard deviation of TAWSS within the vessel was analyzed with the staining results and pathological features. Since the onset of atherosclerosis cannot be explained by a single factor, the aim was to find the correlation between the thickness of atherosclerotic plaques and inflammatory factors through standard deviation analysis. As a result, the gap between low WSS and high WSS widened as the interval between weeks in the atherosclerosis mouse model increased. This finding not only linked the occurrence of atherosclerosis to WSS differences but also provided a connection to the causes of vulnerable plaques.

Keywords: atherosclerosis; plaque formation; computational fluid dynamics (CFD); wall shear stress (WSS); ApoE-KO mice; standard deviation

1. Introduction

Atherosclerosis is a systemic disease characterized by the formation of plaque within the inner lining of arteries, leading to inflammation. The accumulation of fatty material in the intima, the inner layer of the artery, leads to the formation of atherosclerotic plaque, which disrupts blood flow and causes thrombus and tissue ischemia [1]. This condition can result in ischemic stroke and heart disease, which remain the leading causes of adult mortality worldwide [2]. Numerous risk factors contribute to the development of atherosclerosis, including high cholesterol, hypertension, obesity, and diabetes [1]. Low WSS is another significant risk factor that promotes the formation and progression of plaque in the arteries due to lipid accumulation, while high WSS can cause damage to the vascular intima and inflammatory reactions that can contribute to the development of vulnerable plaque [3]. Vulnerable plaque is where a fibrous cap with inflammatory onset exists within a lipid rich core [4]. Thus, WSS is associated with the genetic expression of inflammatory biomarkers such as vascular cell adhesion molecule-1(VCAM-1), nuclear factor kappa-light-chain-enhancer of activated B cells (NF-κB), cluster of differentiation 31 (CD31), alpha-smooth muscle actin (α-SMA), etc. [3]. Since hemodynamic factors such as WSS and bio-inflammatory factors, along with systemic risk factors such as high-fat diet or obesity, are linked to progressive arterial injury and subsequent atherosclerosis, understanding these risk factors and their roles in the development of atherosclerosis is crucial for developing prevention and treatment [5–7].

CFD is a powerful tool for analyzing fluid flow, such as blood flow in this case [8]. CFD simulations enable the prediction of vascular diseases by analyzing aspects of blood flow and vascular geometry that are difficult to replicate in vivo [9]. Different from angiography or computed tomography, CFD analysis can identify hemodynamic changes before the formation of plaque. This method allows for predicting the progression of plaque using hemodynamic parameters [10]. WSS refers to the frictional stress exerted on the vessel wall. When frictional stress is lowered, substances such as lipid and cholesterol can accumulate on the inner wall of blood vessels, which is associated with the onset of plaque formation [6]. This experiment specifically employed the Bird–Carreau model, which uses non-Newtonian flow behavior in calculations [11].

In this study, ApoE-KO mice were used as an in vivo animal model of the formation of atherosclerosis. The lack of apolipoprotein E leads to the accumulation of cholesterol in the bloodstream and results in low lipoprotein clearance [12]. Since the disruption of blood flow and oscillatory WSS are associated with the formation of atherosclerosis, partial ligation of the left carotid artery (LCA) was applied to the mice to induce inflammation and block blood flow [13]. Additionally, the mice were fed a high-fat diet to promote acute plaque formation [14]. The blood flow was measured through MRI to confirm the disruption occurrence on the partially ligated LCA (Figure 1A–C). To observe the relationships between high cholesterol in the bloodstream, the increased expression of inflammatory factors, and the thickness of the intima at the bifurcation and middle part of the LCA with WSS, CFD analysis (Figure 1D) was conducted [8]. ApoE-KO mice were divided into three groups for 1 week, 2 weeks, and 4 weeks. The mice were examined to analyze WSS through CFD and biological factors that influence the development of atherosclerosis. Along with WSS, inflammatory bio-factors and pathological characteristics were identified to establish their relationship in atherosclerosis. Through CFD, an increase in WSS was observed, along with the dispersion and widening gap between low and high WSS over weeks. An increase in inflammatory biomarkers and the thickness of atherosclerotic plaques was also confirmed, establishing a correlation. Since the development of atherosclerosis is influenced by multiple factors, the goal was to simulate and visualize WSS within the vessels and align it with pathological causal relationships. Therefore, as a novel approach, the relative differences in shear stress within the vessel wall were compared to examine factors contributing to the development of atherosclerosis, such as vessel wall thickness and inflammatory substances, at different time intervals.

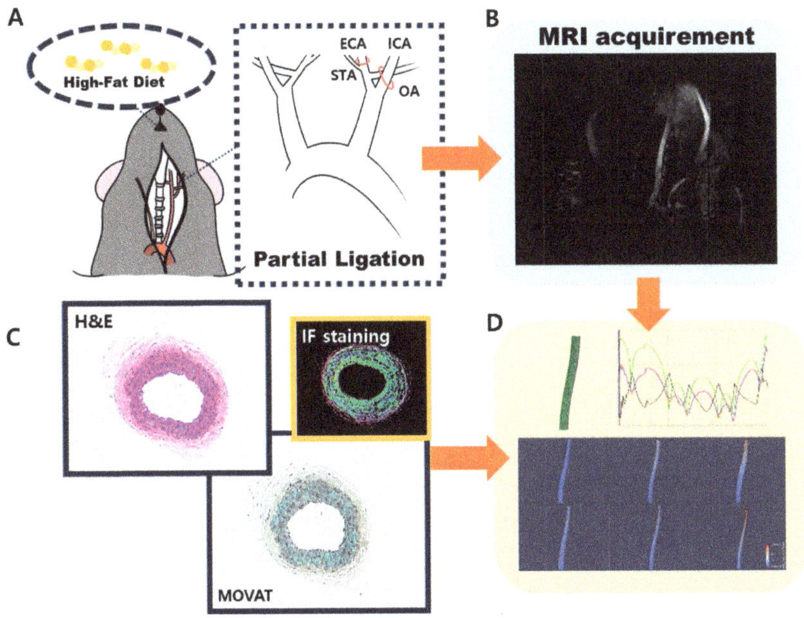

Figure 1. Scheme of WSS evaluation acquisition of ApoE-KO mice atherosclerosis model. (**A**) Partially ligated ApoE-KO mice fed a high-fat diet were developed as an atherosclerosis model. To confirm disrupted blood flow, (**B**) MRI images were acquired, along with (**C**) H&E, Movat staining, and IF staining images. Based on these results, (**D**) a 3D reconstruction of the carotid artery was performed to evaluate WSS.

2. Results

2.1. Assessment of Atherosclerosis Formation via MRI and Histological Staining

A partially ligated LCA disrupts the blood flow, and it can be confirmed by MRI. MRI is a non-invasive imaging technique that uses magnetic field gradients to obtain signals based on blood flow velocity [15]. In this experiment, the TOF mode was applied for blood flow measurement. TOF is commonly used in angiology to visualize blood vessels and blood flow dynamics without the use of contrast agents. Since a magnetic gradient produces a stronger signal in blood fluid than in the surrounding tissue, blood vessels can be easily visualized. To confirm the disruption of blood flow, partially ligated ApoE-KO mice with a high-fat diet underwent MRI imaging in the TOF mode. The mice were observed on a weekly basis. In the 1-week group, blood flow was observed in the LCA. However, in the 4-week group, a longer period of partial ligation and high-fat diet than the 1-week group contributed to the progression of atherosclerotic plaques, reducing blood flow, which was confirmed by MRI. The bloodstream became increasingly obstructed as the duration of ligation and high-fat diet in the mice lengthened, especially when comparing the mice from the 1-week group to those from the 4-week group, the blood disruption is shown to be significantly different (Figure 2A). This can probably be attributed not only to the disruption of blood flow caused by ligation but also to changes in blood flow due to the progression of atherosclerotic plaque. After MRI imaging, the mice were sacrificed, and then histological staining of the carotid artery samples was performed.

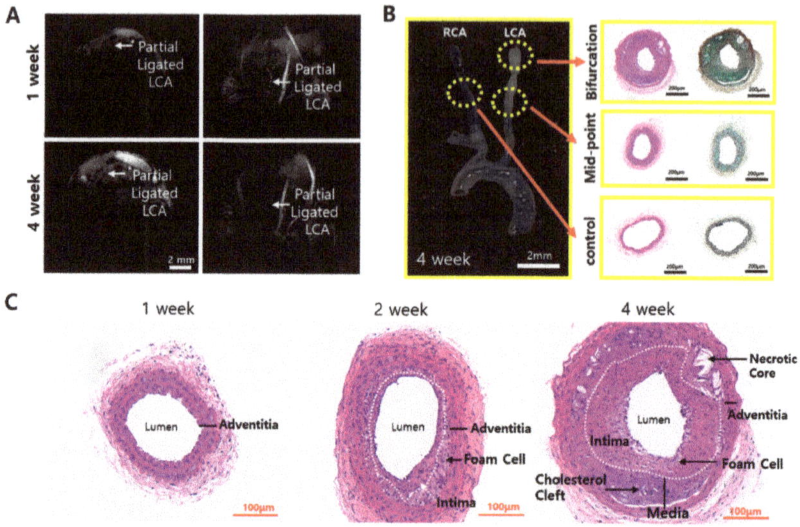

Figure 2. Blood flow disrupt confirmation through MRI TOF mode and histological staining of carotid artery. (**A**) Cross-sectioned MRI image and lateral MRI image of 1- and 4-week partial ligated ApoE-KO mice. Partial ligated LCA are indicated as white arrows in MRI images. (**B**) The excised sample of 4-week mice and H&E and MOVAT staining images of the cross-sectioned tissue at the partial ligation site (bifurcation), the midpoint, and the RCA without partial ligation as control. (**C**) H&E staining results of 1-, 2-, and 4-week LCA. Pathological features are marked in the image.

For H&E and MOVAT staining, plaque formation was observed in areas pathologically predicted to have lesions, as shown in Figure 2B. Atherosclerotic characteristics such as necrotic cores and foam cells appeared in the pathological staining, since foam cells are a major source of necrotic cores in the atherosclerosis plaque [16,17]. Figure 2C shows the 1-, 2-, and 4-week H&E staining results. Pathological features of plaque were not observed in the 1-week group mice samples. However, in the 2-week and 4-week group mice samples, the intima thickened, and foam cells began to appear. In the 4-week group samples, necrotic cores, along with foam cells and cholesterol clefts, were observed. Additionally, the intima appeared to be significantly thickened.

2.2. Immunofluorescence Staining Evaluation for Inflammation Marker

As plaque formation begins, the gene expression of inflammatory bio-factors increases, and it can be visualized through IF staining with target antibodies for the biomarkers. VCAM-1, NF-κB, CD31, and α-SMA were chosen for this experiment. VCAM-1 is one of the crucial molecules that contribute to the formation of atherosclerosis, becoming activated on the surface of arterial endothelial cells [18]. NF-κB is a transcription factor that shows increased expression when stimulated by low WSS on the inner side of the vessel [19]. NF-κB is also involved in general inflammatory responses [20]. CD31, known as platelet endothelial cell adhesion molecule-1(PECAM-1), expresses on the surface of endothelial cells, acting as a signaling receptor and stimulating the expression of inflammatory molecules on atherosclerosis lesions [21]. In addition, smooth muscle cells (SMCs) proliferate during the formation of atherosclerotic plaque, leading to intimal thickening and a change in their phenotype [22]. Since α-SMA is expressed in SMCs, atherosclerotic lesions should contain α-SMA as the intima thickens. As IF staining was conducted, the results are shown in Figure 3. The expression of NF-κB (red) increased in the 4-week mice group compared to the 1-week and 2-week mice groups, as shown in Figure 3A–C with an arrow indication. As the plaque thickened, the inflammatory response was activated, which can be confirmed by the expression level of NF-κB (Figure 3C). However, there was no significant difference in the expression levels of VCAM-1 (green). In Figure 3D–F, the expression of CD31 (red) is shown on the inner side of the intima in endothelial cells in the 4-week mice LCA while CD31 is less shown in the 1- and 2-week mice LCA. On the other hand, α-SMA (green) is shown in all 1-, 2-, and 4-week mice models, and the expression of α-SMA tends to be concentrated towards the intima, where plaque is formed. Through IF staining, it is confirmed that the inflammatory response occurred around atherosclerosis plaque. Additionally, it was confirmed that mice subjected to prolonged partial ligation and a high-fat diet had thicker plaques and atherosclerotic lesions, which corresponded with an increased expression of biomarkers.

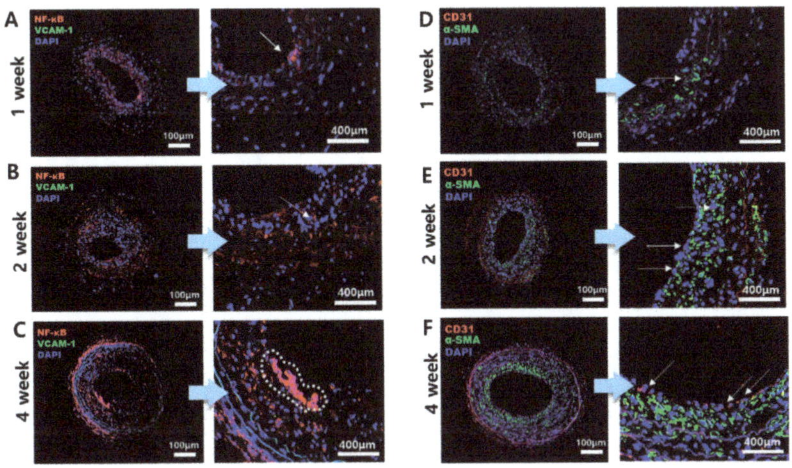

Figure 3. IF performed on the bifurcation part of the LCA. The samples were double-stained with VCAM-1 and NF-κB as one set, and CD31 and α-SMA as another set. (**A–C**) represent the 1-, 2-, and 4-week IF staining results for VCAM-1 (green) and NF-κB (red) in the LCA bifurcation. (**D–F**) show the staining results for CD31 (red) and α-SMA (green) in the LCA bifurcation, respectively. The arrows and dotted lines in the magnified images of each figure indicate the fluorescence biomarker. The arrows in Figures (**A–C**) represent NF-κB (red). The arrows in the magnified images of Figures (**D–F**) represent CD31 (red). For VCAM-1 (green), no significant observations were made, and α-SMA (green) was well visualized in Figures (**D–F**).

2.3. Wall Shear Stress Acquirement

To reconstruct the blood vessels, cross-sectional images of the ligated carotid artery and vessel images obtained from MRI were used to model the 3D structure of the ligated left carotid artery. The 3D images of the blood vessels were reconstructed to match the appearance of atherosclerotic plaques observed at 1-week, 2-week, and 4-week intervals in mice. This reconstruction reflected the narrowed internal diameter of the atherosclerotic arteries, allowing for CFD analysis. The blood flow inlet was set at the midpoint of LACE, and the outlet was set at the bifurcation. In Figure 4A, the blood flow was applied to the 3D remodeled LCA to measure WSS. The results of the blood flow simulation using fluid dynamics showed that WSS was higher at the bifurcation in the ligated mice at 1-week, 2-week, and 4-week intervals. As shown in Figure 4A, the areas with high WSS are shown in red, and in the mouse model with partial ligation and a high-fat diet for about 4 weeks, the WSS was relatively higher at the bifurcation compared to the midpoint of the vessel. Furthermore, in the 2-week mouse model, WSS also increased compared to the 1-week model. This indicates that the areas where atherosclerotic plaques are expected to form show higher WSS depending on the duration of the experiment. However, atherosclerosis formation is dependent on the low WSS [3,23].

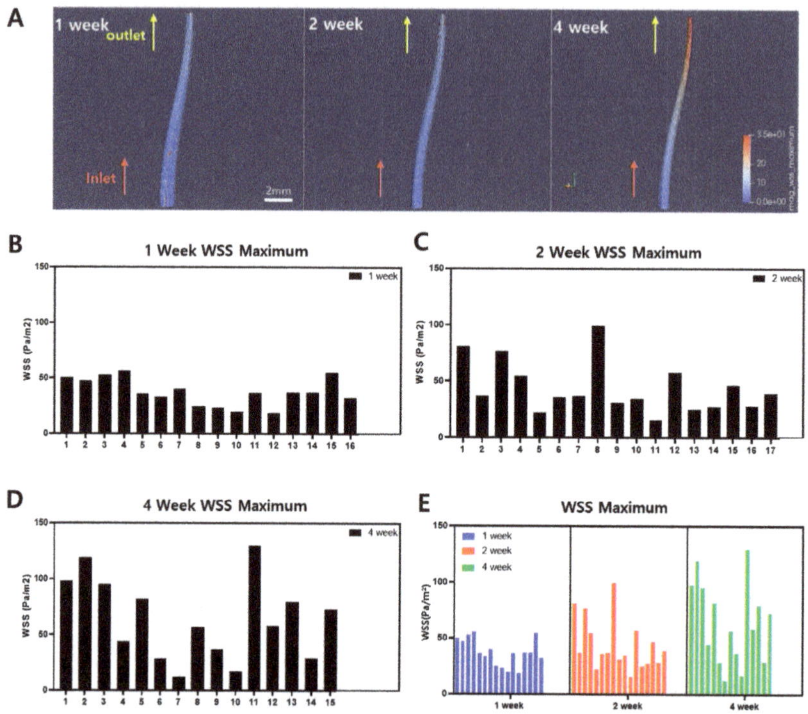

Figure 4. A 3D construction of the left carotid artery from the midpoint of LCA to bifurcation of the partial ligation part with WSS evaluation. (**A**) 3D image of LCA with WSS distribution; the red part refers to high WSS, where the blue part refers to low WSS. (**B–E**) are maximum WSS graphs for 1-, 2-, and 4-week mice in all groups, respectively.

The maximum WSS within the blood vessels of the 1-, 2-, and 4-week mice groups are shown in Figure 4B–D. The general tendency of WSS increases by the duration of the experiment regardless of some mice in the 1-week group showing high WSS and some mice in the 4-week group showing low WSS. This tendency is summarized in Figure 4E, where the maximum WSS of all groups of mice is presented in the graph. Since these results differ from the existing findings that atherosclerosis is caused by low WSS, TAWSS was compared for further analysis [24].

2.4. The Correlation between Wall Shear Stress and Atherosclerotic Lesions

ApoE-KO mice with partial ligation and a high-fat diet were observed at 1-week, 2-week, and 4-week intervals; the CFD model shows WSS values for each interval. High WSS was observed in the partially ligated region, specifically under the bifurcation area of the LCA, as shown in Figure 4A. However, previous studies often indicate that low WSS influences the formation of atherosclerotic plaques [3,23]. Thus, this experiment was approached from the perspective that WSS can be relative to each point of the inner vessel surface. In the development of atherosclerosis, WSS does not have a specific threshold value [25]. Low WSS is one of the contributing factors to the development of atherosclerosis, but it does not have an absolute value [26]. Therefore, the WSS values at each point on the inner surface of the vessel obtained through CFD can be observed using standard deviation, which allows for the relative comparison of WSS. Atherosclerotic lesions can be relatively identified as increasing in the graph of the area excluding the inner mass of the vessel in Figure 5B, as well as in the fluorescence intensity graph in Figure 5D. As the atherosclerotic plaques progress, inflammatory biomarkers increase, leading to stronger fluorescence intensity and an increase in the entire vessel containing the atherosclerotic plaque.

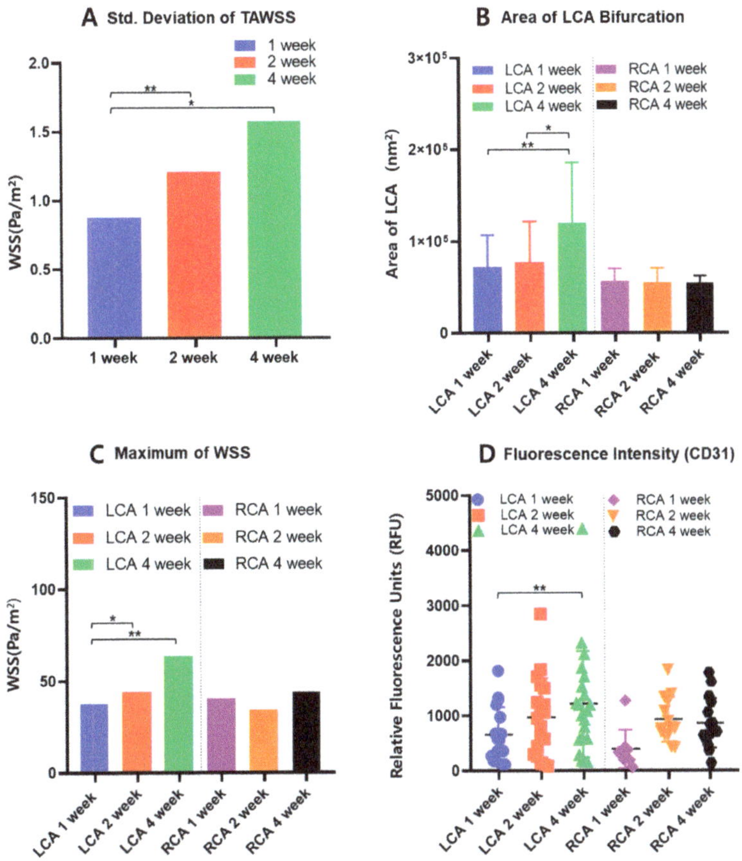

Figure 5. Summary of (**A**) standard deviation of TAWSS, (**B**) area, (**C**) maximum WSS, and (**D**) fluorescence intensity for LCA and RCA (p value < 0.01 ** and <0.05 *).

Comparing the graphs of RCA and LCA for weeks 1, 2, and 4 at the same time, there was a difference in tendency between groups, as summarized in Figure 5B–D. The LCA confirms that WSS increases as weeks 1, 2, and 4 pass. In the case of the RCA, the WSS increases, but not as dramatically as in the LCA. Nevertheless, the RCA also shows an increase, which indicates that the high-fat diet fed to ApoE-KO mice caused stenosis without artificial ligation of the vessel [14]. It can be concluded that vascular stenosis can be caused by many factors, not just shear stress within the vessel [6,7].

As an analytical approach to interpreting WSS and atherosclerosis, the WSS at each point within the vessel were examined. If the deviation of WSS is large, it indicates a significant difference in WSS values within the vessel, which could predict the development of atherosclerosis. A larger standard deviation indicates a wider distribution of low and high WSS values within the vessel. The standard deviation of each group of ApoE mice is shown in Figure 5A. According to Table 1, the mean value and standard deviations for the area and maximum WSS of the LCA, standard deviation of TAWSS, and fluorescence intensity for the 1-, 2-, and 4-week mice are summarized. All values show an increasing trend over time. The standard deviation of TAWSS tended to increase with the duration of the mice survival. Therefore, the large standard deviation in TAWSS, which represents the average WSS value over one blood flow cycle, shows greater disparity between low WSS and high WSS areas. This could lead to endothelial dysfunction and low-density lipoprotein (LDL) plaque deposition. A greater disparity in WSS within the blood vessel indicates the presence of relatively low WSS [24]. This can lead to blood flow stasis, which in turn can cause atherosclerosis [6,24,27]. With standard deviation of TAWSS differences increasing at 1-week, 2-week, and 4-week intervals, the area of the LCA was compared in Figure 5B. The area of the LCA showed an increase over the weeks, confirming that low WSS influences plaque formation. The average LCA area of the 4-week mice group has increased by 66.31% from the 1-week mice group and 38.16% from 2-week mice. This significant increase shows the relationship between the relatively high or low WSS contributing to the thickened plaque within the vessel [3].

Table 1. Summary of LCA evaluation in area of LCA, maximum WSS, TAWSS, and fluorescence intensity.

Parameter (Mean ± SD)	1 Week (n = 16)	2 Weeks (n = 15)	4 Weeks (n = 17)
Area of LCA (nm^2)	$7.21 \times 10^4 \pm 3.41 \times 10^4$	$8.68 \times 10^4 \pm 4.43 \times 10^4$	$12.00 \times 10^4 \pm 6.59 \times 10^4$
Maximum WSS (Pa/m^2)	39.73 ± 12.23	44.11 ± 23.68	63.96 ± 36.73
Std. Deviation of TAWSS	0.8773	1.2056	1.5787
Fluorescence Intensity (RFU)	$6.00 \times 10^2 \pm 4.99 \times 10^2$	$9.68 \times 10^2 \pm 7.88 \times 10^2$	$12.1 \times 10^2 \pm 10.7 \times 10^2$

In addition, to elucidate the correlation between high WSS and inflammatory substances, the results of IF were quantified by the intensity of fluoresce. As shown in Figure 4A, the area of high WSS is under the ligation part, and, therefore, the presence of inflammatory biomarkers indicates the plaque progression. Table 2 shows that the average fluorescence intensity of CD31, an inflammatory biomarker, increased by 101.67% in the 4-week group compared to the 1-week group and 25.00% in the 2-week group. In addition, the average of the maximum WSS of the vascular model increased over time by 60.99% in the 4-week group compared to the 1-week group and 45.00% in the 2-week group. These results indicate that the presence of high WSS in the blood vessels leads to a more active inflammatory response, and the areas with relatively low WSS are continuously at an increased risk of plaque formation and atherosclerosis [24,28].

Table 2. The percentage change in parameter from 1 week to 4 weeks and from 2 weeks to 4 weeks.

Parameter (Mean ± SD)	From 1 Week	From 2 Weeks
Area of LCA (nm^2) (%)	66.44	38.25
Maximum WSS (Pa/m^2) (%)	60.99	45.00
Std. Deviation of TAWSS (%)	79.95	30.95
Fluorescence Intensity (%)	101.67	25.00

3. Discussion

There are many factors that contribute to the development of atherosclerosis, including wall shear stress, blood viscosity, blood pressure, and blood LDL cholesterol. In addition, high blood pressure can continuously damage the arterial walls [24]. Obesity, diabetes, and smoking can also be significant causes. However, physically low WSS in the arteries is known to be a major contributor to atherosclerotic plaque formation, so this study focused on WSS [6]. An animal model in which three of the four branches of the left common carotid artery are ligated is a classic experimental design to induce low WSS [29]. Ligation of three branches inevitably increases the area of recirculating blood flow in front of the ligation site, which increases the area with low WSS and high oscillatory shear index (OSI) [24]. This leads to plaque formation and atherosclerosis progression [6,24,27]. As atherosclerotic plaque forms, the inflammatory response can accelerate and worsen the symptoms of atherosclerosis [30,31]. In the development of atherosclerosis, low WSS can expose the arterial wall, increasing intercellular permeability and leading to the occurrence of atherosclerosis in these areas [32,33]. Additionally, it can be affected by the vasoactive substances released by endothelial cells [31]. On the other hand, high shear stress causes rapid cytoskeletal remodeling in endothelial cells and activates the signaling pathway for nitric oxide and prostacyclin, which can be protective to the atherosclerosis [34–36]. However, other studies suggest that high WSS affects the formation of high-risk plaques [28]. Therefore, the relationship between low WSS and high WSS in the development of stenosis along with various biomarkers and factors were examined to better understand atherosclerosis.

In this experiment, high WSS was primarily observed in ApoE-KO mice models with severe atherosclerosis through CFD simulation. When partially ligated ApoE-KO mice were subjected to a high-fat diet for 4 weeks, MRI imaging and histopathological staining techniques revealed that the severity of atherosclerotic lesions tended to increase with the duration of the survival. Regarding MRI imaging, the mice at 1 and 4 weeks showed that the blood flow was becoming increasingly obstructed. Additionally, tissues were extracted and subjected to H&E or MOVAT staining. It was observed that the vascular walls thickened, and necrotic core, lipid core, or plaque formation occurred progressively each week. However, it is difficult to attribute these findings solely to the partial ligation of the LCA and the high-fat diet, since WSS is one of the hemodynamic parameters that can be changed during the stenotic progress. Therefore, the 3D model using MRI images was constructed and then used for CFD analysis to calculate and compare the WSS in each section within the blood vessel.

The primary purpose of CFD in this study was to observe changes in WSS with the progression of atherosclerosis [8]. CFD simulations showed that WSS tended to increase over time at sites where partial ligation and high-fat diets were maintained, and higher WSS was observed at sites of branch ligation due to the formation of atherosclerotic plaques beneath these sites. Although high WSS can be a protective factor, it can also affect vulnerable plaques [28]. This is consistent with the existing understanding that high WSS may promote the expression of inflammatory factors in the chronic progression of atherosclerosis; however, high WSS alone does not fully explain plaque-induced changes in the vessel lumen, which is one of the main causes in the early stages of atherosclerosis. Analyzing only the mean of the maximum WSS may explain the risk of inflammatory factors but not the plaque formation associated with low WSS. To compensate, we analyzed the standard deviation of carotid artery thickness and TAWSS together to investigate how different patterns of WSS are associated with the progression of atherosclerosis. Standard deviation measures the variability of data, with a high standard deviation indicating greater variability in WSS. The analysis showed that the 4-week group had a high standard deviation, while the 1-week group had a relatively low standard deviation. To account for this trend, we compared the thickness of the carotid arteries and found that the area of the atherosclerotic plaque increased over time. Consequently, a higher variance indicates a higher probability of co-existing high WSS and low WSS within the blood vessel, which can indirectly be associated with the development of atherosclerosis and the formation of vulnerable atherosclerotic plaques.

As atherosclerosis progresses, the expression of various inflammatory factors and endothelial cell-related markers increases [30]. Therefore, IF staining was performed as well, targeting inflammatory biomarkers and endothelial markers such as VCAM-1, NF-κB, CD31, and α-SMA in samples from mice with advanced atherosclerosis. The results showed a higher expression pattern of these markers in samples with severe atherosclerotic plaques, which is consistent with the findings of previous studies [25]. Additionally, the fluorescence intensity from the IF images was quantified and represented. These values were then compared with the maximum WSS to observe the trend. Higher WSS was associated with increased fluorescence intensity. Therefore, it was observed that various inflammatory markers tend to aggregate due to the high WSS caused by strong pressure within the narrowed blood vessels where atherosclerosis has developed [3].

However, a limitation of this experiment is that it did not include factors other than shear stress in the vessel wall. Although atherosclerosis mainly developed in the ligated left carotid artery, atherosclerosis was also found in the un-ligated right common carotid artery, showing that shear stress in the vessel wall is not the only factor in the development of atherosclerosis [6,7]. Atherosclerosis is caused by a combination of factors, including blood viscosity, blood pressure, and structural problems in the blood vessels. However, our experiments were designed to induce low wall shear, so the focus of the study is on wall shear, which needs further study in combination with other factors [29]. Also, we used surgical methods and dietary interventions to create a model of acute atherosclerosis. The observation was conducted over a short period of 1, 2, and 4 weeks, dividing the subjects into small groups. Therefore, while only the tendency showing an increase in atherosclerotic plaques with the increase in TAWSS deviation, or the fluorescence intensity at the bifurcation where maximum WSS occurs, was confirmed, other variables related to the hemodynamics or vascular morphology of each mouse were not considered. Since there were cases where severe plaque formation occurred in mice at 1 week, and cases where significant atherosclerosis did not develop in mice at 4 weeks, these results might be due to individual differences. Therefore, to investigate the correlation in much more detail, a longer duration when creating the atherosclerosis model might be required to obtain a clearer tendency. Moreover, further research on the proximal part of the carotid artery ligation is needed. Ligation of three of the top four branches of the LCA results in stagnant blood flow and increased pressure loading proximal to the ligation [29]. This stagnation of blood flow leads to an enlargement of the recirculating region of blood flow and an increase in the low WSS and OSI regions, which are commonly believed to coincide with plaque-producing regions, which may lead to the progression of atherosclerosis [6,24,27,29]. Finally, the 3D remodeling of the vessel did not include the STA, ECA, ICA, and OA upper part of ligation, which means the shear stress effects to those parts were not considered. Consequently, accurate comparisons of low WSS and plaque formation areas might not be accomplished. Regardless of individual differences and 3D remodeling limitation, the comparison of the standard deviation of TAWSS to the area of atherosclerosis was a new approach to understanding the relationship between WSS and atherosclerotic plaque. This method can provide a new analytical perspective.

4. Experimental Method

4.1. Development of an Atherosclerosis Mouse Model

Eight-week-old C57BL/6 ApoE -/- male mice from Jackson Laboratory were used as an atherosclerosis model. For the partial ligation of the carotid artery (Figure 1A), the mice were placed under respiratory anesthesia with 2.0% isoflurane [12]. The external carotid artery (ECA), internal carotid artery (ICA), and occipital artery (OA), which branch from the LCA, were ligated, while the superior thyroid artery (STA) remained open [37]. The mice were then separated into three groups for the development of atherosclerosis: 1 week, 2 weeks, and 4 weeks. All mice were fed a high-fat diet (VHFD 60 kcal% fat #D12492, Research Diets) after the partial ligation of the LCA. MRI imaging was performed before sacrifice for blood flow measurement. All animal experiments were conducted in accordance with the guidelines and regulations set forth by the Asan Medical Center Institutional Animal Care and Use Committee (IACUC no. 2020-02-153)

4.2. Blood Flow Measurement through MRI

A time-of-flight (TOF) mode MRI was conducted on mice after partial ligation surgery and before their scarification (Figure 1B). This process was performed under respiratory anesthesia with 2.0% isoflurane at room temperature (24 °C). The 9.4 T/160 mm animal MR system (Agilent Technologies, Santa Clara, CA, USA) was used to obtain MRI images depicting blood flow. A 64 mm transmit/receive volume coil was used, and 16 cross-sectional slices were acquired [38].

4.3. Histological and Immunofluorescence Evaluation

For H&E staining and MOVAT (Figure 1C), the samples were made into paraffin blocks and cross sectioned. Both staining methods were followed using procedures from previous studies [37]. For immunofluorescence (IF) evaluation, inflammatory biomarkers NF-κB (Anti-NF-κB p65, Abcam, Cambridge, UK), CD31, VCAM-1 (VCAM-1 Monoclonal Antibody, Invitrogen, Waltham, MA, USA), and α-SMA (Abcam ab5693) were chosen. The samples prepared in paraffin blocks were deparaffinized in xylene (Junsei Chemical, Tokyo, Japan). In accordance with the primary antibody, secondary antibodies Alexa Fluor 488 (Invitrogen) and Alexa Fluor 555 (Invitrogen) were used for fluorescence tagging. DAPI was applied before fluorescent imaging. A confocal laser scanning microscope (LSM780; Carl Zeiss, Oberkochen, Germany) was used for fluorescent image acquisition.

4.4. Carotid Artery 3D Reconstruction

4.4.1. Segmentation of Inner Vessel Cross-Section

Cross-sectional images of H&E-stained carotid artery vessels were collected to refine the inputs and outputs of the 3D model. These high-resolution images were extracted using Slide Viewer v2.7, a digital slide viewing software that standardizes the scale of all vessel cross-sectional images. The extracted images were then imported into the Segment Anything Model (SAM) API developed by Meta AI via the Python library. This API utilizes the SAM model of ViT-H to extract masks corresponding to the inner cross-sections of the vessels. These masks are used as input and output surfaces of blood flow when building the 3D model of the vessel.

4.4.2. 3D Modeling

To determine the WSS applied to the vessel wall, a structured simulation approach was employed, beginning with the modeling of the left carotid artery 3D structure using MRI data (Figure 1D). The segmentation was performed using ITK-SNAP v4.0.1, a software tool designed for this purpose, allowing for accurate reconstruction of the artery's geometric shape. A 3D model of the blood vessels was created by establishing the baseline of the curvature and thickness of the blood vessels and connecting the post-processed cross sections to the beginning and end of the blood vessels. After obtaining the ratio of the actual length of the left carotid artery specimen to the Blender modeling scale, we created a 3D model based on the ratio of all the samples. This process ensured that the detailed anatomical features were preserved and accurately represented.

4.5. Simulation

4.5.1. Blood Vessel and Flow

For the already-formed 3D model using MRI data, the junction of the left common carotid artery and the aorta was set as the inlet of the fluid, and the area just before the division of the upper branches of the LCA was set as the outlet. The vessel wall was set as a rigid body, and the blood flow was set as laminar [39]. We set the fluid to a non-Newtonian fluid and the transport model to Bird–Carreau. The blood flow was given a velocity boundary condition based on the heart pulse, and three pulses were simulated over 2.7 s [25]. These simulations were executed using SimFlow v5.0 based on OpenFOAM v2212, which allowed us to simulate fluid dynamics. Post-processing of the simulation results was conducted using ParaView v5.12.0. This software enabled the creation of detailed visualizations of the blood flow patterns and the WSS distribution along the vessel wall, providing valuable insights into the hemodynamic environment within the carotid artery.

4.5.2. Statistical Analysis

Finally, the simulation data were analyzed using Prism v8, a statistical software tool. This step involved creating graphs and charts to quantitatively represent the WSS values, helping to identify key trends and patterns that contribute to a better understanding of the impact of hemodynamic forces on the vessel wall. The p-value was <0.05, which means our results have statistical significance.

5. Conclusions

Atherosclerosis is an inflammatory response due to plaque formation within arteries, leading to ischemic stroke and heart disease [3]. It is influenced by factors like hyperlipidemia, hypertension, obesity, diabetes, smoking, and WSS. Understanding its mechanisms is crucial for prevention and treatment of atherosclerosis. CFD simulates WSS and hemodynamic changes for analysis of the correlation between contributing factors [8]. In this study, ApoE-KO mice subjected to partial ligation and a high-fat diet at 1-week, 2-week, and 4-week intervals were used as an atherosclerosis model. CFD analysis was conducted, and carotid artery blood flow reconstructed via MRI was compared to inflammatory factors and pathological staining. This analytical approach compared the standard deviation of WSS at each point within the vessel wall with staining results and pathological features. It is found that as the interval between weeks increased, the gap between low and high WSS widened, linking the occurrence of atherosclerosis to WSS differences and vulnerable plaque formation.

Author Contributions: Conceptualization, J.K.K.; methodology, M.C. and J.K.K.; investigation, M.C.; data curation, J.S.H. and K.R.K.; writing—original draft preparation, M.C.; writing—review and editing, J.S.H., K.R.K. and J.K.K.; visualization, M.C. and J.S.H.; supervision, J.K.K.; project administration, J.K.K.; funding acquisition, J.K.K. All authors have read and agreed to the published version of the manuscript.

Funding: The study was supported in part by the Ministry of Science, ICT, and Future Planning (MSIP) through the National Research Foundation of Korea (NRF) under Grant 2018R1A5A2020732. Additionally, it was supported by a grant from the Korea Health Technology R&D Project through the Korea Health Industry Development Institute (KHIDI), funded by the Ministry of Health and Welfare, Republic of Korea, under Grant HI22C1374, and by grants from the Asan Institute for Life Sciences, Asan Medical Center, Seoul, Korea, under Grant 2023IP0071.

Institutional Review Board Statement: All animal experiments were approved by the institutional animal care and use committee of the Asan Institute for Life Sciences, Asan Medical Center (approval no. 2020-02-153) following the Laboratory Animal Act of the Republic of Korea.

Informed Consent Statement: Not applicable.

Data Availability Statement: All data are contained within the article.

Conflicts of Interest: The authors declare no conflicts of interest.

References

1. Libby, P.; Buring, J.E.; Badimon, L.; Hansson, G.K.; Deanfield, J.; Bittencourt, M.S.; Tokgözoğlu, L.; Lewis, E.F. Atherosclerosis. *Nat. Rev. Dis. Primers* **2019**, *5*, 56. [CrossRef] [PubMed]
2. Naghavi, M.; Wang, H.; Lozano, R.; Davis, A.; Liang, X.; Zhou, M.; Vollset, S.E.; Abbasoglu Ozgoren, A.; Abdalla, S.; Abd-Allah, F.; et al. Global, regional, and national age-sex specific all-cause and cause-specific mortality for 240 causes of death, 1990–2013: A systematic analysis for the Global Burden of Disease Study 2013. *Lancet* **2015**, *385*, 117–171. [CrossRef]
3. Zhou, M.; Yu, Y.; Chen, R.; Liu, X.; Hu, Y.; Ma, Z.; Gao, L.; Jian, W.; Wang, L. Wall shear stress and its role in atherosclerosis. *Front. Cardiovasc. Med.* **2023**, *10*, 1083547. [CrossRef] [PubMed]
4. Vorster, M.; Maes, A.; van de Wiele, C.; Sathekge, M. Gallium-68 PET: A Powerful Generator-based Alternative to Infection and Inflammation Imaging. *Semin. Nucl. Med.* **2016**, *46*, 436–447. [CrossRef]
5. Gąsecka, A.; Rogula, S.; Szarpak, Ł.; Filipiak, K.J. LDL-Cholesterol and Platelets: Insights into Their Interactions in Atherosclerosis. *Life* **2021**, *11*, 39. [CrossRef]
6. Moerman, A.M.; Korteland, S.; Dilba, K.; van Gaalen, K.; Poot, D.H.J.; van Der Lugt, A.; Verhagen, H.J.M.; Wentzel, J.J.; van Der Steen, A.F.W.; Gijsen, F.J.H.; et al. The Correlation Between Wall Shear Stress and Plaque Composition in Advanced Human Carotid Atherosclerosis. *Front. Bioeng. Biotechnol.* **2022**, *9*, 828577. [CrossRef]
7. Çinar, Y.; Şenyol, A.M.; Duman, K. Blood viscosity and blood pressure: Role of temperature and hyperglycemia. *Am. J. Hypertens.* **2001**, *14 Pt 1*, 433–438. [CrossRef]
8. Peiffer, V.; Sherwin, S.J.; Weinberg, P.D. Does low and oscillatory wall shear stress correlate spatially with early atherosclerosis? A systematic review. *Cardiovasc. Res.* **2013**, *99*, 242–250. [CrossRef]

9. Zeng, D.; Ding, Z.; Friedman, M.H.; Ethier, C.R. Effects of cardiac motion on right coronary artery hemodynamics. *Ann. Biomed. Eng.* **2003**, *31*, 420–429. [CrossRef]
10. Chaichana, T.; Sun, Z.; Jewkes, J. Computational fluid dynamics analysis of the effect of plaques in the left coronary artery. *Comput. Math. Methods Med.* **2012**, *2012*, 504367. [CrossRef]
11. Domurath, J.; Saphiannikova, M.; Férec, J.; Ausias, G.; Heinrich, G. Stress and strain amplification in a dilute suspension of spherical particles based on a Bird–Carreau model. *J. Nonnewton Fluid. Mech.* **2015**, *221*, 95–102. [CrossRef]
12. Sasso, G.L.; Schlage, W.K.; Boué, S.; Veljkovic, E.; Peitsch, M.C.; Hoeng, J. The Apoe$^{-/-}$ mouse model: A suitable model to study cardiovascular and respiratory diseases in the context of cigarette smoke exposure and harm reduction. *J. Transl. Med.* **2016**, *14*, 146. [CrossRef] [PubMed]
13. Nam, D.; Ni, C.-W.; Rezvan, A.; Suo, J.; Budzyn, K.; Llanos, A.; Harrison, D.; Giddens, D.; Jo, H. Partial carotid ligation is a model of acutely induced disturbed flow, leading to rapid endothelial dysfunction and atherosclerosis. *Am. J. Physiol. Heart Circ. Physiol.* **2009**, *297*, H1535–H1543. [CrossRef] [PubMed]
14. Li, X.; Wang, C.; Tan, H.; Cheng, L.; Liu, G.; Yang, Y.; Zhao, Y.; Zhang, Y.; Li, Y.; Zhang, C.; et al. Gold nanoparticles-based SPECT/CT imaging probe targeting for vulnerable atherosclerosis plaques. *Biomaterials* **2016**, *108*, 71–80. [CrossRef] [PubMed]
15. Klein, W.M.; Bartels, L.W.; Bax, L.; Van der Graaf, Y.; Mali, W.P.T.M. Magnetic resonance imaging measurement of blood volume flow in peripheral arteries in healthy subjects. *J. Vasc. Surg.* **2003**, *38*, 1060–1066. [CrossRef]
16. Gui, Y.; Zheng, H.; Cao, R.Y. Foam Cells in Atherosclerosis: Novel Insights Into Its Origins, Consequences, and Molecular Mechanisms. *Front. Cardiovasc. Med.* **2022**, *9*, 845942. [CrossRef]
17. Cuerrier, C.M.; Chen, Y.-X.; Tremblay, D.; Rayner, K.; McNulty, M.; Zhao, X.; Kennedy, C.R.J.; de BelleRoche, J.; Pelling, A.E.; O'Brien, E.R. Chronic over-expression of heat shock protein 27 attenuates atherogenesis and enhances plaque remodeling: A combined histological and mechanical assessment of aortic lesions. *PLoS ONE* **2013**, *8*, e55867. [CrossRef]
18. Hu, C.; Peng, K.; Wu, Q.; Wang, Y.; Fan, X.; Zhang, D.-M.; Passerini, A.G.; Sun, C. HDAC1 and 2 regulate endothelial VCAM-1 expression and atherogenesis by suppressing methylation of the GATA6 promoter. *Theranostics* **2021**, *11*, 5605–5619. [CrossRef]
19. Sorescu, G.P.; Sykes, M.; Weiss, D.; Platt, M.O.; Saha, A.; Hwang, J.; Boyd, N.; Boo, Y.C.; Vega, J.D.; Taylor, W.R.; et al. Bone morphogenic protein 4 produced in endothelial cells by oscillatory shear stress stimulates an inflammatory response. *J. Biol. Chem.* **2003**, *278*, 31128–31135. [CrossRef]
20. Lawrence, T. The nuclear factor NF-kappaB pathway in inflammation. *Cold Spring Harb. Perspect. Biol.* **2009**, *1*, a001651. [CrossRef]
21. Goel, R.; Schrank, B.R.; Arora, S.; Boylan, B.; Fleming, B.; Miura, H.; Newman, P.J.; Molthen, R.C.; Newman, D.K. Site-specific effects of PECAM-1 on atherosclerosis in LDL receptor-deficient mice. *Arter. Thromb. Vasc. Biol.* **2008**, *28*, 1996–2002. [CrossRef] [PubMed]
22. Hao, H.; Gabbiani, G.; Bochaton-Piallat, M.L. Arterial smooth muscle cell heterogeneity: Implications for atherosclerosis and restenosis development. *Arter. Thromb. Vasc. Biol.* **2003**, *23*, 1510–1520. [CrossRef] [PubMed]
23. Teng, Z.; Wang, S.; Tokgoz, A.; Taviani, V.; Bird, J.; Sadat, U.; Huang, Y.; Patterson, A.J.; Figg, N.; Graves, M.J.; et al. Study on the association of wall shear stress and vessel structural stress with atherosclerosis: An experimental animal study. *Atherosclerosis* **2021**, *320*, 38–46. [CrossRef] [PubMed]
24. DiCarlo, A.L.; Holdsworth, D.W.; Poepping, T.L. Study of the effect of stenosis severity and non-Newtonian viscosity on multidirectional wall shear stress and flow disturbances in the carotid artery using particle image velocimetry. *Med. Eng. Phys.* **2019**, *65*, 8–23. [CrossRef]
25. Suo, J.; Ferrara, D.E.; Sorescu, D.; Guldberg, R.E.; Taylor, W.R.; Giddens, D.P. Hemodynamic shear stresses in mouse aortas: Implications for atherogenesis. *Arter. Thromb. Vasc. Biol.* **2007**, *27*, 346–351. [CrossRef]
26. Hartman, E.M.J.; De Nisco, G.; Gijsen, F.J.H.; Korteland, S.-A.; van der Steen, A.F.W.; Daemen, J.; Wentzel, J.J. The definition of low wall shear stress and its effect on plaque progression estimation in human coronary arteries. *Sci. Rep.* **2021**, *11*, 22086. [CrossRef]
27. Nguyen, K.T.; Clark, C.D.; Chancellor, T.J.; Papavassiliou, D.V. Carotid geometry effects on blood flow and on risk for vascular disease. *J. Biomech.* **2008**, *41*, 11–19. [CrossRef]
28. Eshtehardi, P.; Brown, A.J.; Bhargava, A.; Costopoulos, C.; Hung, O.Y.; Corban, M.T.; Hosseini, H.; Gogas, B.D.; Giddens, D.P.; Samady, H. High wall shear stress and high-risk plaque: An emerging concept. *Int. J. Cardiovasc. Imaging* **2017**, *33*, 1089–1099. [CrossRef]
29. Paszkowiak, J.J.; Dardik, A. Arterial wall shear stress: Observations from the bench to the bedside. *Vasc. Endovasc. Surg.* **2003**, *37*, 47–57. [CrossRef]
30. Hansson, G.K. Inflammation, Atherosclerosis, and Coronary Artery Disease. *N. Engl. J. Med.* **2005**, *352*, 1685–1695. [CrossRef]
31. Schmitt, M.M.; Megens, R.T.; Zernecke, A.; Bidzhekov, K.; Akker, N.M.V.D.; Rademakers, T.; Van Zandvoort, M.A.; Hackeng, T.M.; Koenen, R.R.; Weber, C. Endothelial junctional adhesion molecule-a guides monocytes into flow-dependent predilection sites of atherosclerosis. *Circulation* **2014**, *129*, 66–76. [CrossRef] [PubMed]
32. Cecchi, E.; Giglioli, C.; Valente, S.; Lazzeri, C.; Gensini, G.F.; Abbate, R.; Mannini, L. Role of hemodynamic shear stress in cardiovascular disease. *Atherosclerosis* **2011**, *214*, 249–256. [CrossRef] [PubMed]
33. Okano, M.; Yoshida, Y. Junction complexes of endothelial cells in atherosclerosis-prone and atherosclerosis-resistant regions on flow dividers of brachiocephalic bifurcations in the rabbit aorta. *Biorheology* **1994**, *31*, 155–161. [CrossRef] [PubMed]

34. Traub, O.; Berk, B.C. Laminar shear stress: Mechanisms by which endothelial cells transduce an atheroprotective force. *Arter. Thromb. Vasc. Biol.* **1998**, *18*, 677–685. [CrossRef]
35. Malek, A.M.; Alper, S.L.; Izumo, S. Hemodynamic shear stress and its role in atherosclerosis. *JAMA* **1999**, *282*, 2035–2042. [CrossRef]
36. Mahmoudi, M.; Farghadan, A.; McConnell, D.R.; Barker, A.J.; Wentzel, J.J.; Budoff, M.J.; Arzani, A. The Story of Wall Shear Stress in Coronary Artery Atherosclerosis: Biochemical Transport and Mechanotransduction. *J. Biomech. Eng.* **2021**, *143*, 041002. [CrossRef]
37. Lee, S.; Jue, M.; Cho, M.; Lee, K.; Paulson, B.; Jo, H.; Song, J.S.; Kang, S.; Kim, J.K. Label-free atherosclerosis diagnosis through a blood drop of apolipoprotein E knockout mouse model using surface-enhanced Raman spectroscopy validated by machine learning algorithm. *Bioeng. Transl. Med.* **2023**, *8*, e10529. [CrossRef]
38. Chae, Y.J.; Kim, K.W.; Kim, M.-H.; Woo, C.-W.; Kim, S.-T.; Kim, J.-W.; Shin, T.-H.; Lee, D.-W.; Kim, J.K.; Choi, Y.; et al. Comparison of the Pharmacokinetics of Gadolinium-Based and Iron Oxide-Based Contrast Agents inside the Lymphatic Structure using Magnetic Resonance Lymphangiography. *Mol. Imaging Biol.* **2024**, *26*, 638–648. [CrossRef]
39. Cebral, J.R.; Yim, P.J.; Löhner, R.; Soto, O.; Choyke, P.L. Blood flow modeling in carotid arteries with computational fluid dynamics and MR imaging. *Acad. Radiol.* **2002**, *9*, 1286–1299. [CrossRef]

International Journal of *Molecular Sciences*

MDPI

Article

Phenotypic, Metabolic, and Functional Characterization of Experimental Models of Foamy Macrophages: Toward Therapeutic Research in Atherosclerosis

Amina Sarah Henni Mansour [1], Mathilde Ragues [1], Julien Brevier [2], Coraline Borowczyk [1], Janaïna Grevelinger [1], Jeanny Laroche-Traineau [1], Johan Garaude [3], Sébastien Marais [4], Marie-Josée Jacobin-Valat [1], Edouard Gerbaud [5], Gisèle Clofent-Sanchez [1] and Florence Ottones [1,*]

1 CRMSB UMR5536, CNRS DR-15, INSB, 33000 Bordeaux, France; sarah.henni-mansour@rmsb.u-bordeaux.fr (A.S.H.M.); mathilde.ragues@rmsb.u-bordeaux.fr (M.R.); coraline.borowczyk@univ-cotedazur.fr (C.B.); janaina.grevelinger@inrae.fr (J.G.); jlaroche@rmsb.u-bordeaux.fr (J.L.-T.); marie-josee.jacobin-valat@rmsb.u-bordeaux.fr (M.-J.J.-V.); gisele.clofent-sanchez@rmsb.u-bordeaux.fr (G.C.-S.)

2 UMR 7252, XLIM, 87060 Limoges, France; julien.brevier@unilim.fr

3 MRGM INSERM U1211, 33076 Bordeaux, France; johan.garaude@u-bordeaux.fr

4 Bordeaux Imaging Center, BIC, UAR 3420, US 4, 33000 Bordeaux, France; sebastien.marais@u-bordeaux.fr

5 Centre de Recherche Cardio Thoracique, INSERM U 1045, 33000 Bordeaux, France; edouard.gerbaud@chu-bordeaux.fr

* Correspondence: florence.ottones@u-bordeaux.fr

Abstract: Different types of macrophages (Mφ) are involved in atherogenesis, including inflammatory Mφ and foamy Mφ (FM). Our previous study demonstrated that two-photon excited fluorescence (TPEF) imaging of NADH and FAD autofluorescence (AF) could distinguish experimental models that mimic the different atherosclerotic Mφ types. The present study assessed whether optical differences correlated with phenotypic and functional differences, potentially guiding diagnostic and therapeutic strategies. Phenotypic differences were investigated using three-dimensional principal component analysis and multi-color flow cytometry. Functional analyses focused on cytokine production, metabolic profiles, and cellular oxidative stress, in LDL dose-dependent assays, to understand the origin of AF in the FAD spectrum and assess FM ability to transition toward an immunoregulatory phenotype and function. Phenotypic studies revealed that FM models generated with acetylated LDL (Mac) were closer to immunoregulatory Mφ, while those generated with oxidized LDL (Mox) more closely resembled inflammatory Mφ. The metabolic analysis confirmed that inflammatory Mφ primarily used glycolysis, while immunoregulatory Mφ mainly depended on mitochondrial respiration. FM models employed both pathways; however, FM models generated with high doses of modified LDL showed reduced mitochondrial respiration, particularly Mox FM. Thus, the high AF in the FAD spectrum in Mox was not linked to increased mitochondrial respiration, but correlated with the dose of oxidized LDL, leading to increased production of reactive oxygen species (ROS) and lysosomal ceroid accumulation. High FAD-like AF, ROS, and ceroid accumulation were reduced by incubation with α-tocopherol. The cytokine profiles supported the phenotypic analysis, indicating that Mox FM exhibited greater inflammatory activity than Mac FM, although both could be redirected toward immunoregulatory functions, albeit to different degrees. In conclusion, in the context of immunoregulatory therapies for atherosclerosis, it is crucial to consider FM, given their prevalence in plaques and our results, as potential targets, regardless of their inflammatory status, alongside non-foamy inflammatory Mφ.

Keywords: atherosclerosis; foamy macrophages; TPEF autofluorescence; phenotype and cytokine profiling; bioenergetic immunometabolism; cellular oxidative stress; ceroids; antioxidant; immunoregulation; diagnostic and therapeutic strategies

1. Introduction

Atherosclerosis, a chronic inflammation of medium- and large-size arteries, is characterized by the accumulation of lipids and immune cells in the artery wall. The retention of Low-Density Lipoproteins (LDL) leads to the formation of fat on the inner surface of the artery, which favors LDL oxidation. Consequently, endothelial cell activation facilitates the massive and persistent recruitment of blood monocytes to the intima, where they differentiate into macrophages (Mφ). Blood monocyte-derived Mφ are implicated in all atherogenesis steps [1–5]. These Mφ are highly heterogeneous and plastic, and this variability is particularly evident in atherogenesis [6]. In response to microenvironmental clues, they can be polarized toward an inflammatory phenotype or become foamy Mφ (FM) after the endocytosis of LDL. Plaque progression might be regulated by the delicate balance between atherogenic and immunoregulatory Mφ [7–11]. The accumulation of inflammatory Mφ and dying FM is a hallmark of vulnerable plaque areas. Inflammatory Mφ are clearly pro-atherogenic and have recently been described as predominantly non-foamy [12]. Some studies suggest that inflammatory Mφ might be induced toward immunoregulatory functions as a therapeutic approach to atherosclerosis [13,14]. A crucial issue is whether other major subsets of atherogenic Mφ, specifically FM, might also be targeted by immunoregulatory therapeutic strategies.

The functional status of FM remains highly controversial. Early publications suggested that FM secrete inflammatory cytokines and metalloproteinases that sustain inflammation [15,16]. Conversely, recent results from single-cell technologies have shown that FM possess a non-inflammatory transcriptomic profile [17–20]. However, single-cell technologies often require cells to be extracted from their microenvironment, which typically results in the loss of FM due to their fragility. Consequently, only a limited number of FM subsets may be analyzed—usually the less foamy ones that are not representative of pathogenic FM. Different FM types exist in atherosclerotic plaques, and their functional status is influenced by various environmental stimuli and the type and quantity of modified LDL trapped within these cells. This was demonstrated by multiplex immunofluorescent and mass spectrometry imaging [21]. Therefore, characterizing the FM panel in plaques is crucial, as FM may exhibit various functional statuses with altered lysosomal function, autophagy, oxidative stress, apoptosis, and necrosis, depending on their lipid load and content [22].

In our previous work, we generated different FM models and analyzed the typical cell surface marker expression patterns associated with inflammatory or immunoregulatory phenotypes using flow cytometry. We found that the different FM models co-express inflammatory and immunoregulatory markers, albeit at low level, and that Two-Photon Excited Fluorescence (TPEF) imaging of NADH and FAD autofluorescence (AF) can distinguish non-foamy inflammatory and immunoregulatory Mφ [23]. This observation was consistent with our initial hypothesis that these two types of Mφ would exhibit distinct optical properties due to the autofluorescence of these cofactors, which are crucial for cellular energy metabolism. Specifically, NADH is primarily produced during glycolysis, while FAD is a key byproduct of mitochondrial oxidative phosphorylation (OXPHOS). It is well established that inflammatory Mφ rely on glycolysis, whereas immunoregulatory Mφ predominantly use OXPHOS pathways to generate the ATP necessary for their functions [24]. However, little was known about the metabolic pathways used by FM. Surprisingly, we observed high AF in both spectra, with particularly elevated FAD-like AF in FM generated with high doses of modified LDL, which was inconsistent with our preliminary metabolism analysis showing low mitochondrial respiration in these macrophages.

In this study, we introduced a broader array of FM models, examining not only the type of LDL (acetylated or oxidized) but also varying doses (low and high). The work presented here has a dual objective. First is to understand why, in TPEF imaging, different FM models exhibit distinct optical properties related to autofluorescence (AF) in the NADH and FAD spectra. In this context, we demonstrated that ceroids are the biological origin of the higher FAD-like AF observed in the Mox model compared to the Mac model. Second is to utilize these results to develop a strategy aimed at restoring atheroprotective functions.

In this paper, we focused on immunoregulation and, for the first time, showed that the dysfunctional state of FM can be alleviated by a treatment combining immunoregulatory cytokines and antioxidants.

To determine whether optical differences correlate with phenotypic and functional differences, we first compared the phenotypes (both surface markers expression and natural AF in the NADH and FAD spectra) of different experimental Mφ models: M1 and M2 models, which mimic inflammatory and immunoregulatory Mφ respectively, and two commonly used models to mimic FM, based on Mφ incubated with oxidized LDL (oxLDL; Mox models) or acetylated LDL (acLDL; Mac models). In-depth analysis of multi-color flow cytometry data provided further insights into each experimental FM model. We used the co-expression of cell surface markers to define different subsets (inflammatory, intermediary, immunoregulatory, undefined), the proportions of which suggested that FM models fall differently along the phenotypic continuum from the inflammatory to immunoregulatory extremes (i.e., M1 and M2 models, respectively). Moreover, three-dimensional Principal Component Analysis (3D-PCA) using both flow cytometry and TPEF data clearly discriminated the different experimental Mφ models, particularly distinguishing the Mac model from the Mox model. We then investigated their functional differences by analyzing cytokine secretion profiles and performing metabolic profiling of the different experimental Mφ models. The results confirmed the link between the signal in the NADH spectrum and the use of the glycolysis pathway in all experimental models. Conversely, we could not establish a link between the FAD spectrum signal and the level of FAD produced by mitochondrial respiration. Specifically, FM models generated with a high oxLDL dose displayed higher FAD-like AF and lower mitochondrial respiration compared to those generated with a high dose of acLDL. This suggested a link between the FAD-like AF and the uptake, degradation, and/or storage of modified LDL by FM. As mitochondrial respiration might be influenced by the LDL type and dose, we hypothesized that the mechanism leading to FAD-like AF might involve lipid peroxidation, oxidative stress, and ceroid formation in Mφ. Thus, we measured Reactive Oxygen Species (ROS) production and cellular ceroids in each experimental model. To confirm the role of oxidative stress in producing FAD-like AF, we investigated the effect of the antioxidant alpha-tocopherol. Lastly, we analyzed the functional state of these models by assessing their ability to be polarized toward immunoregulatory Mφ, measuring CD206 surface expression, cytokine secretion profiles, and oxygen consumption. The lower ability of Mox FM, compared to Mac FM, to be polarized highlighted the more dysfunctional state of the Mox models. Overall, this work provides new insights into the functional discrepancies between commonly used FM models and discusses their potential for developing new therapeutic approaches based on the induction of immunoregulatory Mφ in atherosclerosis.

2. Results

2.1. Phenotypes of the Different Experimental Models of Mφ

- Single-marker flow cytometry analysis and Two-Photon Excited Fluorescence (TPEF) imaging of NADH and FAD suggest differences between the Mox and Mac models

In a previous study, we obtained flow cytometry and TPEF data from different Mφ models (M1, M2, and Foamy macrophages (FM)) that mimic the main Mφ types found in atherosclerotic plaques and showed that these experimental models could be distinguished by TPEF imaging [23]. Here, we focused on the comparison of different FM models generated using 50 µg/mL of oxLDL (Mox50) or acLDL (Mac50), respectively. First, we observed that both Mox50 and Mac50 models displayed a low Mean of Fluorescence Intensity (MFI) for the typical immunoregulatory CD206 marker, compared with the M2 model, and for the typical inflammatory CD86 and CD40 markers, compared with the M1 model (Figure 1A). However, the Percentage of Cells Positive (PCP) for CD86 in the Mox50 model was closer to the M1 model. Similarly, the PCP for CD206 in the Mac50 model was closer to the M2 model (Figure 1B). We observed no difference of the PCP CD40 between the different models. The optical features of the Mac50 model were not different from those of M1 and M2 Mφ. Conversely, the Mox50 model presented distinct optical features from all the other models, except for the NADH autofluorescence (AF) level that was similar to that of M1 cells. To note, the AF percentage in the FAD spectrum was higher in the Mox50 model than in M1, in M2, and also Mac50 cells (Figure 1C).

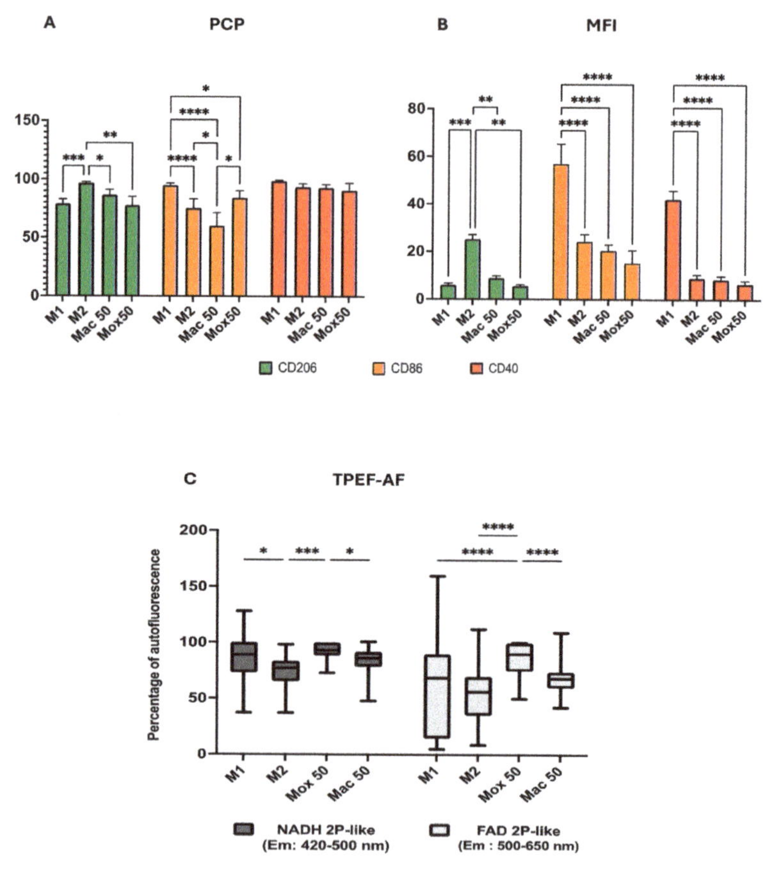

Figure 1. Phenotype comparison of the different experimental models of Mφ: M1, M2, and FM generated with 50 μg/mL of oxLDL (Mox50) or with 50 μg/mL of acLDL (Mac50). (**A**) Mean Fluorescence Intensity (MFI) of CD206, CD86, and CD40 (representing the mean level of expression of each marker at the cell surface); (**B**) Percentage of Cells Positive (PCP) for CD206, CD86, and CD40. (**A**,**B**): data obtained using experimental models derived using blood samples from different donors (n = 5 for Mox, n = 7 for Mac, and n = 13 for M1 and M2) after immunostaining using anti-CD86 and anti-CD206 antibodies. (**C**) FAD and NADH autofluorescence (AF) from TPEF imaging in the NADH spectrum (excitation at 760 nm and detection at 420–500 nm) and FAD spectrum (excitation at 860 nm and detection at 500–650 nm). Normalization was performed for each donor using the maximal value obtained for the experimental model Mox50 as the 100% reference. Data were from n = 8 different donors for all models. * p-value < 0.05; ** p-value < 0.01; *** p-value < 0.001 and **** p-value < 0.0001.

Altogether, these results **highlight the differences between FM models obtained with oxLDL and acLDL. Specifically, Mac50 Mφ are closer to M2 Mφ, and Mox50 Mφ are closer to M1 Mφ.**

- Multicolor flow cytometry analysis of M1- and M2-specific surface marker co-expression suggests that Mox Mφ have more inflammatory features than Mac Mφ.

To thoroughly compare the FM model phenotypes, we classified cells in each model in four different sub-populations (see Methods): $CD86^{-}CD206^{-}$ ("indeterminate" Mφ), $CD86^{-}CD206^{+}$ ("immunoregulatory" Mφ), $CD86^{+}CD206^{+}$ ("intermediate" Mφ), and $CD86^{+}CD206^{-}$ ("inflammatory" Mφ) (Figure 2). This analysis showed that M1 and M2 polarization resulted in a change of the percentage of each subpopulation and also in the MFI level for CD86 and CD206. M1 polarization was characterized by a reduction of the immunoregulatory (green pie) subpopulations and an increase of the inflammatory (red pie) and intermediate (orange pie) subpopulations, compared with M2. Moreover, in the M1 condition, the expression of CD86 (M1 marker) was increased in the inflammatory and intermediate subsets (MFI of 36.2 and 43) (rings in Figure 2). Conversely, in the M2 condition, the percentage of inflammatory cells was decreased, the percentage of immunoregulatory was increased, and intermediate and immunoregulatory cells strongly expressed CD206 (MFI of 17 and 27) compared with the other experimental conditions.

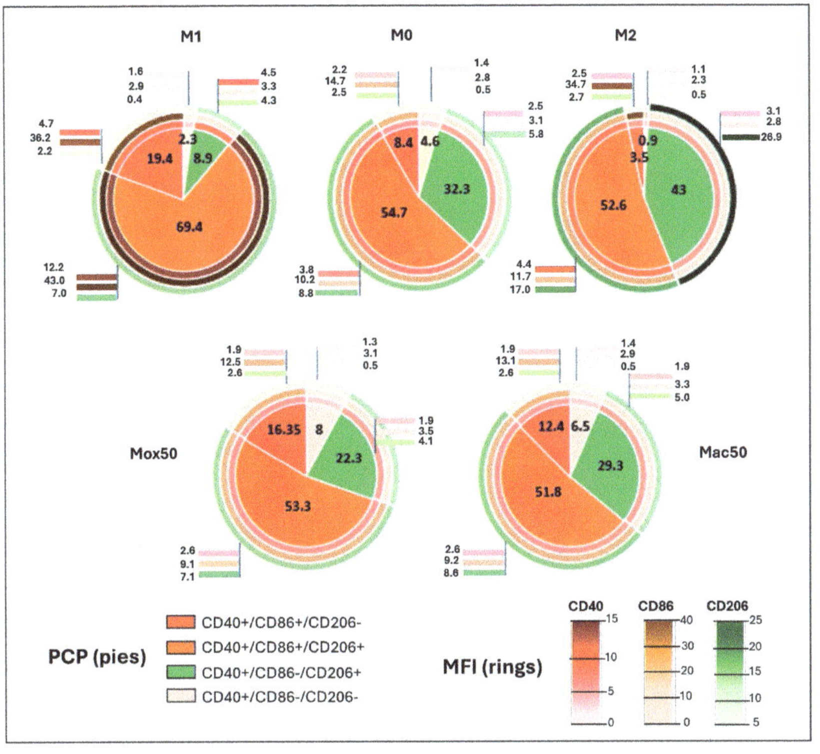

Figure 2. Characterization of the M1, M0, M2, Mox50, and Mac50 models using flow cytometry analysis. Pie charts show the percentage of $CD86^{+}/CD206^{-}$, $CD86^{+}/CD206^{+}$, $CD86^{-}/CD206^{+}$, and $CD86^{-}/CD206^{-}$ subsets for each experimental condition. The M0 model, which corresponds to unstimulated control Mφ, shows, as expected, intermediate percentages of the $CD86^{+}/CD206^{-}$ and $CD86^{-}/CD206^{+}$ subpopulations compared to the two extremes of the continuum, the M1 and M2 models. The outer colored rings indicate the mean fluorescence intensity of CD86 and CD206 using the shown color gradient scale. Data are the mean values of three donors (all cells expressed CD40).

Comparison of the data for the different FM models showed low expression of M1 and M2 markers without differences between Mox and Mac Mφ, except for the CD206 level that was higher in the Mac50 intermediate subset. Furthermore, the percentage of inflammatory cells was lower and the percentage of the immunoregulatory subset was higher in Mac50 than in Mox50 FM. Thus, this multi-marker analysis confirmed that **Mac50 Mφ are closer to M2 Mφ and Mox50 Mφ are closer to M1 Mφ.**

Altogether, these flow cytometry data suggest that our FM models fit differently in the phenotypic continuum going from the inflammatory to immunoregulatory extremes.

- The 3D-PCA of TPEF and flow cytometry data show clear differences between the Mox and Mac models

To better assess the differences among FM models, we performed 3D-PCA with all collected data (PCP, MFI, and AF values) (Figure 3A) and only with PCP and AF data (Figure 3B). The results for the M1 (red), M2 (green), Mox50 (orange), and Mac50 (yellow) models, represented by confidence ellipses, showed that these populations were clearly separated. The opposite polarization of M1 and M2 Mφ also was clearly visible as well as the spatial separation of the FM models from M1 and M2 cells (Figure 3A). The 3D-PCA performed using only the PCP+AF data highlighted the closer proximity of the Mac50 model with M2 (partial overlap of the green and yellow confidence ellipses) (Figure 3B). The segregation or overlap of the confidence ellipses corresponding to the various experimental conditions can be readily visualized in the 3D video representations generated from captured images, provided in Supplementary Figure S1A,B. The contribution of each individual parameter to the principal components is detailed in Supplementary Figure S2A,B.

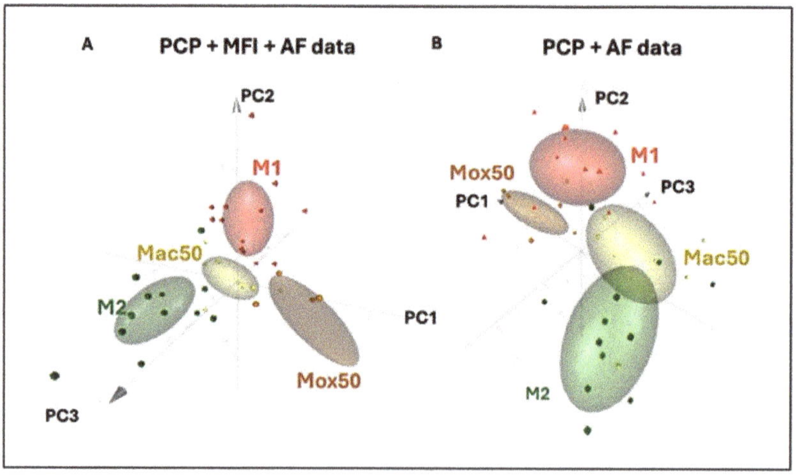

Figure 3. Discrimination of the M1, M2, Mac50, and Mox50 Mφ models using 3D-PCA. (**A**) The 3D-PCA with the PCP, AF, and MFI data and (**B**) 3D-PCA with PCP and AF data. Data obtained from different donors (n = 5 for Mox, n = 7 for Mac and n = 13 for M1 and M2). See Supplemental Figures S1A,B and S2A,B.

The 3D-PCA analysis showed clear differences between FM models: the Mac50 model is closer to M2 Mφ, whereas the Mox50 model is clearly distinct from all the other models.

2.2. Functional Comparison of the Experimental Mφ Models

- Cytokine quantification confirms the phenotype differences between Mox and Mac Mφ

To assess whether the slight phenotypic differences observed between Mac and Mox Mφ translated into functional differences, we assessed the cytokine secretion profiles of the different experimental models. We quantified inflammatory cytokines (IL-18, IL-1β, and IL-6) and IL-10, an immunoregulatory cytokine (Figure 4).

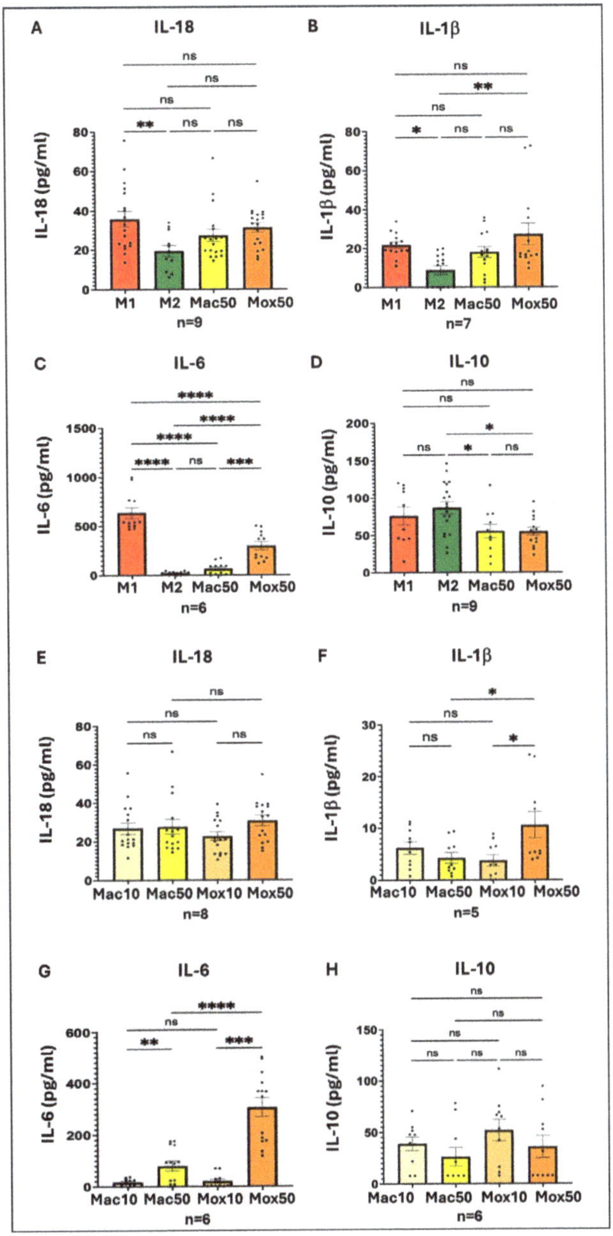

Figure 4. Quantification of the cytokines secreted in the culture supernatant of the different experimental models of Mφ. (**A**) Interleukin-18 (IL-18); (**B**) Interleukin-1β (IL-1 β); (**C**) Interleukin-6 (IL-6); and (**D**) Interleukin-10 (IL-10) in the M1, M2, Mac50, and Mox50 models. Data obtained from different donors (n = 9 for IL-18, n = 7 for IL-1β, n = 6 for IL-6, and n = 9 for IL-10). (**E**) IL-18; (**F**) IL-1β; (**G**) IL-6; and (**H**) IL-10 in the Mac10, Mac50, Mox10, and Mox50 models. Data obtained from different donors (n = 8 for IL-18, n = 5 for IL-1β, n = 6 for IL-6, and n = 6 for IL-10). ns = p-value > 0.05; * p-value < 0.05; ** p-value < 0.01; *** p-value < 0.001 and **** p-value < 0.0001.

As expected, secretion of inflammatory cytokines was higher in the reference inflammatory M1 model than in the M2 model (Figure 4A–C). The inter-individual variations among donors did not allow appreciating fine variations of cytokine production. IL-18 was similarly produced by Mac50 and Mox50 cells (Figure 4A). Conversely, IL-1β secretion was similar in Mox50 Mφ and the M1 model and was significantly higher than in the M2 model. The wide inter-individual variations of IL-1β production in Mac50 cells did not allow differentiating these Mφ from the two extreme models of the M1/M2 continuum (Figure 4B). Remarkably, IL-6 production was higher in the Mox50 model than in M2 and Mac Mφ (no significant difference between these last models) (Figure 4C). For these experiments, we generated more FM models using low doses (10 μg/mL) of oxLDL (Mox10) and acLDL (Mac10). This allowed showing that the production of inflammatory cytokines was influenced by the oxLDL dose. Indeed, IL-1β and IL-6 production was higher in the Mox50 than in the Mox10 model (Figure 4F,G). On the other hand, IL-10 production was lower in the FM models than in M2 Mφ and not significantly different from M1 Mφ. Altogether, these data suggest that the Mox50 model includes more inflammatory Mφ than the Mac50 model. These results confirmed that **Mox50 Mφ are closer to M1 Mφ and Mac50 Mφ are closer to M2 Mφ.**

- Metabolism studies show clear differences between the Mox and Mac models

As inflammatory cells usually produce ATP via the glycolysis pathway, we first compared the bioenergetic metabolic profile of the Mox50 model and the M0, M1 and M2 models. To this aim, we quantified (1) Oxygen Consumption Rate (OCR), which reflects the mitochondrial respiration flux; (2) ExtraCellular Acidification Rate (ECAR), which reflects the glycolytic flux; and (3) mitochondrial versus non mitochondrial ATP production.

Figure 5A shows a representative OCR measurement using the Seahorse technology. OCR values were lower in the Mox50 model compared with the other Mφ models and also with the Mac models (Figure 5B,C), indicating that the high AF observed in the FAD spectrum in Mox50 may not be related to the FAD produced by the mitochondrial respiration. In addition, comparison of the FM models obtained with two different concentrations of modified LDL indicated that the OCR values (and thus mitochondrial respiration) decreased with higher concentrations (Figure 5C). Conversely, ECAR values were higher in the Mox50 than M0 and M2 and even M1 models (Figure 5D). The ECAR values in the Mox50 and Mac50 models were similar and higher than those in Mox10 and Mac10, respectively (Figure 5E). Lastly, quantification of mitochondrial and non-mitochondrial ATP production (Figure 5F) confirmed that the Mox50 model uses mainly the glycolytic pathway.

The finding that Mox50 Mφ display high FAD AF but low mitochondrial respiration suggests that **the signal observed in the FAD spectrum does not rely only on FAD produced by the OXPHOS pathway**, particularly in the FM models generated using the higher oxLDL concentration.

2.3. *Determination of the Biological Origin of the High FAD-like AF in Mox50 Mφ*

- The FAD AF is influenced by the LDL dose and is higher in Mox than in Mac Mφ

The AF emitted in the FAD spectrum measured by TPEF was significantly higher in the Mox50 than in the Mac50 model and also the M2 model (Figure 6A,B), unlike what was observed for the OCR values (Figure 4B,C). This suggested that the AF observed in the FAD spectrum was due to another molecule. The level of this FAD-like AF was also significantly higher in Mox50 Mφ than in Mox10 Mφ and decreased when α-tocopherol (an antioxidant) was simultaneously used with oxLDL (Figure 6C,D).

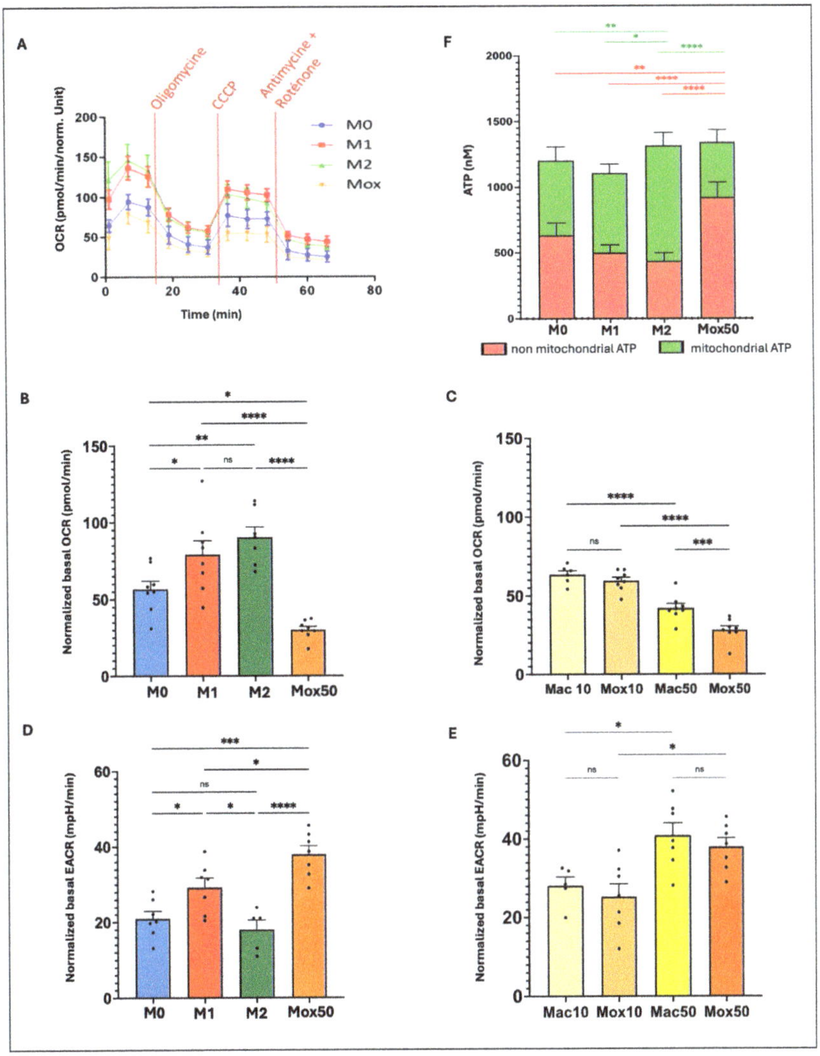

Figure 5. Oxygraphy measurement and ATP production in the different Mφ models. (**A**) Basal Oxygen Consumption Rate (OCR) (basal respiration, ATP-linked respiration, maximal respiratory capacity, and reserve capacity) in M0, M1, M2, and Mox50 cells (representative results; n = 8 different donors). (**B**) Basal OCR in M0, M1, M2, and Mox50 cells (n = 8 donors). (**C**) Basal OCR in Mac10, Mac50, Mox10, and Mox50 cells (n = 8 donors). (**D**) ExtraCellular Acidification Rate (ECAR) indicative of the level of glycolytic flux in M0, M1, M2, and Mox50 cells (n = 7 donors). (**E**) ECAR in Mac10, Mac50, Mox10, and Mox50 cells (n = 7 donors). (**F**) ATP-linked to mitochondrial respiration (light green) versus non-mitochondrial ATP production (light red) in M0, M1, M2, and Mox50 cells (n = 8 donors). Statistical comparisons between experimental conditions are represented by green stars for mitochondrial ATP and red stars for non-mitochondrial ATP. ns = p-value > 0.05; * p-value < 0.05; ** p-value < 0.01; *** p-value < 0.001 and **** p-value < 0.0001.

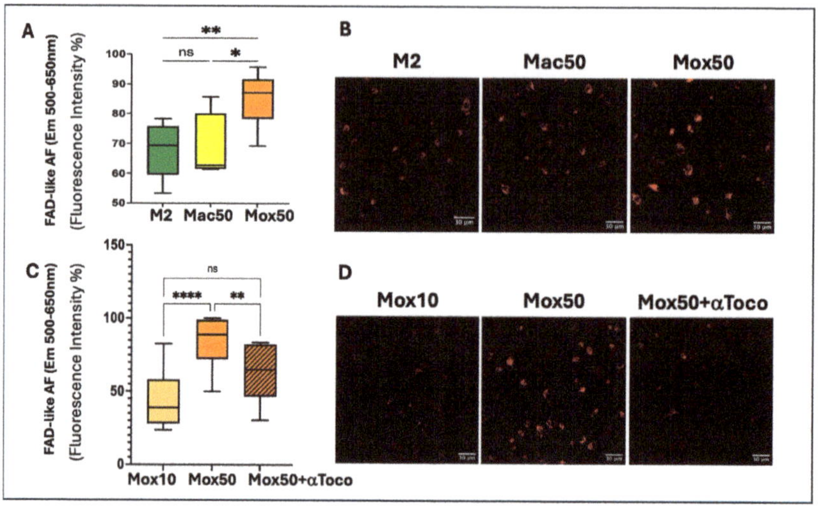

Figure 6. The AF in the FAD spectrum is linked to LDL handling and oxidative stress. (**A**) Quantification of FAD-like AF (λ_{Em}= 500–650 nm) in M2, Mac50, and Mox50 cells (n = 8). (**B**) Representative TPEF images of one donor (n = 8) in the M2, Mac50, and Mox50 conditions. (**C**) Quantification of AF emission in the FAD spectrum (Em 500–650 nm) in the Mox10, Mox50, and Mox50 + α-tocopherol conditions (n = 4). (**D**) Representative TPEF images of one donor (n = 3), in the Mox10, Mox50, and Mox50 + α-tocopherol conditions. ns = p-value > 0.05; * p-value < 0.05; ** p-value < 0.01; **** p-value < 0.0001.

As the AF signal intensity was proportional to the oxLDL concentration used to generate the Mox models and was significantly decreased by α-tocopherol, we hypothesized that **the AF signal in the spectrum of FAD might be linked to oxLDL uptake and the subsequent cellular oxidative stress.** Therefore, we quantified ROS production in the Mox and Mac models (with and without α-tocopherol) and compared the lysosomal accumulation of ceroids in both models.

- The levels of ROS and cellular ceroids are higher in Mox than in Mac Mφ

To investigate the implication of cellular oxidative stress, we evaluated ROS production in the different FM models in the presence or absence of α-tocopherol. ROS production was higher in the Mox than in the Mac models (Figure 7A) and was decreased by co-incubation with α-tocopherol (Figure 7B,C). As oxidative stress may result in lipid peroxidation and lysosomal accumulation of ceroids, we quantified ceroids in the different models using a derivative of Sudan Black, SenTraGor™®, which binds specifically to cellular ceroids. As observed for the FAD-like AF, the level of ceroids was higher in Mox50 than in Mac50 and Mox10 cells (Figure 7D) and markedly decreased in the presence of α-tocopherol (all models) (Figure 7E,F).

Altogether, in Mox50, the AF signal (λ_{Em}= 500–650 nm) and ceroid presence decreased when FM were generated in the presence of the antioxidant α-tocopherol that limited ROS production in these cells. These results support the hypothesis that ceroids are the biological origin of the FAD-like AF signal in our FM models. This was further supported by the colocalization of SenTraGor™®-positive ceroids with LAMP2, a lysosome marker (Figure 8).

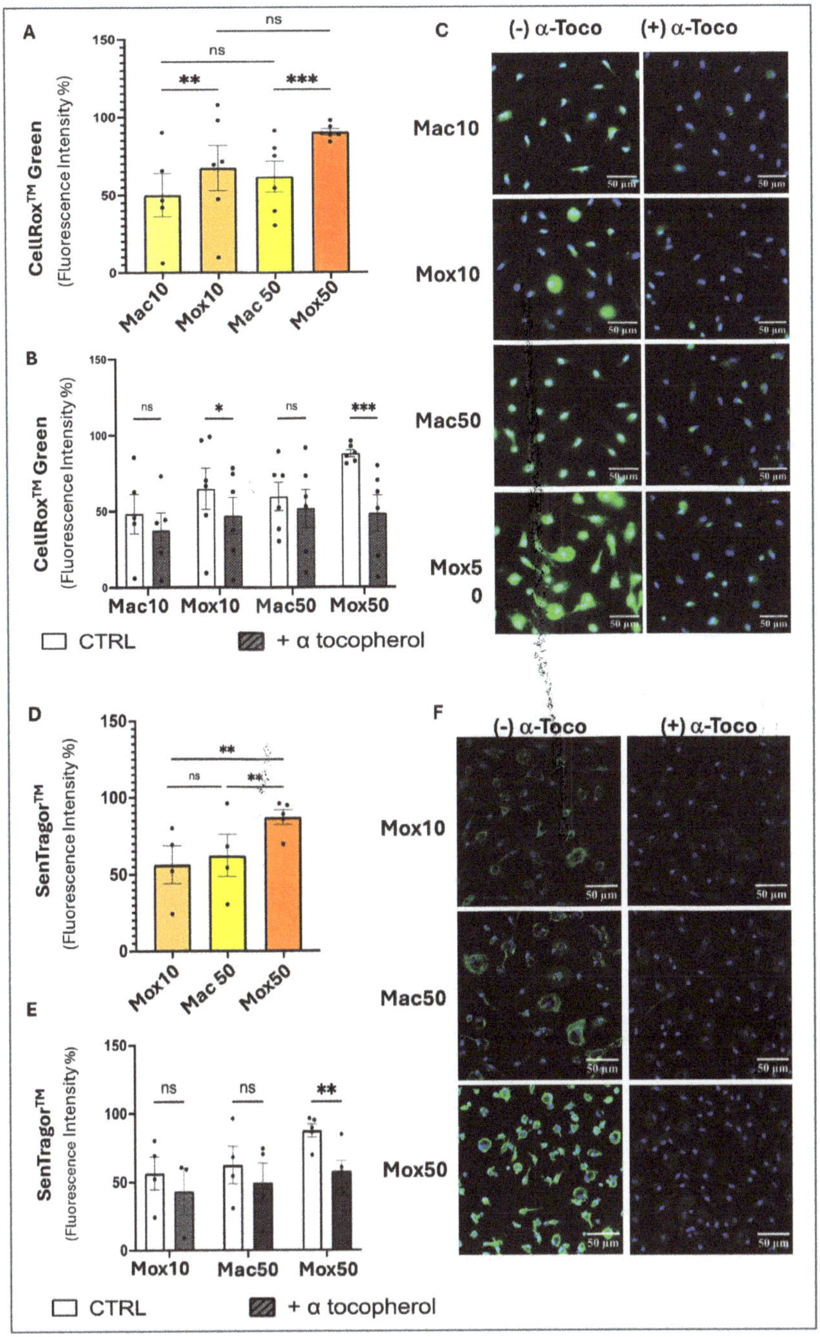

Figure 7. Detection of cellular reactive oxygen species (ROS) and ceroids. (**A**) Quantification of ROS level in the different experimental models of FM (Mac10, Mox10, Mac50, Mox50) after labeling with CellROX (n = 6 donors) (expressed as percentage of the maximal fluorescence intensity observed in the Mox50 models for each donor). (**B**) Quantification of ROS in the different models (Mox10, Mox50, Mac10, Mac50) obtained in the presence or absence of the antioxidant α-tocopherol (n = 6 donors). (**C**) Fluorescence microscopy images of the different models (Mox10, Mox50, Mac10, Mac50) after

CellROX labeling (n = 6 donors). (**D**) Quantification of the SenTraGor$^{TM®}$ fluorescence intensity in the different FM models (Mox10, Mac50, Mox50) (n = 6 donors). (**E**) Quantification of SenTraGor$^{TM®}$ fluorescence intensity in the presence or absence of the antioxidant α-tocopherol (n = 6 donors). (**F**) Confocal microscopy images of the different models generated in the presence or absence of α-tocopherol and labeled with SenTraGor$^{TM®}$ (n = 6 donors). ns = *p*-value > 0.05; * *p*-value < 0.05; ** *p*-value < 0.01; *** *p*-value < 0.001.

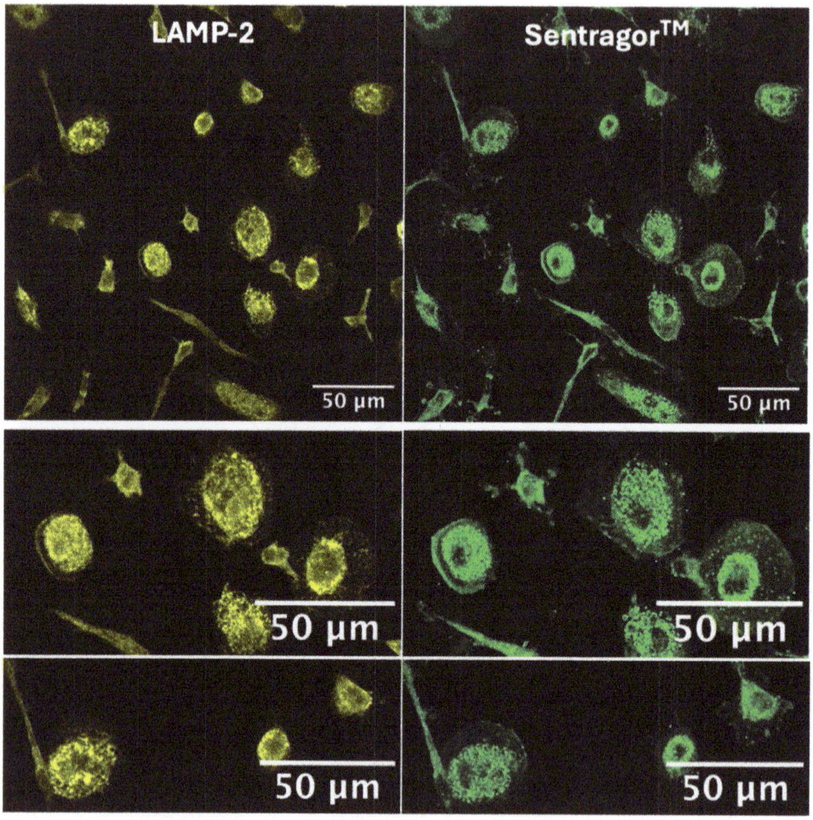

Figure 8. Colocalization of ceroids and LAMP-2 (lysosomal marker) in the Mox50 model (representative images obtained from one donor, n = 3, with a Leica TCS SP5 microscope).

All these findings support the conclusion that Mφ in the Mox model exhibit a more inflammatory profile compared to those in the Mac model. Additionally, these Mφ are in a more dysfunctional state, as evidenced by reduced mitochondrial respiration, increased oxidative stress, and ceroid accumulation, indicating lysosomal dysfunction.

2.4. *Evaluation of the Effects of α-Tocopherol and/or Type-2 Cytokine Cocktail on the Phenotypes and Functions of These FM Models*

- The antioxidant α-tocopherol influences the energetic metabolism in both FM models

To determine whether decreasing the cellular oxidative stress could modify the energetic pathways in both FM models, we generated FM models in the presence of α-tocopherol and used oxygraphy. The basal OCR values were increased in both Mac and Mox models generated by co-incubation with modified LDL and α-tocopherol compared with models generated by incubation with modified LDL alone. Notably, the effect was more pronounced when acLDL were used at a low dose, suggesting that cell dysfunction is more severe (and therefore more difficult to restore) with oxLDL (regardless of the dose) and with a high dose of acLDL (Figure 9A). The antioxidant treatment had no effect on the level of glycolysis in the cells, except for a slight increase of glycolysis in the Mac10 cells (Figure 9B).

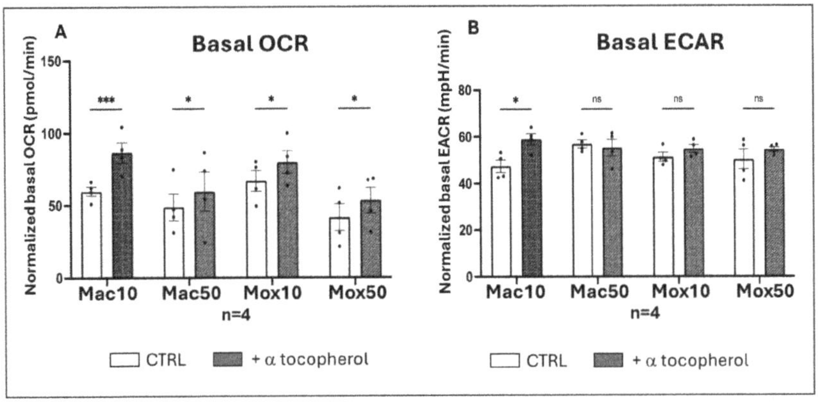

Figure 9. Oxygraphy measurement in the different FM models generated in the absence or in the presence of α-tocopherol. (**A**) Basal Oxygen Consumption Rate (OCR) indicative of the level of basal mitochondrial respiration in Mac10, Mac50, Mox10, and Mox50 Mφ incubated or not with α-tocopherol (n = 4 donors), (**B**) Basal ExtraCellular Acidification Rate (ECAR) indicative of the level of glycolytic flux in Mac10, Mac50, Mox10, and Mox50 Mφ incubated or not with α-tocopherol (n = 4 donors). ns = *p*-value > 0.05; * *p*-value < 0.05; *** *p*-value < 0.001.

The restoration of Mφ mitochondrial respiration using α-tocopherol suggests that the diminution of ceroids in atherosclerotic plaques observed in vivo after α-tocopherol treatment [25] might be partly linked to the metabolic shift of cells toward the energetic pathway preferentially used by immunoregulatory M2.

- A type-2 cytokine cocktail induces the M2 phenotype in Mac and Mox Mφ.

To address the capacity of FM to be polarized toward the M2 phenotype, we generated Mac and Mox models by co-incubating cells with a cocktail of type-2 cytokines (IL-4 and IL-13) and LDL for 48 h ("Polarization") or added the cocktail for 48 h after the 48 h incubation with LDL ("Delayed polarization"). In this case, the medium was changed before incubation with the cytokine cocktail. Then, we evaluated CD206, CD86, and CD40 cell surface expression (Figure 10). We calculated the fold induction of each marker in a specific experimental condition compared to the control condition (unstimulated Mφ). We observed a significant increase in CD206 cell surface expression in all FM models incubated with the cytokine cocktail during LDL uptake (Figure 10A) and afterward (Figure 10B). This suggests that both Mac and Mox models might switch to the M2 phenotype. The increase was lower with the higher doses of modified LDL (Figure 10A). In addition, when stimulation with the cytokines was performed after incubation with LDL (thus, when cells had become FM), CD206 expression increase was significantly lower in the Mox models than in the Mac models (Figure 10B). CD86 expression did not vary significantly after co-incubation with LDL and the cytokine cocktail (Figure 10C), but slightly increased in all FM models when polarization was induced after LDL uptake by Mφ (Figure 10D). CD40 expression was not affected by both polarization protocols (Figure 10E,F).

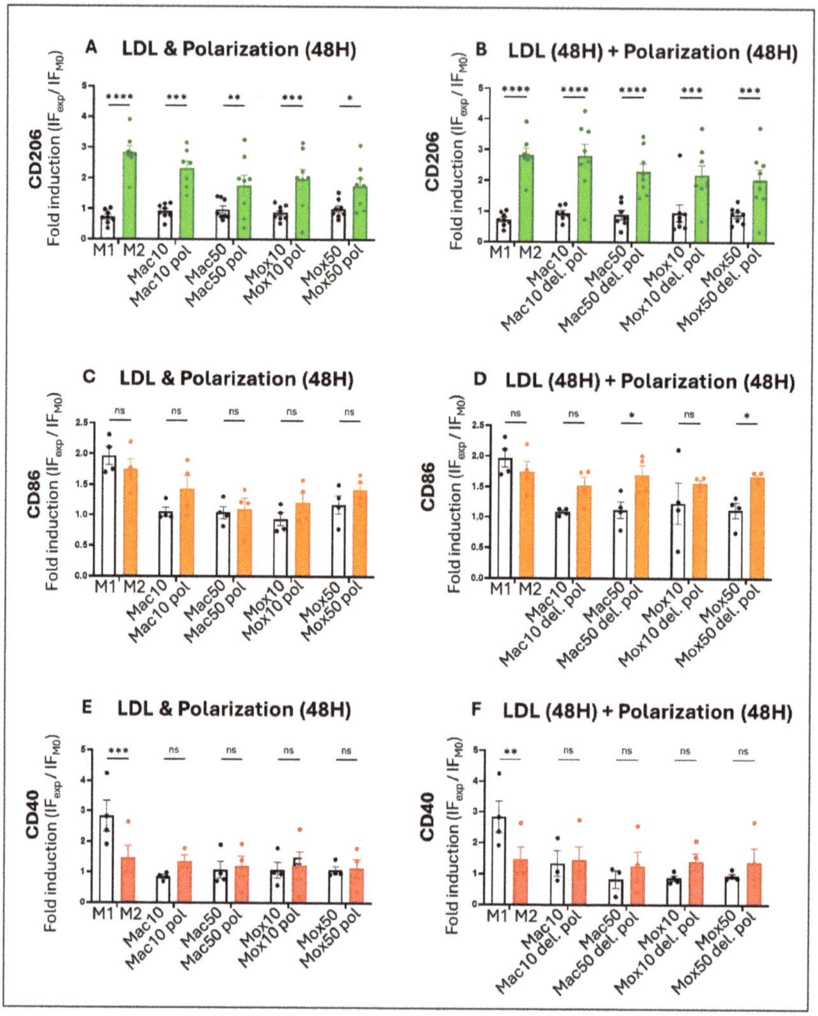

Figure 10. Fold induction of the different surface markers (MFI of the marker in the experimental condition divided by its MFI in the control condition, M0 = unstimulated Mφ) for the 'Polarization' protocol (stimulation with the cytokine cocktail added simultaneously with oxLDL/acLDL for 48 h): (**A**) CD206 (n = 8 donors); (**C**) CD86 (n = 4 donors); and (**E**) CD40 (n = 4 donors), or for the 'Delayed Polarization' protocol (treatment with oxLDL/acLDL for 48 h, followed by the cytokine cocktail for 48 h after changing the medium): (**B**) CD206 (n = 8 donors); (**D**) CD86 (n = 4 donors); and (**F**) CD40 (n = 4 donors). Here 'Mac/Mox' models were named 'Mac/Mox pol' (for polarization) when the cytokine cocktail was added during LDL incubation or 'Mac/Mox del. pol' (for delayed polarization) when the cytokine cocktail was added after the incubation with LDL, once the cells had already become FM. ns = p-value > 0.05; * p-value < 0.05; ** p-value < 0.01; *** p-value < 0.001 and **** p-value < 0.0001.

In either case (polarization or delayed polarization), the different experimental conditions can be classified along the inflammatory-to-immunoregulatory continuum (or the "M1-to-M2 polarization continuum") depending on the CD206 fold induction (Figure 11). This classification clearly showed that all the cells treated with cytokines with or without α-tocopherol expressed CD206 at the same level than the reference M2 condition. Addition of α-tocopherol (always in the first 48 h of incubation with LDL) did not induce any additional effect compared with the cocktail of cytokines alone (added at the same time, Figure 11A, or after the LDL, Figure 11B).

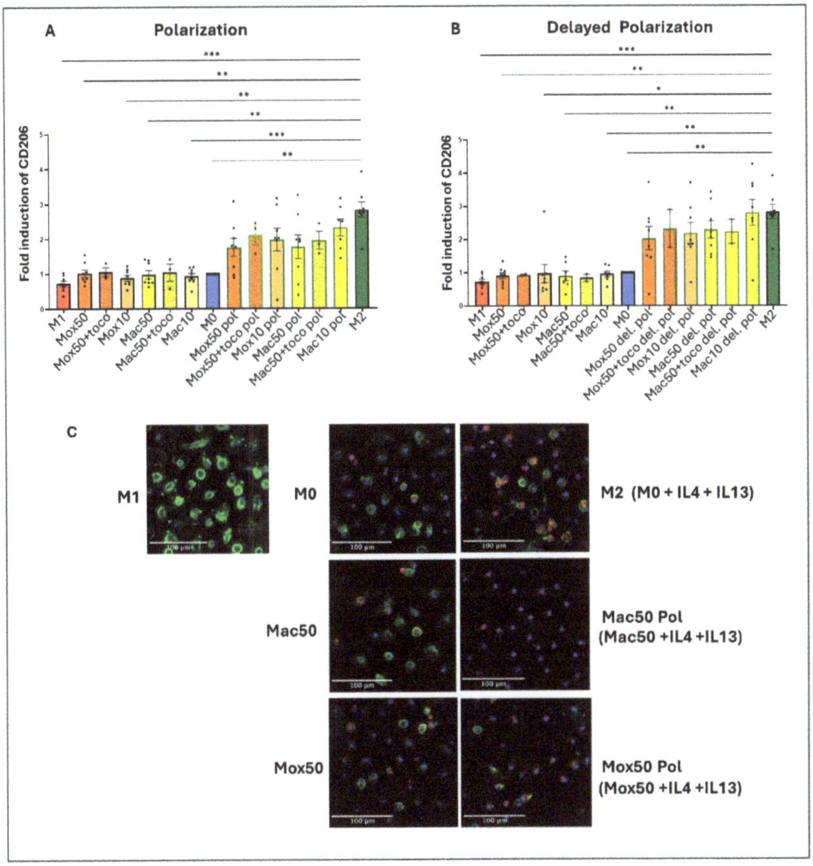

Figure 11. Degree of polarization (represented by the fold induction of CD206) according to the experimental conditions: (**A**) for the 'Polarization' protocol, where the cytokine cocktail, alone or with α-tocopherol, is added simultaneously with oxLDL/acLDL for 48 h, and (**B**) for the 'Delayed Polarization' protocol, when oxLDL/acLDL alone or in combination with α-tocopherol was added for 48 h, followed (after changing the medium) by the cytokine cocktail for 48 h. The Mac/Mox models were named 'Mac/Mox pol' (for polarization) when the cytokine cocktail (to induce polarization) was added during LDL incubation, or 'Mac/Mox del. pol' (for delayed polarization) when the cytokine cocktail was added after incubation with LDL, once the cells had already become FM. Data for the histograms were obtained by automated quantification of the CD40 and CD206 fluorescence signals in the imaged cells (representative images obtained from one donor, n = 4). (**C**) Images of Mφ obtained after a 48 h incubation with ac/oxLDL alone, or in combination with the cytokine cocktail. * p-value < 0.05; ** p-value < 0.01; *** p-value < 0.001.

To illustrate this experiment, some representative images are shown in Figure 11C. M1 cells strongly expressed CD40 (in green) and weakly expressed CD206 (in red). Conversely, M2 cells strongly expressed CD206 and weakly expressed CD40. Regarding FM models, CD206 expression was also clearly increased in both Mac and Mox models by using the cytokine treatment (Figure 11C).

Altogether, these findings demonstrated that Mac and Mox Mφ can be polarized toward an M2-like phenotype.

- The type-2 cocktail might induce immunoregulatory functions

To determine whether the different FM models can be polarized toward M2-like functions, we quantified the cytokines secreted by Mox50 and Mac50 Mφ following stimulation, as previously described. The secretion of IL-10 by both Mac50 and Mox50 cells was significantly increased compared to untreated cells only after co-incubation with LDL and the cytokine cocktail (Figure 12A), but not after stimulation of cells that were already differentiated into FM (Figure 12B).

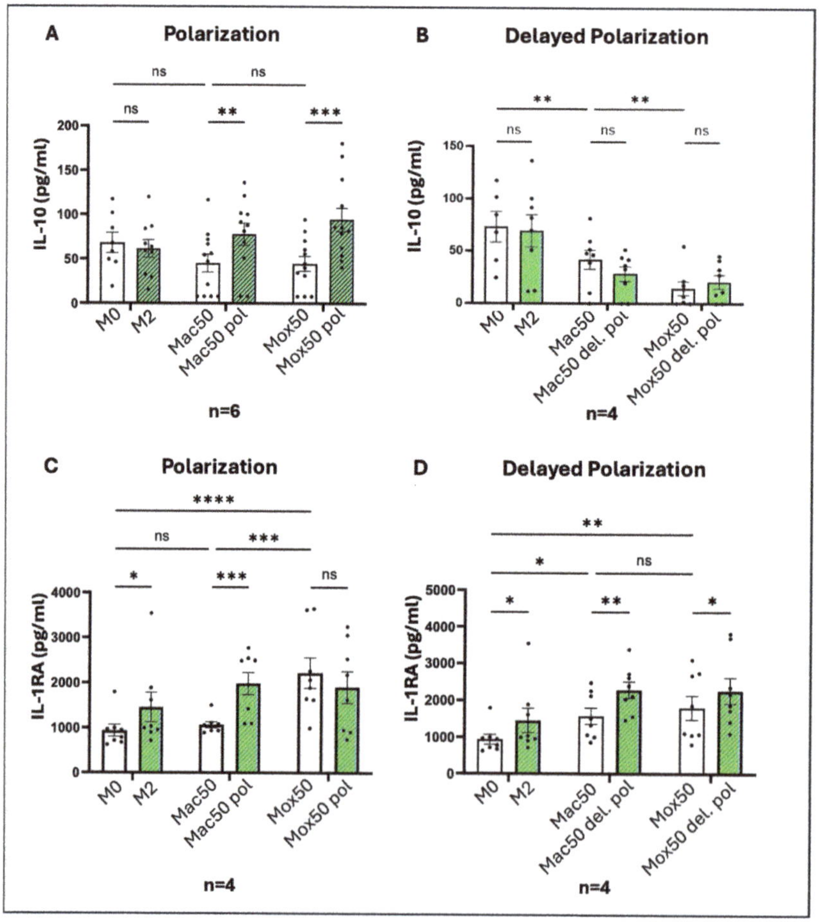

Figure 12. Quantification of the production of type-II cytokines after treatment with the immunoregulatory cytokine cocktail. IL-10 production in the Mac50 and Mox50 models: (**A**) stimulated with the cytokine cocktail added simultaneously with oxLDL/acLDL (polarization) (n = 6 donors), or (**B**) stimulated with the cytokine cocktail added after the incubation with modified LDL (delayed polarization) (n = 4 donors); IL1-RA production in the Mac50 and Mox50 models: (**C**) stimulated with the cytokine cocktail added simultaneously with oxLDL/acLDL, or (**D**) stimulated with the cytokine cocktail added after incubation with modified LDL (delayed polarization) (n = 4 donors). ns = p-value > 0.05; * p-value < 0.05; ** p-value < 0.01; *** p-value < 0.001 and **** p-value < 0.0001.

We also measured the secretion of IL-1RA, another immunoregulatory cytokine. Basal production of IL-1RA was notably high in Mox50 cells, significantly higher than in Mac50 and M2 cells. Consequently, we only observed an increase in IL-1RA secretion in Mac50 cells after co-incubation with LDL and the type-II cytokine cocktail (Figure 12C). In contrast, when the cytokine cocktail was added after LDL, we saw a significant increase in IL-1RA production in both models, though the increase was less pronounced in Mox50 Mφ (Figure 12D).

These results showed that both models can be polarized toward immunoregulatory functions, with the lower reactivity of Mox FM reflecting their more dysfunctional state.

- Incubation with the type-2 cytokine cocktail and α-tocopherol reduces drastically IL-6 production by Mox50 cells

Mox50 Mφ generated in the presence of oxLDL combined with IL-4 and IL-13 exhibited significantly reduced IL-6 production compared to Mφ treated with oxLDL alone (Figure 13). This effect was further enhanced when α-tocopherol was also added, resulting in IL-6 levels comparable to those seen in Mac50 Mφ (whose IL-6 production was similar to the M2 model shown in Figure 4C). These findings suggested that **the cytokine cocktail effectively reduces the inflammatory profile of Mox50** Mφ.

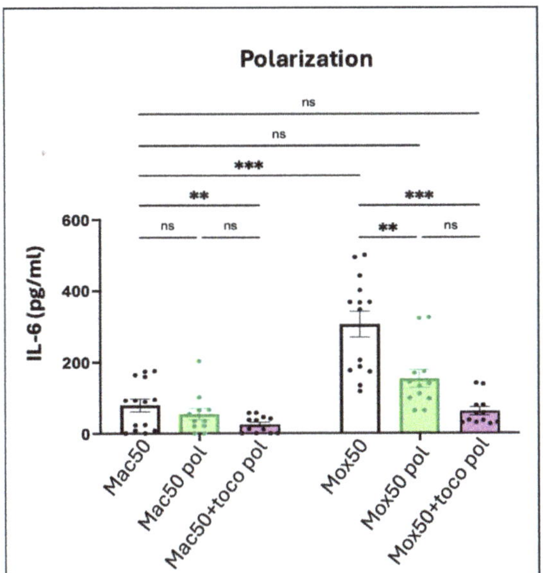

Figure 13. Quantification of IL-6 production in the Mac50 and Mox50 models stimulated with the cytokine cocktail, added simultaneously with oxLDL/acLDL, with or without α-tocopherol (n = 6 donors). Cells were incubated with acLDL/oxLDL (Mac50/Mox50), with acLDL/oxLDL + IL-4 + IL-13 (Mac50/Mox50 pol) or with acLDL/oxLDL + α-tocopherol + IL-4 + IL-13 (Mac50/Mox50 + toco pol). ns = p-value > 0.05; ** p-value < 0.01; *** p-value < 0.001.

3. Discussion

Recent advances in cytometry by time of flight and single-cell RNA sequencing have revealed the presence of numerous distinct Mφ subsets within plaques. This diversity can be attributed to the high plasticity of Mφ, fostered by microenvironmental cues. These subsets can be broadly classified into pro-atherogenic Mφ (including non-foamy inflammatory Mφ and dysfunctional Mφ) and anti-atherogenic Mφ (including non-foamy immunoregulatory Mφ). Foamy macrophages (FM) have long been considered as a key feature of atherosclerotic plaques, being abundant in vulnerable plaques during disease progression.

Traditionally, FM were categorized as inflammatory M1-like cells. However, Chinetti-Gbaguidi et al. [26] proposed the existence of various FM types, and Medbury et al. observed that FM can display heterogeneity and co-express both M1 and M2 markers, such as CD86 and CD206 [27]. More recent single-cell analyses identified FM as M2-like immunoregulatory cells [17–20]. Despite these insights, single-cell analyses may miss fragile FM subpopulations due to the limitations of cell extraction methods. Goossens et al. [21] utilized ex vivo multispectral imaging to map FM phenotypes in tissue samples, identifying several FM subsets, including one correlated with the TREM2^{hi} FM subset identified by single-cell RNA sequencing [28]. Nevertheless, the specific roles of each FM subset remain unclear. FM likely represent a complex population with diverse functions, including some involved in lipid clearance or plaque progression.

In our previous study, we discriminated inflammatory and immunoregulatory Mφ using TPEF imaging of NADH and FAD, which are produced in the glycolysis and OXPHOS pathways, respectively. At that time, the energetic metabolism pathway associated with FM was unknown. Using FM models made with acLDL and oxLDL (Mac and Mox models), we observed unexpectedly high TPEF imaging signals in the FAD spectrum, particularly in Mox FM. Additionally, the expression levels of CD86 and CD206 in Mox were lower compared to those in the M1 and M2 models, respectively.

Our multi-marker analysis revealed key differences between the Mac and Mox FM models. Mox FM had a higher percentage of the CD86$^+$/CD206$^-$ subset and a lower percentage of the CD86$^-$/CD206$^+$ subset compared to Mac FM. The NADH AF signal in Mox FM was similar to that in M1 Mφ, associated with a very high AF signal in the FAD spectrum. The 3D-PCA of flow cytometry and TPEF data suggested that Mac FM are closer to M2 cells, while the Mox model is distinct from all the other experimental models. Overall, the Mac and Mox FM models differ in surface marker expression and endogenous natural AF, allowing us to distinguish various Mφ types using 3D-PCA.

We then investigated the functional and energetic metabolic profiles of the Mac and Mox models using low (10 μg/mL: Mac10, Mox10) or high doses (50 μg/mL: Mac50, Mox50) of modified LDL.

Cytokine secretion comparison has focused on three inflammatory cytokines and two immunoregulatory cytokines. The inflammatory cytokines, IL-1β, IL-6, and IL-18, are recognized as key drivers of the athero-inflammatory process [29–31], two of which, IL-1β and IL-6, are already the targets of therapeutic strategies [32–34]. We also chose to quantify the immunoregulatory cytokines, IL-10, which has shown strong potential as a therapeutic target [35–37] and IL-1RA, an antagonist of IL-1 even if its therapeutic application in cardiovascular diseases remains unproven [38].

Cytokine quantification in Mox and Mac models revealed that both FM models produced high levels of the inflammatory cytokines IL-18 and IL-1β, similar to M1. Compared to Mac cells, Mox50 cells produced significantly more IL-6 but less IL-10. The inflammatory state of Mox models was dose-dependent, with higher IL-1β and IL-6 production in Mox50 than Mox10. This cytokine profiling confirmed that the Mox50 model contains more inflammatory cells than the Mac50 model.

These findings align with our metabolic analyses. Inflammatory Mφ primarily rely on glycolysis, whereas immunoregulatory Mφ depend more on mitochondrial respiration. The Mox50 model exhibited higher glycolysis and lower mitochondrial respiration than the M1 model, indicating a metabolic similarity to inflammatory Mφ. The Mac50 model also relied on glycolysis. These results suggest that the AF observed in the NADH spectrum in both Mox50 and Mac50 models is likely due to NADH produced during glycolysis. Conversely, the Mox50 model showed reduced mitochondrial respiration and higher FAD-like AF compared with the Mac50 model, ruling out the possibility that the strong AF in the FAD spectrum originated from mitochondrial FAD production. Furthermore, the FAD-like AF signal was higher and mitochondrial respiration was lower in the Mox50 model compared with the Mox10 model. The increased FAD-like AF and reduced mitochondrial respiration in Mox50 cells led us to hypothesize that this AF is associated with a more pronounced dysfunctional state in Mox50 Mφ.

To address this question, we compared ROS production and lysosomal ceroid accumulation across the different FM models. Ceroids are aggregates of oxidized proteins and lipids with natural AF that overlaps with the FAD spectrum. Mox cells are associated with dysfunctional lysosomes, leading to ceroid deposition and impaired cholesterol efflux [39,40], mitophagy, and autophagy, along with inflammation, senescence. and apoptosis [22]. A recent study from Albaghdadi M.S. et al. [25] highlighted ceroid as a key source of near-infrared autofluorescence (NIRAF) in human atherosclerosis and demonstrated that oxLDL induces (NIRAF), oxidative stress, and production of lipid peroxidation products in Mφ, which were decreased by a treatment with antioxidants (α-tocopherol and N-acetylcysteine (NAC). In accordance with their study, our results showed that ROS production and ceroid accumulation were higher in Mox50 cells. Antioxidant α-tocopherol reduced FAD-like AF, ROS production, and ceroid accumulation in the Mox50 model, suggesting a connection between this AF and oxLDL handling. Additionally, the comparison of different lipid types and doses showed that they may induce Mφ with varying functional profiles. The Mox50 model may represent FM with more severe dysfunction due to impaired oxLDL handling, resulting in higher cellular stress, ROS production, and lysosomal accumulation of ceroids. This underscores the importance of developing different experimental models to mimic different plaque FM subsets. While these models may imperfectly replicate plaque Mφ, they could represent Mφ with varying lipid loads and dysfunction levels, which may be used to explore therapeutic approaches aimed at restoring atheroprotective functions, such as blocking inflammation, promoting cholesterol efflux, or inducing immunoregulation.

The effects of acLDL and oxLDL on cholesterol metabolism in Mφ have been extensively studied by other groups. OxLDL induces more severe lysosomal damage compared to acLDL. While acLDL is efficiently hydrolyzed and allows cholesterol efflux, oxLDL is less effectively degraded, leading to cholesterol accumulation, crystal formation, and altered lysosomal pH. This disruption impairs lysosomal hydrolase activity, causing significant lysosomal dysfunction marked by increased ceroid formation [40–45]. These findings are consistent with our AF and SenTraGor® imaging results, indicating that oxLDL is associated with greater functional impairment of lysosomes than acLDL. Although cholesterol efflux is a well-established therapeutic approach to ameliorating the condition of FM, our study deliberately focused on an alternative strategy involving the induction of immunoregulation in FM.

We thus assessed whether the different FM models (Mox10, Mac10, Mox50, and Mac50 cells) could be polarized toward an immunoregulatory profile using immunoregulatory cytokines (IL-4 and IL-13) according to two protocols: (1) co-incubation of Mφ with modified LDL and the cytokine cocktail ("polarization") to mimic Mφ that have recently infiltrated the intima and are being exposed to both oxLDL and therapeutic treatment, and (2) initial incubation with modified LDL, followed by cytokine stimulation ("Delayed Polarization") to mimic the effect of the treatment on Mφ that have already taken up modified LDL and are potentially dysfunctional. In some experiments, α-tocopherol was added to the modified LDL to test whether this antioxidant could improve the functional state of FM and enhance their response to the immunoregulatory treatment.

CD206 expression was significantly increased in all FM models incubated with the cytokine cocktail, both during and after LDL uptake. IL-10 secretion increased significantly when cytokines were added during LDL incubation, but not after FM formation, suggesting that established FM may be less amenable to M2 polarization. The high IL-10 production in M1 Mφ (and also in unstimulated M0 Mφ) was unexpected, although it has been previously observed in a similar M1 model [45].Therefore, we measured the production of IL-1RA, another well-known immunoregulatory cytokine. IL-1RA production increased in the Mac50 model when the cytokine cocktail was added early, but not in the Mox50 model. This lack of increase in the Mox50 model may be due to already high levels of IL-1RA present in untreated Mox50 cells. Sequential incubation (LDL first, followed by cytokine stimulation) increased IL-1RA in both models, but to a lesser extent in Mox50, suggesting greater dysfunction and reduced potential for immunoregulatory polarization. IL-6 production in Mox50 cells decreased with cytokine treatment, and α-tocopherol addition further reduced it to levels similar to Mac50 and M2 conditions, indicating that α-tocopherol may alleviate inflammation and dysfunction caused by high oxLDL concentration. Further comparative studies with antioxidants with superior efficacity, such as probucol, could provide insights into more effective treatments [46].

In summary, our study provides insights into the functional profiles of FM models and their potential use in screening drugs with anti-inflammatory or immunoregulatory effects. Both acLDL- and oxLDL-induced FM models could serve as useful tools for evaluating drugs, as they may reflect FM at an early or late stage, respectively. The choice of the model should align with the conceptual framework and experimental objectives. The Mac model could be more suitable for evaluating whether drugs or biologics (e.g., therapeutic antibodies) can repolarize early FM to an immunoregulatory phenotype. The Mox50 model, representing a more advanced stage of FM, might be used to assess therapeutics aimed at restoring cholesterol efflux and reversing LDL handling dysfunction.

4. Materials and Methods

4.1. Monocyte Isolation, Differentiation, and Stimulation to Generate the Experimental Models of Mφ

Monocytes were negatively selected (PAN BioTech kit, Miltenyi Biotec, Paris, France) from peripheral blood mononuclear cells (PBMC) isolated using Ficoll-Paque Premium 1.073 density gradient (GE Healthcare, Strasbourg, France) from blood samples of healthy donors (Etablissement Français du Sang (EFS) of Bordeaux, Bordeaux, France). A quantity of 3–5 × 10^5 purified monocytes/mL were seeded on round glass coverslips (for cell imaging) in 12-well plates and differentiated into monocyte-derived macrophages by 5–6-day culture in complete medium (RPMI-1640 medium (Dutscher, Bernolsheim, France) with 10% heat-inactivated AB human serum (Dutscher), 100 U/mL penicillin (Dutscher), and 100 µg/mL streptomycin (Dutscher)) containing 20 ng/mL recombinant human (rh) M-CSF (Miltenyi Biotec). Half of the medium was replaced with fresh medium once during culture. After the differentiation period, cultures were rested for 24 h (complete medium without M-CSF) before a 48 h incubation with the following: (1) 20 ng/mL of rhIFN-γ (Miltenyi Biotec) plus 100 pg/mL of lipopolysaccharide (LPS) (cell culture-suitable, γ-irradiated, BioXtra LPS, Sigma Aldrich) for the classically activated M1 model; (2) 20 ng/mL of rhIL-4 and rhIL-13 (Miltenyi Biotec) for the alternatively activated M2 model; (3) 10 and 50 µg/mL of human oxLDL (Thermo Fischer Scientific France, Illkirch-Graffenstaden, France) for the Mox10 and Mox50 models; (4) 10 and 50 µg/mL of human acLDL (Thermo Fischer Invitrogen) for the Mac10 and Mac50 models. In some experiments, α-tocopherol (Sigma Aldrich, St-Quentin-Fallavier, France) was added in combination with LDL. In some experiments (polarization assays), 20ng/mL of both IL-4 and IL-13, with or without 1 mM α-tocopherol, were combined with modified LDL for a 48 h stimulation before assessing CD206 surface marker expression or cytokine production.

4.2. TPEF Data Acquisition

Three-dimensional autofluorescence (AF) images were acquired with a Leica TCS SP5 system (Leica Microsystems, Mannheim, Germany) using the two-photon excitation fluorescence (TPEF) modality and analyzed as described previously [23,47]. Briefly, imaging in the NADH fluorescence spectral band was performed at 760 nm excitation and 420–500 nm detection. Imaging in the FAD fluorescence spectral band was performed at 860 nm excitation and 500–650 nm detection. Taking advantage of intrinsic optical sectioning of two-photon excitation, the AF volume densities of individual cells were extracted in both spectral bands.

4.3. Combined Analysis of Flow Cytometry and TPEF Data Using 3D-PCA

Starting from previously acquired flow cytometry data and TPEF data [23], the phenotypes of the FM models Mac and Mox were compared to those of the reference models. Fifteen parameters were considered: for TPEF data, NADH and FAD AF, Optical Redox Ratio parameter (which represents the [FAD AF]/[NADH AF] ratio) and for flow cytometry data, Positive Cell percentage (PCP) and Mean Fluorescence Intensity (MFI) of the following markers: CD86, CD40, and CD197 (M1 markers), and CD206, CD200R, and CD163 (M2 markers). PCP and MFI were considered first for each marker individually, then in the four defined subsets: $CD86^+/CD206^-$, $CD86^+/CD206^+$, $CD86^-/CD206^+$, and $CD86^-/CD206^-$. MFI, PCP, and AF data were also used as quantitative variables in an original 3D-PCA performed using the FactomineR and pca3d packages in the R software 4.4.1. Experimental conditions served as categorical (qualitative) variable. The mean value for a sample was taken for each variable analyzed in the 3D-PCA. As all markers were not labeled in all flow cytometry acquisitions, missing values (~10% of the whole data) for the corresponding flow cytometry variable were inferred using the missDMA R package before 3D-PCA [48]. This package handles missing values by statistical analysis and then 3D-PCA can be performed with all samples, despite the presence of few missing data. Retaining only the first two dimensions of the PCA was insufficient to adequately capture the variability within the dataset. However, the first three dimensions accounted for approximately 75% of the total inertia and were deemed sufficient to represent the majority of the dataset's variability. Visualizing three dimensions on a two-dimensional plane typically necessitates the presentation of multiple 2D plots, which individually fail to clearly convey the spatial relationships between different experimental conditions. Consequently, a 3D plot was generated, despite its potential to be somewhat challenging for initial interpretation. To enhance visualization, we provided rotating animated GIFs in Supplementary Figure S1A,B. Moreover, enhanced versions of these figures (Supplementary Figure S2A,B) are included, which further depict the contributions of individual variables to the three principal components. The ellipsoids drawn in the plots represent the dispersion of data points corresponding to each experimental condition, with approximately 80% of the measurements falling within these ellipsoids.

4.4. Metabolic Characterization of the Macrophage Experimental Models by Extracellular Flux Analysis

The bioenergetic profiles of the macrophage models were investigated using a Seahorse Bioscience XF96 Extracellular Flux Analyzer (Agilent, Santa Clara, CA, USA) that allows the simultaneous kinetic measurements of Oxygen Consumption Rate (OCR) and ExtraCellular Acidification Rate (ECAR), which reflect respiration and glycolysis, respectively. Cells were plated on 96-well custom plates designed for use with the analyzer (50,000 cells/well) and grown to confluence in complete medium. Then, the different macrophage models were generated as previously described. The day before the assay, the calibration plate was incubated (overnight) with water without CO_2 for probe hydration. The next day, water was replaced with Seahorse calibration medium (Agilent Seahorse XF-calibrant, Agilent) at 37 °C without CO_2 for 30 min. Before the experiment, the growth medium was removed, and cells were washed and incubated at 37 °C without CO_2 in warm enriched Seahorse medium (Seahorse XF medium, 11 mM glucose, 2 mM glutamine, 1 mM pyruvate, 2% BSA with pH adjusted to 7.4) for 1 h. Once the calibration completed, the "Mito Stress" assay was performed by sequential addition of four compounds: 1 µM oligomycin (inhibitor of ATP synthesis), 2 µM carbonyl cyanide 4-(trifluoromethoxy) phenylhydrazone (uncoupling agent), 1 µM rotenone/antimycin A (inhibitors of complex I and complex III of the respiratory chain, respectively). The instrument was set to acquire consecutive measurements for 1 h with mixing in between. Data were analyzed using the Wave Desktop software 2.6.1. The Agilent Seahorse XF Real-time ATP rate assay was performed to measure the rate of ATP production from the two key energy pathways, simultaneously in live macrophages using a label-free technology that delivers a dynamic picture of the cell bioenergetics with indicators of the glycolysis and respiration contribution.

4.5. ROS Detection

ROS accumulation was assessed with CellROX® Green (Cat. No.C10444, Thermo Fisher Scientific France) a fluorogenic, ROS-sensitive dye. The reagent measures superoxide (O_2^-) and hydroxyl radical ($^{\bullet}OH$) in living cells. This dye becomes fluorescent upon binding to DNA after being oxidized, allowing ROS quantification. CellROX® Green Reagent was added directly to the medium at a final concentration of 5 µM per well and incubated at 37 °C for 30 min. Cells were then fixed with 4% paraformaldehyde solution in PBS for 15 min. After two washes with 1X PBS, 4′,6-diamino-2-phenylindole (DAPI) dihydrochloride (Thermo Fisher Scientific) was used as nuclear counterstain at a concentration of 0.47 µM (Thermo Fisher Scientific). After one wash with 1X PBS 0.1X, the samples were mounted on a slide with Prolong medium (Prolong Diamond Antifade 5, Thermo Fisher Scientific). Excitation and emission were 485 and 520 nm. Fluorescence was measured within 24 h after staining. Images were obtained using a Leica DMI8 inverted camera fluorescence microscope with a 63X/1.4 oil objective at the Bordeaux Imaging Center (BIC). Fluorescence intensity was quantified automatically by the FIJI software 2.14.0.

4.6. Ceroid Staining

Ceroids were detected using a hybrid immunochemical/immunofluorescence assay based on GL13, a lipophilic, biotin-linked Sudan Black-B (SBB) analog (SenTraGorTM®) (P.Galanis & Co_Lab Supplies, Athens, Greece) [49]. Staining was performed according to the manufacturer's protocol. Briefly, the reagent was dissolved in 3.75 mL absolute ethanol and incubated in 56 °C water for 120 min. The dissolved dye was kept in the original vial and sealed with parafilm to avoid evaporation of ethanol and stored at room temperature in the dark. Cells were washed twice with 10X PBS, once with 50% ethanol, then once with 70% ethanol at room temperature for 5 min. The SenTraGor® reagent was then filtered using a 0.22 µm filter and added to cells at a concentration of 8.2 mmol/L. After 8 min, cells were washed four times with 50% ethanol, four times with PBS, and then incubated with 0.5%Triton X-100 in 10X PBS for 3 min. This allowed visualizing ceroid staining after removal of other neutral lipids. Then, a rabbit anti-biotin (600–401-098, Rockland Immunochemicals) antibody was used at a concentration of 2.6 µg/mL to directly detect biotin in the SenTraGor® reagent. After incubation with the antibody at 4 °C overnight, cells were washed with 1X PBS three times before incubation with the goat anti-rabbit secondary antibody coupled to Alexa Fluor 488 (ab150077, Abcam, Amsterdam, Netherlands) at a concentration of 2 µg/mL. To show that ceroids are formed in lysosomes, LAMP2 (a lysosome marker) was simultaneously detected using a rat anti-LAMP2 antibody (ab13524, Abcam) at a concentration of 10 µg/mL after saturation in 10% AB serum, 0.1% Tween-20, and 0.1% Triton X-100 at room temperature for 30 min. A goat anti-rat secondary antibody coupled to Cy5 (ab6565, Abcam) was used at a concentration of 2 µg/mL for LAMP2 revelation. After five washes with 1X PBS and 1 wash with 0.1X PBS, Prolong medium (Prolong Diamond Antifade 5, Thermo Fisher Scientific France) containing 2 µg/mL DAPI dihydrochloride (Thermo Fisher Scientific France) was used for mounting the glass coverslips onto slides before imaging with a confocal laser scanning microscope (TCS SP5 multiphoton confocal microscope, Leica Microsystems, Mannheim Germany), with the following wavelengths of excitation and emission, Ex 633 nm/Em 650–750 nm, Ex 488 nm/Em 500–550 nm, and Ex 405/Em 415–460 nm, to detect the fluorescence of LAMP2, ceroids, and DAPI, respectively, in addition to the contrast phase acquisition. Image analysis and fluorescence quantification were performed with the FIJI software 2.14.0)

4.7. Polarization Assay

Two protocols of polarization were established: In the first one, Mφ were treated for 48 h with modified LDL and a type-II cytokine cocktail. Alternatively, Mφ were incubated 48 h with modified LDL first, then the cell medium was changed and the cytokine cocktail was added for another 48 h. Following these two polarization processes, phenotypic and functional polarization of Mφ compared to M1 and M2 models and to untreated controls (LDL alone, without adding cytokines) was addressed. In some experiments, α-tocopherol was also added during the incubation with LDL. After stimulation, supernatants were collected and human ELISA kits IL-10 (KE00170-96T), IL-6 (KE00139), IL-18 (KE00193), IL-1β (KE0021) (Proteintech™ Planegg-Martinsried, Germany) and IL-1RA (KAC1181) from Invitrogen, Thermo Fisher Scientific France) were used according to the manufacturer's instructions. Cells were washed and fixed with 4%PFA, incubated for 20 min in a blocking buffer composed of 1X PBS, 10% FBS, 1% BSA, 0.3M glycine, and 0.1% Tween-20, and stained with an anti-CD40 antibody (rabbit anti-human AB224639, Abcam, and a secondary goat anti-rabbit Alexa 488 antibody: Ex 495/Em 519 nm, AB150077, Abcam), or an anti-CD86 antibody (rabbit anti-human Alexa Fluor® 488: Ex 495/Em 519 nm, ab290990, Abcam), and anti-CD206 antibody (mouse anti-human CD206-Coralite: Ex 593/Em 614 nm, 2A6A10, Thermo Fisher Scientific France). After mounting the coverslips on glass slides in a suitable medium (Prolong Diamond Antifade, Thermo Fisher Scientific) containing 0.47 μM DAPI (Thermo Fisher Scientific France), immunofluorescence images were acquired with the Leica DMI8 (Microsystems, Mannheim Germany), inverted camera system using a 63X/1.4 oil objective at the Bordeaux Imaging Center ((BIC), Bordeaux, France). The TRITC, FITC, and DAPI filters were used. Z-stacks were acquired using 1 μm optical sections. The images were analyzed with FIJI 2.14.0. Brightness and contrast were standardized for all representative images. A program that automates a series of commands on FIJI 2.14.0 (macro) was used for the quantification of fluorescence intensities in the two channels.

4.8. Statistical Analysis

Statistical tests and data graphs were performed with the GraphPad Prism 10.0.2 software (GraphPad software). Outliers in each dataset were not considered when data for one experimental condition was missing; mixed-effects models were used to handle the absences and ensure the robustness of the analysis. We primarily applied one-way repeated measures ANOVA for experiments involving a single factor (Figures 4, 5B–E, 7A,D and 11A,B) and two-way ANOVA for experiments involving multiple factors (Figures 1, 5F, 7B,E, 9, 10, 12 and 13). One-way ordinary ANOVA was used for Figure 6. Most ANOVAs were conducted using repeated measures to account for the structure of the data. The resulting histograms represent the mean ± SEM and the *p*-values were considered significant at alpha of 0.05. (NS = p-value > 0.05; * p-value < 0.05; ** p-value < 0.01; *** p-value < 0.001 and **** p-value < 0.0001).

5. Future Directions

We plan to use these models to screen human antibodies for their therapeutic potential: we will compare Mφ status before and after treatment with these antibodies and assess their functional polarization to an immunoregulatory profile. Nevertheless, other therapies focusing on immunoregulation, such those involving cytokines or other M2-promoting agents, can also be considered if properly targeted, thereby minimizing systemic effects while directly modulating Mφ within the plaques. Gene therapy approaches using viral vectors or lipid-based nanoparticles to deliver genes encoding these cytokines to Mφ could also enhance their polarization toward the M2 phenotype. Additionally, drugs already used clinically, such as PPARγ agonists (e.g., pioglitazone), which promote anti-inflammatory gene expression and enhance cholesterol efflux, reducing foam cell formation, could be redesigned or adapted to specifically target Mφ within atherosclerotic plaques. Nanoparticles and liposomes can also be engineered to carry immunomodulatory agents to these macrophages, ensuring targeted and enhanced delivery while minimizing side effects. The administration of these treatments, whether intravenously or locally, could be combined with existing therapies like statins to provide a more comprehensive approach to managing atherosclerosis, potentially reducing plaque progression and cardiovascular risk.

In another study, we are considering exploring nanoparticles loaded with ApoA1 and biomimetics acceptors such as reconstituted HDL to induce cholesterol efflux and using TPEF imaging to monitor changes in the FAD-like AF signal, which would indicate improvements in cholesterol management. In this therapeutic strategy, we plan to provide a thorough characterization of our FM models. This includes understanding the mechanisms driving their lipid uptake and trafficking, such as the levels of free cholesterol and cholesterol esters, the activity of enzymes like ACAT1, and the expression of surface receptors such as ABCA1 (ATP-binding cassette, sub-family A, member 1) and ABCG1 (ATP-binding cassette, sub-family G, member 1). This comprehensive analysis will be essential for comparing the ability of these models to efflux cholesterol in the presence of the acceptors that will be designed in our future studies.

From a diagnostic perspective, TPEF imaging of NADH and FAD-like AF may be valuable for assessing plaque vulnerability. Developing an endoscopic fiber for optical imaging could enable in vivo distinction of pro-atherogenic and anti-atherogenic Mφ to assess coronary plaque vulnerability.

6. Limitations of the Study

The aim of experimental FM models is to mimic the FM found in atherosclerotic plaques; however, it is challenging to perfectly replicate all Mφ subpopulations and their interactions. The models characterized in this study represent different positions on the continuum between inflammatory and immunoregulatory Mφ and may represent FM subsets with varying levels of lipid accumulation, as recently identified ex vivo. Despite their limitations, these models are valuable for studying LDL handling dysfunction and screening new therapeutic tools, such as antibodies and/or drugs that can induce immunoregulation or restore cholesterol management and efflux. The characterization of scavenger receptors, cholesterol efflux capacity, and lipid content in these models is necessary for better understanding and future applications.

7. Conclusions

Our study demonstrates that cellular NADH and FAD-like autofluorescence (AF) primarily reflect different features of Mφ metabolism and dysfunction. Specifically, NADH AF indicates glycolytic activity, while FAD-like AF correlates with lysosomal ceroid accumulation, a marker of oxidative stress and dysfunctional lipid handling.

The use of 3D-Principal Component Analysis (3D-PCA) has proven to be an innovative approach for distinguishing between different Mφ models based on their functional phenotypes. This technique allows for the effective distinction of Mφ based on their inflammatory versus immunoregulatory characteristics, as well as their autofluorescence profiles associated with energetic and lipid metabolism.

In our models, Mac and Mox FM exhibit distinct phenotypic and functional profiles along the inflammatory-to-immunoregulatory continuum. The Mox model, aligning more closely with inflammatory Mφ, is characterized by elevated FAD-like AF, increased reactive oxygen species (ROS) production, and higher ceroid accumulation. In contrast, the Mac model is more representative of immunoregulatory Mφ, showing a less pronounced inflammatory profile and lower levels of dysfunction.

Both FM models demonstrated potential for polarization toward an immunoregulatory profile through treatment with IL-4 and IL-13. Notably, the inflammatory profile of Mox50 macrophages was significantly attenuated by this cytokine cocktail, with additional improvement observed when α-tocopherol was included, suggesting a potential therapeutic avenue for mitigating Mφ dysfunction.

These findings underscore the relevance of both FM models for studying the mechanisms underlying dysfunctional LDL handling and for developing and testing new therapeutic interventions. Both models are valuable for assessing new drugs and therapeutic strategies designed to reduce inflammation, enhance cholesterol efflux, and restore Mφ function in the context of atherosclerosis. The Mac model may be particularly useful for evaluating treatments aimed at promoting immunoregulation, while the Mox model offers insights into advanced stages of dysfunction and oxidative stress.

Supplementary Materials: The following supporting information can be downloaded at: https://www.mdpi.com/article/10.3390/ijms251810146/s1.

Author Contributions: A.S.H.M., M.R., J.G. (Janaïna Grevelinger), J.G. (Johan Garaude), C.B., J.L.-T. and F.O. performed the in vitro experiments and data analysis. A.S.H.M., M.R. and S.M. performed the images acquisition and J.B. performed image data analysis and 3D-PCA. J.B., A.S.H.M., M.-J.J.-V., E.G., G.C.-S. and F.O. designed the study. G.C.-S., J.B., E.G. and F.O. wrote the grant applications. G.C.-S. and F.O. were involved in the project administration and supervision. A.S.H.M., G.C.-S. and F.O. were involved in writing the manuscript. All authors have read and agreed to the published version of the manuscript.

Funding: This study was supported by the Fédération Française de Cardiologie, the French National Research Agency (ANR) [ANR-19-CE19-0019] and [ANR-22-CE09-0001], and the European Union [HORIZON-EIC-2023-PATHFINDEROPEN-01, HORIZON EIC Grants#101130308] and was conducted in the framework of the University of Bordeaux's France 2030 program RRI "IMPACT" that received financial support from the French government.

Institutional Review Board Statement: All work with human tissues was approved by the local Ethics committee (Comité de Protection des Personnes Sud-Ouest et Outre Mer) and the French Research Ministry (Authorization number DC-2016-2724).

Informed Consent Statement: Not applicable.

Data Availability Statement: Data is contained within the article or Supplementary Material.

Acknowledgments: We would like to thank Xavier Noguès, who contributed to the statistical analysis of experiments, and the students who contributed to the experiments (Noam Prudhomme, Valentine Galibert, Simon Ferrer, and Marine Guilmois).

Conflicts of Interest: The authors declare they do not have anything to disclose regarding conflicts of interest with respect to this manuscript.

References

1. Falk, E. Pathogenesis of Atherosclerosis. *J. Am. Coll. Cardiol.* **2006**, *47*, C7–C12. [CrossRef] [PubMed]
2. Libby, P.; Hansson, G.K. Inflammation and Immunity in Diseases of the Arterial Tree: Players and Layers. *Circ. Res.* **2015**, *116*, 307–311. [CrossRef] [PubMed]
3. Flynn, M.C.; Pernes, G.; Lee, M.K.S.; Nagareddy, P.R.; Murphy, A.J. Monocytes, Macrophages, and Metabolic Disease in Atherosclerosis. *Front. Pharmacol.* **2019**, *10*, 666. [CrossRef] [PubMed]
4. Biessen, E.A.L.; Wouters, K. Macrophage Complexity in Human Atherosclerosis: Opportunities for Treatment? *Curr. Opin. Lipidol.* **2017**, *28*, 419–426. [CrossRef] [PubMed]
5. Peterson, K.R.; Cottam, M.A.; Kennedy, A.J.; Hasty, A.H. Macrophage-Targeted Therapeutics for Metabolic Disease. *Trends Pharmacol. Sci.* **2018**, *39*, 536–546. [CrossRef]
6. Colin, S.; Chinetti-Gbaguidi, G.; Staels, B. Macrophage Phenotypes in Atherosclerosis. *Immunol. Rev.* **2014**, *262*, 153–166. [CrossRef]
7. Cho, K.Y.; Miyoshi, H.; Kuroda, S.; Yasuda, H.; Kamiyama, K.; Nakagawara, J.; Takigami, M.; Kondo, T.; Atsumi, T. The Phenotype of Infiltrating Macrophages Influences Arteriosclerotic Plaque Vulnerability in the Carotid Artery. *J. Stroke Cerebrovasc. Dis.* **2013**, *22*, 910–918. [CrossRef]
8. Lee, C.W.; Hwang, I.; Park, C.-S.; Lee, H.; Park, D.-W.; Kang, S.-J.; Lee, S.-W.; Kim, Y.-H.; Park, S.-W.; Park, S.-J. Macrophage Heterogeneity of Culprit Coronary Plaques in Patients with Acute Myocardial Infarction or Stable Angina. *Am. J. Clin. Pathol.* **2013**, *139*, 317–322. [CrossRef]
9. Stöger, J.L.; Gijbels, M.J.J.; van der Velden, S.; Manca, M.; van der Loos, C.M.; Biessen, E.A.L.; Daemen, M.J.A.P.; Lutgens, E.; de Winther, M.P.J. Distribution of Macrophage Polarization Markers in Human Atherosclerosis. *Atherosclerosis* **2012**, *225*, 461–468. [CrossRef]
10. Feig, J.E.; Parathath, S.; Rong, J.X.; Mick, S.L.; Vengrenyuk, Y.; Grauer, L.; Young, S.G.; Fisher, E.A. Reversal of Hyperlipidemia with a Genetic Switch Favorably Affects the Content and Inflammatory State of Macrophages in Atherosclerotic Plaques. *Circulation* **2011**, *123*, 989–998. [CrossRef]

11. Peled, M.; Fisher, E.A. Dynamic Aspects of Macrophage Polarization during Atherosclerosis Progression and Regression. *Front. Immunol.* **2014**, *5*, 579. [CrossRef] [PubMed]
12. Kim, K.; Shim, D.; Lee, J.S.; Zaitsev, K.; Williams, J.W.; Kim, K.-W.; Jang, M.-Y.; Jang, H.S.; Yun, T.J.; Lee, S.H.; et al. Transcriptome Analysis Reveals Non-Foamy Rather than Foamy Plaque Macrophages Are Pro-Inflammatory in Atherosclerotic Murine Models. *Circ. Res.* **2018**, *123*, 1127–1142. [CrossRef] [PubMed]
13. Lin, P.; Ji, H.-H.; Li, Y.-J.; Guo, S.-D. Macrophage Plasticity and Atherosclerosis Therapy. *Front. Mol. Biosci.* **2021**, *8*, 679797. [CrossRef]
14. Nagenborg, J.; Goossens, P.; Biessen, E.A.L.; Donners, M.M.P.C. Heterogeneity of Atherosclerotic Plaque Macrophage Origin, Phenotype and Functions: Implications for Treatment. *Eur. J. Pharmacol.* **2017**, *816*, 14–24. [CrossRef]
15. Hayes, E.M.; Tsaousi, A.; Di Gregoli, K.; Jenkinson, S.R.; Bond, A.R.; Johnson, J.L.; Bevan, L.; Thomas, A.C.; Newby, A.C. Classical and Alternative Activation and Metalloproteinase Expression Occurs in Foam Cell Macrophages in Male and Female ApoE Null Mice in the Absence of T- and B-Lymphocytes. *Front. Immunol.* **2014**, *5*, 537. [CrossRef]
16. Newby, A.C.; George, S.J.; Ismail, Y.; Johnson, J.L.; Sala-Newby, G.B.; Thomas, A.C. Vulnerable Atherosclerotic Plaque Metalloproteinases and Foam Cell Phenotypes. *Thromb. Haemost.* **2009**, *101*, 1006–1011.
17. Vallejo, J.; Cochain, C.; Zernecke, A.; Ley, K. Heterogeneity of Immune Cells in Human Atherosclerosis Revealed by scRNA-Seq. *Cardiovasc. Res.* **2021**, *117*, 2537–2543. [CrossRef]
18. Willemsen, L.; de Winther, M.P. Macrophage Subsets in Atherosclerosis as Defined by Single-Cell Technologies. *J. Pathol.* **2020**, *250*, 705–714. [CrossRef] [PubMed]
19. Depuydt, M.A.C.; Prange, K.H.M.; Slenders, L.; Örd, T.; Elbersen, D.; Boltjes, A.; de Jager, S.C.A.; Asselbergs, F.W.; de Borst, G.J.; Aavik, E.; et al. Microanatomy of the Human Atherosclerotic Plaque by Single-Cell Transcriptomics. *Circ. Res.* **2020**, *127*, 1437–1455. [CrossRef]
20. Fernandez, D.M.; Rahman, A.H.; Fernandez, N.F.; Chudnovskiy, A.; Amir, E.-A.D.; Amadori, L.; Khan, N.S.; Wong, C.K.; Shamailova, R.; Hill, C.A.; et al. Single-Cell Immune Landscape of Human Atherosclerotic Plaques. *Nat. Med.* **2019**, *25*, 1576–1588. [CrossRef]
21. Goossens, P.; Lu, C.; Cao, J.; Gijbels, M.J.; Karel, J.M.H.; Wijnands, E.; Claes, B.S.R.; Fazzi, G.E.; Hendriks, T.F.E.; Wouters, K.; et al. Integrating Multiplex Immunofluorescent and Mass Spectrometry Imaging to Map Myeloid Heterogeneity in Its Metabolic and Cellular Context. *Cell Metab.* **2022**, *34*, 1214–1225.e6. [CrossRef] [PubMed]
22. Marques, A.R.A.; Ramos, C.; Machado-Oliveira, G.; Vieira, O.V. Lysosome (Dys)Function in Atherosclerosis—A Big Weight on the Shoulders of a Small Organelle. *Front. Cell Dev. Biol.* **2021**, *9*, 658995. [CrossRef] [PubMed]
23. Borowczyk, C.; Laroche-Traineau, J.; Brevier, J.; Jacobin-Valat, M.-J.; Marais, S.; Gerbaud, E.; Clofent-Sanchez, G.; Ottones, F. Two-Photon Excited Fluorescence (TPEF) May Be Useful to Identify Macrophage Subsets Based on Their Metabolic Activity and Cellular Responses in Atherosclerotic Plaques. *Atherosclerosis* **2020**, *309*, 47–55. [CrossRef] [PubMed]
24. Liu, Y.; Xu, R.; Gu, H.; Zhang, E.; Qu, J.; Cao, W.; Huang, X.; Yan, H.; He, J.; Cai, Z. Metabolic Reprogramming in Macrophage Responses. *Biomark. Res.* **2021**, *9*, 1. [CrossRef]
25. Albaghdadi, M.S.; Ikegami, R.; Kassab, M.B.; Gardecki, J.A.; Kunio, M.; Chowdhury, M.M.; Khamis, R.; Libby, P.; Tearney, G.J.; Jaffer, F.A. Near-Infrared Autofluorescence in Atherosclerosis Associates With Ceroid and Is Generated by Oxidized Lipid-Induced Oxidative Stress. *Arterioscler. Thromb. Vasc. Biol.* **2021**, *41*, e385–e398. [CrossRef] [PubMed]
26. Chinetti-Gbaguidi, G.; Baron, M.; Bouhlel, M.A.; Vanhoutte, J.; Copin, C.; Sebti, Y.; Derudas, B.; Mayi, T.; Bories, G.; Tailleux, A.; et al. Human Atherosclerotic Plaque Alternative Macrophages Display Low Cholesterol Handling but High Phagocytosis Because of Distinct Activities of the PPARγ and LXRα Pathways. *Circ. Res.* **2011**, *108*, 985–995. [CrossRef]
27. Medbury, H.J.; Williams, H.; Fletcher, J.P. Clinical Significance of Macrophage Phenotypes in Cardiovascular Disease. *Clin. Transl. Med.* **2014**, *3*, e63. [CrossRef]
28. Zernecke, A.; Winkels, H.; Cochain, C.; Williams, J.W.; Wolf, D.; Soehnlein, O.; Robbins, C.S.; Monaco, C.; Park, I.; McNamara, C.A.; et al. Meta-Analysis of Leukocyte Diversity in Atherosclerotic Mouse Aortas. *Circ. Res.* **2020**, *127*, 402–426. [CrossRef]
29. Mallat, Z.; Corbaz, A.; Scoazec, A.; Besnard, S.; Lesèche, G.; Chvatchko, Y.; Tedgui, A. Expression of Interleukin-18 in Human Atherosclerotic Plaques and Relation to Plaque Instability. *Circulation* **2001**, *104*, 1598–1603. [CrossRef]
30. González, L.; Rivera, K.; Andia, M.E.; Martínez Rodriguez, G. The IL-1 Family and Its Role in Atherosclerosis. *Int. J. Mol. Sci.* **2022**, *24*, 17. [CrossRef]
31. Katkenov, N.; Mukhatayev, Z.; Kozhakhmetov, S.; Sailybayeva, A.; Bekbossynova, M.; Kushugulova, A. Systematic Review on the Role of IL-6 and IL-1β in Cardiovascular Diseases. *J. Cardiovasc. Dev. Dis.* **2024**, *11*, 206. [CrossRef] [PubMed]
32. Grebe, A.; Hoss, F.; Latz, E. NLRP3 Inflammasome and the IL-1 Pathway in Atherosclerosis. *Circ. Res.* **2018**, *122*, 1722–1740. [CrossRef] [PubMed]
33. Abbate, A.; Toldo, S.; Marchetti, C.; Kron, J.; Van Tassell, B.W.; Dinarello, C.A. Interleukin-1 and the Inflammasome as Therapeutic Targets in Cardiovascular Disease. *Circ. Res.* **2020**, *126*, 1260–1280. [CrossRef] [PubMed]
34. Hartman, J.; Frishman, W.H. Inflammation and Atherosclerosis: A Review of the Role of Interleukin-6 in the Development of Atherosclerosis and the Potential for Targeted Drug Therapy. *Cardiol. Rev.* **2014**, *22*, 147–151. [CrossRef]
35. Mallat, Z.; Besnard, S.; Duriez, M.; Deleuze, V.; Emmanuel, F.; Bureau, M.F.; Soubrier, F.; Esposito, B.; Duez, H.; Fievet, C.; et al. Protective Role of Interleukin-10 in Atherosclerosis. *Circ. Res.* **1999**, *85*, e17–e24. [CrossRef]

36. Xu, S.; Zhang, J.; Liu, J.; Ye, J.; Xu, Y.; Wang, Z.; Yu, J.; Ye, D.; Zhao, M.; Feng, Y.; et al. The Role of Interleukin-10 Family Members in Cardiovascular Diseases. *Int. Immunopharmacol.* **2021**, *94*, 107475. [CrossRef]
37. Han, X.; Kitamoto, S.; Wang, H.; Boisvert, W.A. Interleukin-10 Overexpression in Macrophages Suppresses Atherosclerosis in Hyperlipidemic Mice. *FASEB J.* **2010**, *24*, 2869–2880. [CrossRef]
38. Tsioufis, P.; Theofilis, P.; Tsioufis, K.; Tousoulis, D. The Impact of Cytokines in Coronary Atherosclerotic Plaque: Current Therapeutic Approaches. *Int. J. Mol. Sci.* **2022**, *23*, 15937. [CrossRef]
39. Jessup, W.; Kritharides, L. Metabolism of Oxidized LDL by Macrophages. *Curr. Opin. Lipidol.* **2000**, *11*, 473–481. [CrossRef]
40. Yancey, P.G.; Jerome, W.G. Lysosomal Cholesterol Derived from Mildly Oxidized Low Density Lipoprotein Is Resistant to Efflux. *J. Lipid Res.* **2001**, *42*, 317–327. [CrossRef]
41. Hoppe, G.; O'Neil, J.; Hoff, H.F. Inactivation of Lysosomal Proteases by Oxidized Low Density Lipoprotein Is Partially Responsible for Its Poor Degradation by Mouse Peritoneal Macrophages. *J. Clin. Investig.* **1994**, *94*, 1506–1512. [CrossRef]
42. Jerome, W.G.; Cox, B.E.; Griffin, E.E.; Ullery, J.C. Lysosomal Cholesterol Accumulation Inhibits Subsequent Hydrolysis Of Lipoprotein Cholesteryl Ester. *Microsc. Microanal.* **2008**, *14*, 138–149. [CrossRef]
43. Dhaliwal, B.S.; Steinbrecher, U.P. Cholesterol Delivered to Macrophages by Oxidized Low Density Lipoprotein Is Sequestered in Lysosomes and Fails to Efflux Normally. *J. Lipid Res.* **2000**, *41*, 1658–1665. [CrossRef]
44. Weiss-Sadan, T.; Maimoun, D.; Oelschlagel, D.; Kaschani, F.; Misiak, D.; Gaikwad, H.; Ben-Nun, Y.; Merquiol, E.; Anaki, A.; Tsvirkun, D.; et al. Cathepsins Drive Anti-Inflammatory Activity by Regulating Autophagy and Mitochondrial Dynamics in Macrophage Foam Cells. *Cell. Physiol. Biochem.* **2019**, *53*, 550–572. [CrossRef]
45. Luque-Martin, R.; Angell, D.C.; Kalxdorf, M.; Bernard, S.; Thompson, W.; Eberl, H.C.; Ashby, C.; Freudenberg, J.; Sharp, C.; Van den Bossche, J.; et al. IFN-γ Drives Human Monocyte Differentiation into Highly Proinflammatory Macrophages That Resemble a Phenotype Relevant to Psoriasis. *J. Immunol.* **2021**, *207*, 555–568. [CrossRef]
46. Toledo-Ibelles, P.; Mas-Oliva, J. Antioxidants in the Fight Against Atherosclerosis: Is This a Dead End? *Curr. Atheroscler. Rep.* **2018**, *20*, 36. [CrossRef]
47. Georgakoudi, I.; Quinn, K.P. Optical Imaging Using Endogenous Contrast to Assess Metabolic State. *Annu. Rev. Biomed. Eng.* **2012**, *14*, 351–367. [CrossRef]
48. Josse, J.; Husson, F. missMDA: A Package for Handling Missing Values in Multivariate Data Analysis. *J. Stat. Softw.* **2016**, *70*, 1–31. [CrossRef]
49. Evangelou, K.; Gorgoulis, V.G. Sudan Black B, The Specific Histochemical Stain for Lipofuscin: A Novel Method to Detect Senescent Cells. *Methods Mol. Biol.* **2017**, *1534*, 111–119. [CrossRef]

International Journal of
Molecular Sciences

MDPI

Article

Nidogen 2 Overexpression Promotes Hepatosteatosis and Atherosclerosis

Ishita Kathuria [1], Aditi Prasad [1], Bal Krishan Sharma [2], Ravi Varma Aithabathula [1], Malvin Ofosu-Boateng [1], Maxwell A. Gyamfi [1], Jianxiong Jiang [1], Frank Park [1], Udai P. Singh [1] and Bhupesh Singla [1,*]

[1] Department of Pharmaceutical Sciences, College of Pharmacy, The University of Tennessee Health Science Center, Memphis, TN 38103, USA; ikathuri@uthsc.edu (I.K.); aprasad9@uthsc.edu (A.P.); raithaba@uthsc.edu (R.V.A.); mofosubo@uthsc.edu (M.O.-B.); mgyamfi@uthsc.edu (M.A.G.); jjiang18@uthsc.edu (J.J.); fpark@uthsc.edu (F.P.); usingh1@uthsc.edu (U.P.S.)

[2] Cancer and Blood Diseases Institute, Cincinnati Children's Hospital Medical Center, Cincinnati, OH 45229, USA; balkrishan.sharma@cchmc.org

* Correspondence: bsingla@uthsc.edu; Tel.: +1-901-448-4135

Abstract: Clinical and genetic studies strongly support a significant connection between nonalcoholic fatty liver disease (NAFLD) and atherosclerotic cardiovascular disease (ASCVD) and identify ASCVD as the primary cause of death in NAFLD patients. Understanding the molecular factors and mechanisms regulating these diseases is critical for developing novel therapies that target them simultaneously. Our preliminary immunoblotting experiments demonstrated elevated expression of nidogen 2 (NID2), a basement membrane glycoprotein, in human atherosclerotic vascular tissues and murine steatotic livers. Therefore, we investigated the role of NID2 in regulating hepatosteatosis and atherosclerosis utilizing Western diet-fed *Apoe*$^{-/-}$ mice with/without *NID2* overexpression. Quantitative real-time PCR confirmed increased *NID2* mRNA expression in multiple organs (liver, heart, kidney, and adipose) of *NID2*-overexpressing mice. Male mice with *NID2* overexpression exhibited higher liver and epididymal white adipose tissue mass, increased hepatic lipid accumulation, and fibrosis. Additionally, these mice developed larger atherosclerotic lesions in the whole aortas and aortic roots, with increased necrotic core formation. Mechanistic studies showed reduced AMPK activation in the livers of *NID2*-overexpressing mice compared with controls, without any effects on hepatic inflammation. In conclusion, these findings suggest that NID2 plays a deleterious role in both hepatosteatosis and atherosclerosis, making it a potential therapeutic target for these conditions.

Keywords: nidogen 2; hepatosteatosis; atherosclerosis; AMPK; NAFLD

1. Introduction

The liver plays a central role in regulating systemic lipid metabolism and maintaining homeostasis. Disruptions in hepatic lipid metabolism lead to NAFLD development. NAFLD comprises a spectrum of pathological changes in the liver, which can be histologically classified into two categories: (a) nonalcoholic fatty liver (NAFL), characterized by lipid accumulation (steatosis) in more than 5% of hepatocytes without signs of hepatocyte injury, and (b) nonalcoholic steatohepatitis (NASH), defined as hepatic steatosis and inflammation, along with hepatocyte injury with or without fibrosis [1,2]. Over the past two decades, the global incidence of NAFLD has increased significantly from 25% to 32% [3], and this trend is expected to continue at an alarming rate. Nonetheless, until recently, there was no Federal Drug Administration (FDA)-approved pharmacological treatment for NAFLD or NASH [4]. In March 2024, the FDA approved Resmetirom, a liver-targeted agonist of thyroid hormone receptor β-selective for treating NASH. Regardless of its benefits, Resmetirom's usage is associated with several side effects, including nausea, diarrhea, gallbladder-related side effects, and drug-induced liver toxicity. Moreover, it is contraindicated in patients with decompensated cirrhosis [5,6]. Given the high prevalence and complications associated with NAFLD, the development of additional novel therapeutic drugs with minimal side effects is essential. In addition, dysregulated hepatic lipid metabolism elevates circulating levels of low-density lipoprotein (LDL) particles, which induces vascular endothelium toxicity, promotes LDL infiltration into the arterial wall, and contributes to plaque formation, thereby linking NAFLD to atherosclerosis development [7]. Since NAFLD shares risk factors such as dyslipidemia, visceral obesity, and insulin resistance with ASCVD, patients with NAFLD are at higher risk for adverse ASCVD events. Notably, ASCVD is recognized as the major cause of death among NAFLD patients, independent of traditional risk factors [8]. However, our knowledge about the endogenous molecular factors and downstream signaling mechanisms responsible for dysregulated hepatic lipid metabolism and their roles in atherosclerotic lesion formation remains limited.

NID2 is a glycoprotein present in the basement membrane, where it interacts with collagen IV, perlecan, and collagen I to stabilize the membrane structure [9]. NID2 expression has been linked to the development of various cancers, including ovarian, lung, gastric, pancreatic, and oral squamous cell carcinoma [10–14]. Additionally, elevated *NID2* mRNA levels have been observed in human atherosclerotic echolucent calcified plaques [15,16], which was further confirmed by a study analyzing publicly available transcriptomic profiles of atherosclerotic arteries from the Gene Expression Omnibus database [17]. Interestingly, in murine models of vascular calcification and neointima formation, NID2 demonstrated a protective role against vascular calcification and helped in promoting the contractile phenotype of vascular smooth muscle cells (VSMCs), respectively [18,19]. This apparent contradiction suggests NID2's diverse role in different cell types and disease models, highlighting the need for further studies. Nevertheless, its role in regulating hepatosteatosis and associated atherosclerosis has never been explored.

In this study, we investigated the role of NID2 in the pathogenesis of NAFLD and atherosclerosis by overexpressing *NID2* using an adeno-associated viral (AAV) vector in $Apoe^{-/-}$ mice and Western diet feeding. We observed that NID2 protein expression is increased in both steatotic livers and atherosclerotic vascular tissues. *NID2* overexpression in male $Apoe^{-/-}$ mice promoted hepatic steatosis, fibrosis, and atherosclerosis development. Interestingly, female mice with or without *NID2*-overexpression exhibited no differences in atherosclerosis development and hepatic fibrosis. Mechanistically, we found attenuated AMPK activation in the livers of *NID2*-overexpressing mice compared with controls, with no effects on hepatic inflammation. These findings provide the first experimental evidence of NID2's detrimental role in the development of NAFLD and atherosclerosis.

2. Results

2.1. Expression of NID2 Protein Is Elevated in Human Atherosclerotic Arteries and Murine Steatotic Livers

A recent RNA-sequencing study reported increased levels of *NID2* mRNA in human carotid artery echolucent plaques, which are lipid-rich lesions and associated with a higher risk of adverse cardiovascular events [16,20,21]. Additionally, a separate study utilizing liquid chromatography–mass spectrometry suggested an association between *NID2* mRNA expression and calcified hard plaques [15]. However, no previous studies have investigated the levels of NID2 protein in non-atherosclerotic and atherosclerotic arteries. Therefore, we performed immunoblotting experiments using tissue lysates from the atherosclerotic inner curvature (IC) of the aorta and non-atherosclerotic descending aorta (DA). The presence and absence of atherosclerosis was confirmed using Oil Red O (ORO) staining of frozen sections, as reported earlier [22]. The results demonstrated significantly elevated NID2 protein expression in atherosclerotic IC compared with non-atherosclerotic DA segments (Figure 1A).

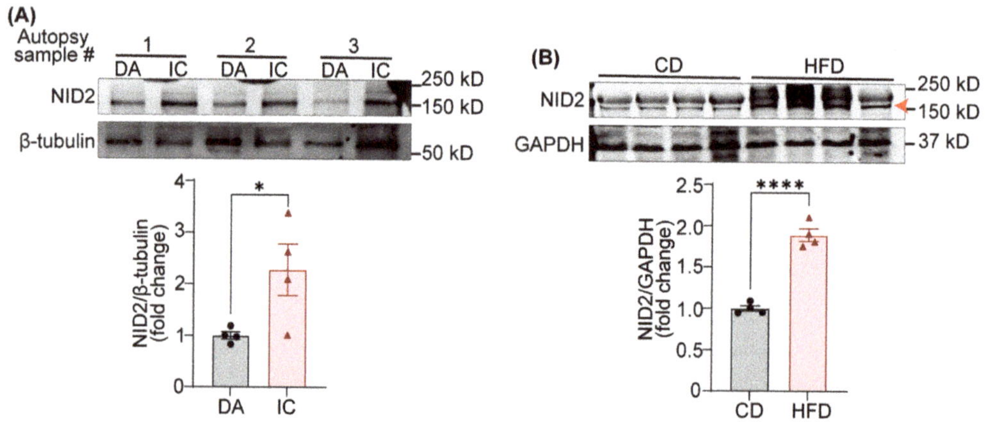

Figure 1. Expression of NID2 protein is elevated in human atherosclerotic arteries and murine steatotic livers. (**A**) Representative western blot images for NID2 and β-tubulin protein expression in human atherosclerotic inner curvature (IC) and non-atherosclerotic descending aorta (DA) vascular tissue. The bar diagram shows mean protein levels expressed as a ratio of NID2 to β-tubulin. (**B**) Representative Western blot images for NID2 (red arrowhead points to the correct band) and GAPDH in the livers of control diet (CD)- and calorie-matched high-fat diet (HFD, 12 weeks)-fed C57BL/6J mice. The bar diagram represents the mean NID2 protein expression ($n = 4$). Statistical analyses were performed using a two-tailed unpaired t-test (**A**,**B**). Data represent mean ± SEM. * $p < 0.05$, and **** $p < 0.0001$.

Hepatosteatosis (deposition of lipids in the liver) is closely linked with the development of atherosclerosis [8,23]. However, no information is available on the expression of NID2 in steatotic livers. To investigate NID2 levels in steatotic livers, we conducted immunoblotting with liver tissue lysates from wild-type (C57BL/6) mice fed a control diet (CD) and calorie-matched high-fat diet (HFD). The hepatosteatosis in HFD-fed mice was confirmed with ORO staining. The immunoblotting data revealed increased hepatic expression of NID2 in HFD-fed mice compared with CD-fed mice, suggesting an association between hepatosteatosis and NID2 protein expression (Figure 1B). Similar results were obtained when NID2 expression in the livers of *Apoe*$^{-/-}$ mice fed regular chow and a Western diet was compared (Supplementary Figure S1). Collectively, these data indicate that NID2 levels are augmented in both atherosclerotic arteries and steatotic livers.

2.2. NID2 Overexpression Enhances Liver and Epididymal White Adipose Tissue Mass in Male Mice

Since our data shown in Figure 1 demonstrated increased NID2 levels in both atherosclerotic arteries and steatotic livers, we next aimed to examine the effects of *NID2* overexpression on the development of hepatosteatosis and atherosclerosis in mice. Therefore, we used male and female *Apoe*$^{-/-}$ mice, a genetic model of both atherosclerosis and NAFLD [24,25]. These mice were injected with either control or *NID2*-AAV intraperitoneally and fed a Western diet for 12 weeks (Figure 2A). The quantitative real-time PCR (qRT-PCR) analysis showed overexpression of *NID2* in various organs, including liver, kidney, epididymal white adipose tissue, and heart of *NID2*-AAV-administered mice compared with control mice (Figure 2B–E). Throughout the 12-week Western diet feeding period, mice were weighed weekly, and no significant differences were observed in body weight between male and female control and *NID2*-overexpressing mice (Supplementary Figures S2 and S3A). However, weight gain was significantly higher in male *NID2*-AAV-injected mice compared with controls (Figure 2F). In addition, plasma total cholesterol, fasting blood glucose, whole-body fat, and lean mass were comparable between the two groups (Figure 2G–I and Supplementary Figure S3B–D). Interestingly, in male *NID2*-AAV-injected mice, mean liver weight (Figures 2J and S4) and epididymal white adipose tissue (epiWAT, Figure 2K) weight were significantly higher in comparison to control mice. However, no such differences were observed in female mice (Supplementary Figure S3E,F). Moreover, spleen weights were not different between the two groups (Figures 2L and S3G). These observations suggest that *NID2* overexpression in male mice increases liver and epididymal white adipose tissue weight but does not affect these parameters in female mice.

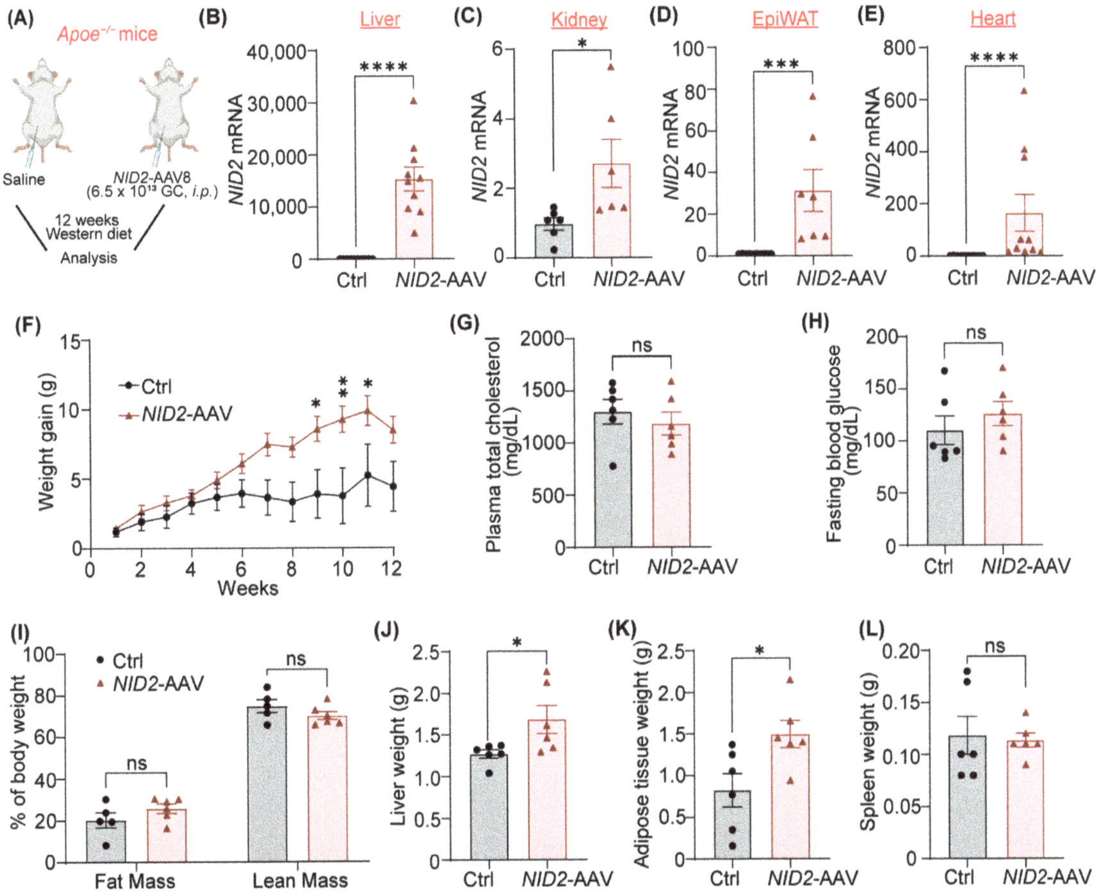

Figure 2. *NID2* overexpression enhances liver and epididymal white adipose tissue mass in male mice. (**A**) The schematic diagram illustrates the experimental plan. *Apoe*$^{-/-}$ mice were injected with control (Ctrl) and *NID2*-AAV intraperitoneally, fed a Western diet for 12 weeks, and analyzed. (**B–E**) Male control and *NID2*-AAV-injected *Apoe*$^{-/-}$ mice were utilized to measure *NID2* mRNA levels in various organs by qRT-PCR at least in duplicate. Bar diagrams represent mRNA expression in the liver (**B**, $n = 10$), kidney (**C**, $n = 6$), epididymal white adipose tissue (EpiWAT, **D**, $n = 7$–10), and heart (**E**, $n = 10$). Bar diagrams show body weight gain (**F**), plasma total cholesterol (**G**), fasting blood glucose (**H**), whole-body fat/lean mass (**I**), liver weight (**J**), adipose tissue weight (**K**), and spleen weight (**L**) ($n = 5$–6). A two-tailed unpaired t-test (**C**,**G–K**), two-tailed unpaired Mann–Whitney test (**B**,**D**,**E**,**L**), and two-way ANOVA followed by Sidak post hoc test for multiple comparisons (**F**) were utilized for statistical analyses. Data represent mean ± SEM. ns: non-significant. * $p < 0.05$, *** $p < 0.001$ and **** $p < 0.0001$.

2.3. NID2 Overexpression in Mice Promotes Hepatic Lipid Accumulation and Fibrosis

Since (a) NID2 expression is elevated in steatotic livers of HFD-fed mice, and (b) *NID2* overexpression increases liver weight in male mice, we investigated the role of NID2 in regulating hepatic steatosis and fibrosis. To begin, we confirmed hepatic NID2 expression in both control and *NID2*-AAV-injected mice using Western blotting. As expected, *NID2*-AAV administration significantly increased NID2 protein (Figure 3A) and mRNA levels (Figure 2B) compared with controls. Next, serial liver sections (paraffin/frozen) from similar regions of livers from male mice were stained with hematoxylin and eosin (H & E), ORO, and Sirius red to visualize lipid droplets, neutral lipid accumulation, and fibrosis, respectively (Figure 3B). These histological analyses demonstrated an increased frequency/size lipid droplets, enhanced lipid deposition, and higher hepatic fibrosis in male *NID2*-AAV-injected mice, in contrast with sex-matched controls (Figure 3B–D). Similar investigations were conducted on female liver samples. *NID2* overexpression significantly increased lipid droplet accumulation and elevated the ORO-positive area; however, no differences in liver fibrosis were found between the two female groups (Supplementary Figure S3H–J).

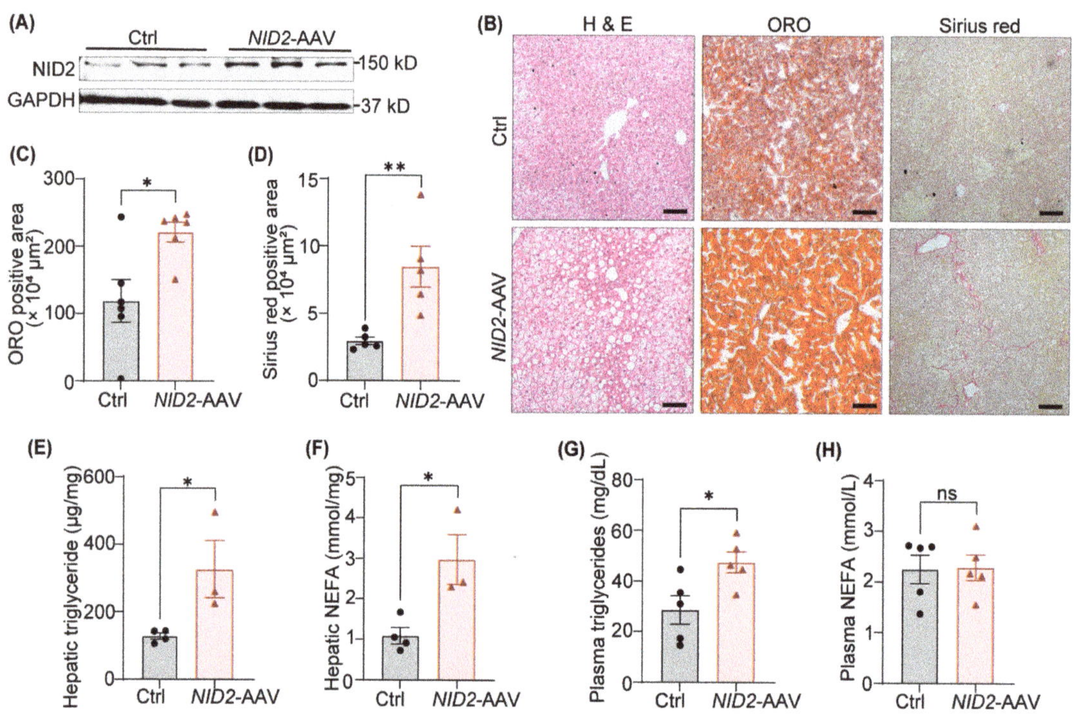

Figure 3. *NID2* overexpression in mice promotes hepatic lipid accumulation and fibrosis. Male $Apoe^{-/-}$ mice were injected with control and *NID2*-AAV intraperitoneally, fed a Western diet for 12 weeks, and analyzed. (**A**) Representative Western blot images for NID2 and GAPDH protein expression in the livers of control and *NID2*-overexpressing mice ($n = 3$). (**B**) Representative images of liver sections stained with H & E (lipid droplets), ORO (neutral lipid accumulation), and Sirius red (fibrosis); scale bar 100 μm. (**C–H**) Bar diagrams represent lipid accumulation (**C**, $n = 6$), fibrosis area (**D**, $n = 5$), hepatic triglyceride (**E**, $n = 3$–4), NEFA levels (**F**, $n = 3$–4), plasma triglyceride (**G**, $n = 5$) and NEFA levels (**H**, $n = 5$), in control and *NID2*-AAV-injected mice. Statistical analyses were performed using a two-tailed unpaired *t*-test (**C–H**). Data represent mean ± SEM. ns: non-significant. * $p < 0.05$, and ** $p < 0.01$.

Hepatosteatosis is marked by the accumulation of triglycerides and the presence of free fatty acids in the liver [26]. Therefore, we next measured triglyceride and non-esterified fatty acid (NEFA) levels in hepatic samples of male mice. Our data showed a significant increase in the levels of hepatic triglyceride and NEFA in *NID2*-overexpressing mice compared with controls (Figure 3E,F). Moreover, plasma triglyceride levels were elevated in *NID2*-AAV-injected mice, while plasma NEFA levels were similar between the two groups (Figure 3G,H). Free fatty acids released by lipolysis in adipose tissues are diverted to the liver, suggesting a pivotal interaction between hepatic metabolism and adipose tissue in the pathogenesis of NAFLD [27]. Additionally, adipocyte hypertrophy has been linked with NAFLD development [28]; therefore, we performed H & E staining of epididymal white adipose tissue and found increased adipocyte size in male *NID2*-AAV-injected mice compared with the control group (Supplementary Figure S5). Altogether, these findings suggest that *NID2* overexpression contributes to hepatic lipid accumulation and fibrosis in male mice.

2.4. NID2 Overexpression Augments Atherosclerosis in Male Hypercholesterolemic Mice

To explore the effects of dysregulated hepatic metabolism on the development of atherosclerosis, we investigated atherosclerotic lesion formation in control and *NID2*-overexpressing *Apoe*$^{-/-}$ mice. In situ images of the aortic arch revealed a larger plaque area in *NID2*-AAV-injected mice compared to control mice (Figure 4A). *En face* ORO staining of whole aorta further confirmed a significant increase in atherosclerosis in male mice with *NID2* overexpression [% plaque area: 12.5 $\pm$ 1.14 (74.09% increase)] compared with controls (7.18 $\pm$ 1.53), indicating a detrimental role for NID2 in the development of atherosclerosis (Figure 4B). Interestingly, no differences in plaque burden were observed in female mice (Supplementary Figure S3K,L). Moreover, H & E staining performed on serial aortic cross-sections (4 sections/mouse, 90–100 µm apart) from male *NID2*-AAV-injected mice demonstrated a significantly higher atherosclerotic lesion area compared with sex-matched control tissue (42.71 $\pm$ 4.09 $\times$ 10^4 µm^2 vs. 27.29 $\pm$ 0.55 $\times$ 10^4 µm^2) (Figure 4C,D). Additional aortic root histological analyses showed increased ORO-positive area (lipid accumulation), reduced collagen (Masson trichrome), and enlarged necrotic area (acellular areas) in *NID2*-overexpressing mice compared with control animals (Figure 4C,E–G). Collectively, these data show that *NID2* overexpression in male hypercholesterolemic mice exacerbates atherosclerotic lesion formation, promotes necrotic core formation, and reduces plaque stability. In contrast, consistent with *en face* ORO staining results, aortic root histology revealed no significant differences in lesion area in female mice (Supplementary Figure S3M).

2.5. NID2 Overexpression Inhibits the Activation of Lipid Metabolism-Related Protein AMPK

Our experiments as shown above revealed that *NID2* overexpression leads to increased hepatosteatosis and atherosclerosis. To uncover the underlying molecular mechanisms by which NID2 regulates hepatic lipid metabolism, we determined the expression of various proteins and genes involved in lipid metabolism and inflammation. Adenosine monophosphate-activated protein kinase (AMPK) serves as a key energy sensor, and its activation by phosphorylation promotes the metabolic switch from an anabolic to a catabolic state, shutting down ATP-dependent synthetic pathways to restore energy balance [29]. When activated, AMPK deactivates acetyl-COA carboxylase (ACC) via phosphorylation at serine 79, reducing the levels of malonyl-CoA, which is a precursor of fatty acid synthesis and an inhibitor of mitochondria fatty acid uptake via carnitine palmitoyltransferase-1 (CPT1) [30,31]. Therefore, we investigated the activation status of AMPK and ACC in liver tissue lysates from control and *NID2*-AAV-injected mice. Western blot analysis demonstrated decreased phosphorylation of AMPK (Thr 172) in *NID2*-overexpressing livers in comparison to control livers (Figure 5A,C). However, there were no significant differences in ACC phosphorylation between the two groups (Figure 5A,B). These results indicate that NID2 may regulate hepatic lipid metabolism by modulating AMPK activation without directly affecting ACC activity.

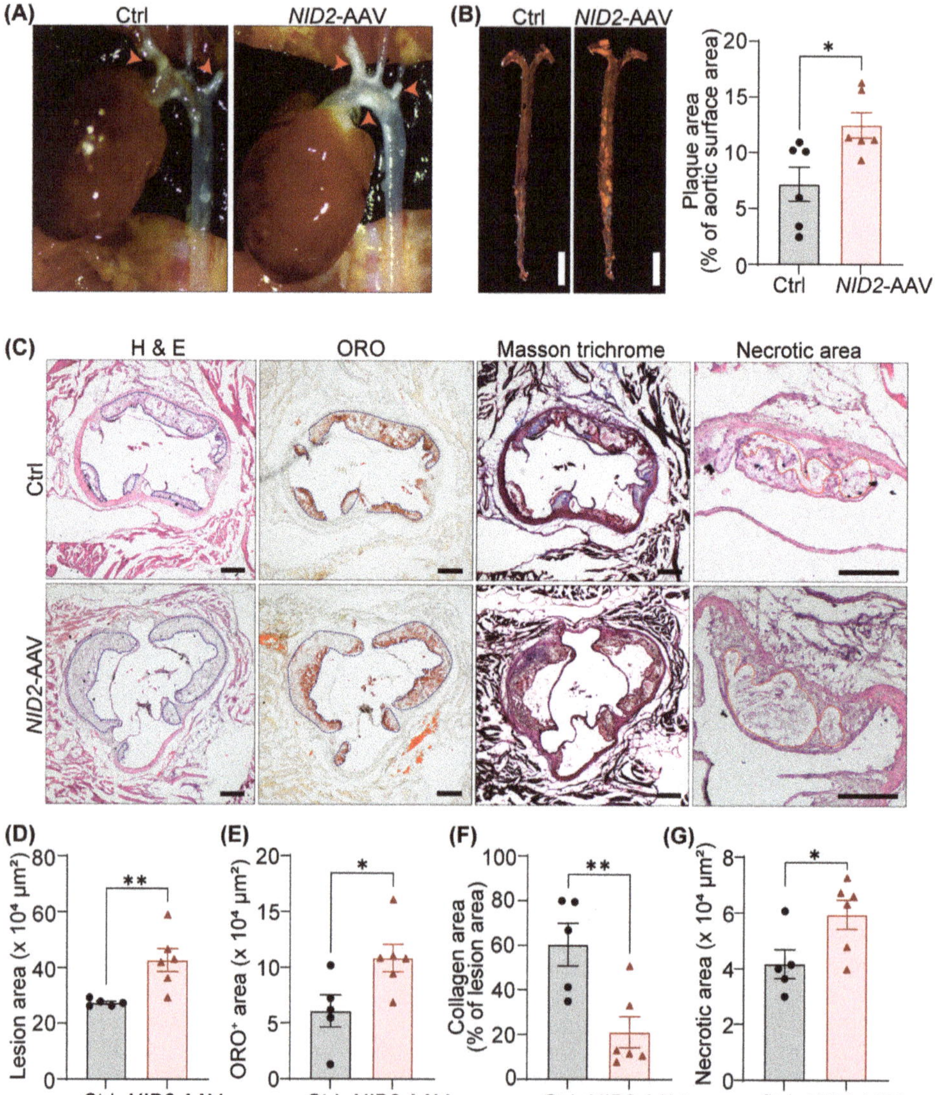

Figure 4. *NID2* overexpression augments atherosclerosis in male hypercholesterolemic mice. Male *Apoe*$^{-/-}$ mice were injected with control (Ctrl) and *NID2*-AAV intraperitoneally, fed a Western diet for 12 weeks and analyzed. (**A**) Representative in situ images of the aortic arch (red arrowheads point to atherosclerotic lesions). (**B**) Representative ORO staining of whole aortas; scale bar 5 mm. The bar diagram represents ORO-positive areas in whole aortas (n = 6). (**C**) Representative images of aortic root cross-sections stained with H & E (lesion area and necrotic core), ORO (lipid accumulation), and Masson's trichrome (collagen content); scale bar 200 μm. (**D–G**) Bar diagrams show lesion area (**D**), lipid deposition (**E**), collagen content (**F**), and necrotic core area (**G**) (n = 5–6). Statistical analyses were performed using a two-tailed unpaired t-test (**B**,**D–G**). Data represent mean ± SEM. * $p < 0.05$, and ** $p < 0.01$.

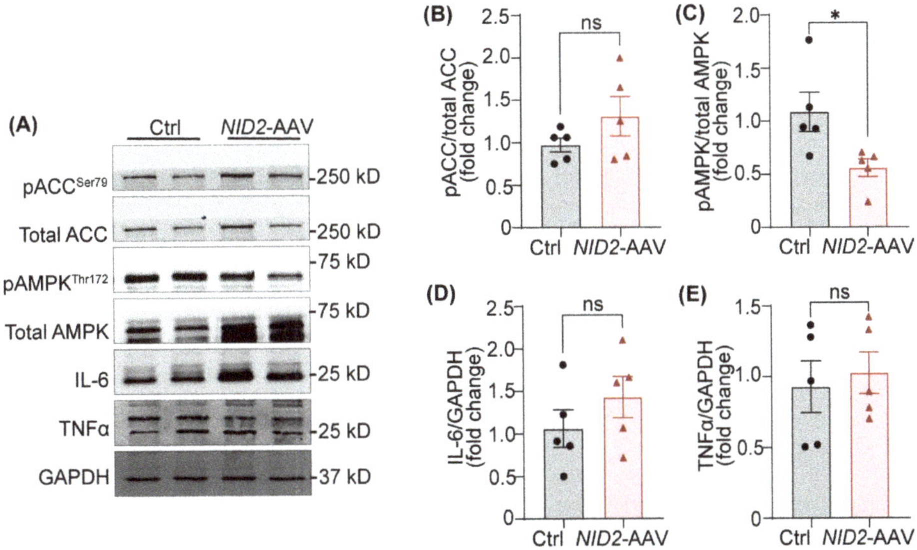

Figure 5. *NID2* overexpression inhibits the activation of the lipid metabolism-related protein AMPK. (**A**) Representative Western blot images for lipid metabolism and pro-inflammatory proteins utilizing liver lysates from control and *NID2*-AAV-injected mice. Bar diagrams represent mean protein expression (**B**,**C**) as the ratios of phospho-total proteins ACC (**B**) and AMPK (**C**), and protein levels of IL-6 (**D**) and TNFα (**E**) ($n = 5$). Statistical analyses were performed using a two-tailed unpaired *t*-test. Data represent mean ± SEM. ns: non-significant. * $p < 0.05$.

Inflammation plays a key role in promoting hepatocyte death and tissue injury in NAFLD [32]. To explore this, we performed qRT-PCR to determine the hepatic mRNA levels of various inflammatory genes including nitric oxide synthase 2 (*Nos2*), tumor necrosis factor alpha (*Tnfa*), and interleukin 6 (*Il6*). However, no significant differences were observed between the groups (Supplementary Figure S6). Consistently, Western blot data exhibited comparable TNFα and IL-6 levels in the livers of control and *NID2*-AAV-injected mice (Figure 5A,D,E). We also investigated the mRNA expression of genes involved in lipid uptake (*Msr1* and *Cd36*), fatty acid synthesis (*Fasn*), fatty acid transport (*Cpt1a*), and fatty acid beta-oxidation (*Ppara*); however, no significant differences were noted. Interestingly, *Ldlr* expression was significantly increased in mice injected with *NID2*-AAV, in contrast to controls (Supplementary Figure S6). Taken together, these results indicate that *NID2* overexpression in male mice may disrupt hepatic lipid metabolism by inhibiting AMPK activation.

3. Discussion

The liver plays a key role in systemic lipid metabolism by regulating the synthesis, uptake, storage, and efflux of cholesterol [8,33]. The prevalent liver disease NAFLD and its inflammatory form NASH are associated with the development of coronary artery calcification, atherosclerotic plaques, and increased carotid intima-media thickness [34,35]. These associations have stimulated interest in identifying the shared molecular mechanisms which drive these liver and vascular diseases. Nevertheless, our knowledge about the intrinsic molecular factors and downstream mechanisms responsible for dysregulated hepatic lipid metabolism and their roles in atherosclerotic lesion formation remains limited. Herein, we investigated the role of NID2 in regulating hepatosteatosis, fibrosis, and atherosclerotic lesion formation. Our results demonstrated (a) elevated NID2 levels in murine steatotic livers and human atherosclerotic vascular tissues, (b) increased hepatic steatosis and fibrosis in *NID2*-overexpressing mice, (c) exacerbated atherosclerosis in mice with *NID2* overexpression, and (d) reduced AMPK activation in the livers of *NID2*-overexpressing mice. Collectively, these findings suggest that NID2 contributes to the progression of both hepatosteatosis and atherosclerosis.

NID2 is a secretory glycoprotein, which is ubiquitously present in the basement membrane (BM) and helps to maintain BM stability [9,36]. Depending on the cell type and disease, NID2 plays both beneficial and detrimental roles. Previous studies have associated NID2 expression with various cancers, including gastric, ovarian, bladder, pancreatic, and esophageal squamous cell carcinoma [11,12,14,37]. Additionally, recent studies have linked *NID2* mRNA levels with human echolucent calcified plaques [15,16]. Further murine studies have identified the role of NID2 in non-atherosclerotic and atherosclerotic vascular calcification [18,38]. Interestingly, Chen et al. recently demonstrated a protective role of NID2 against aortic calcification induced by 5/6 nephrectomy, cholecalciferol-overload, and $CaCl_2$ administration [18]. However, its role in regulating hepatosteatosis and atherosclerosis remains unknown. To address this gap, firstly, we investigated the expression of NID2 protein in human atherosclerotic arterial tissues and murine steatotic livers. Consistent with upregulated *NID2* expression in non-atherosclerotic and atherosclerotic calcified vascular tissues, increased NID2 protein expression was observed in atherosclerotic arteries and steatotic livers [15,16]. To explore NID2's role in these diseases, we induced AAV-mediated overexpression of the *NID2* gene in *Apoe*-deficient mice. AAVs are widely used tools in research for their ability to efficiently transduce various cell types, allow long-term gene expression, and avoid integration into the host genome, reducing the risk of mutagenesis. Furthermore, this approach facilitates the rapid generation of mouse models without the need of breeding for several generations.

One of our notable observations was the significant increase in liver and EpiWAT weight in male mice overexpressing *NID2* compared to controls. This increase in liver weight, a hallmark of hepatosteatosis [39], indirectly suggests that NID2 may exacerbate hepatic fat accumulation in males following Western diet feeding. The lack of difference in plasma cholesterol, fasting glucose, and body fat composition between the groups indicates that NID2's effects on liver and epiWAT mass are independent of systemic metabolic changes, such as overall cholesterol or glucose regulation. Interestingly, female mice did not exhibit any differences in liver or adipose tissue weights despite *NID2* overexpression, which points to a protective sex hormone/chromosome-regulated mechanism in females or a differential response to *NID2* overexpression. Future studies are warranted to determine the mechanisms of observed sex-specific responses.

Our data demonstrate that *NID2* overexpression in male mice promotes hepatic steatosis, as evidenced by increased triglyceride, NEFA levels, and ORO staining of liver frozen sections, as well as increased plasma triglycerides. These findings are consistent with previous studies that implicate lipid dysregulation as a characteristic of NAFLD [40,41]. While plasma NEFA levels did not differ between control and *NID2*-overexpressing mice, the elevated hepatic NEFA levels suggest that NID2 may alter the balance between hepatic lipid uptake and secretion. Free fatty acids, primarily derived from lipolysis in adipose tissue, are known to be transported to the liver, where they contribute to the pathogenesis of NAFLD [42]. In this context, the increased adipocyte size observed in *NID2*-overexpressing male mice further supports the link between adipose tissue dysfunction and hepatic lipid accumulation, a well-established mechanism in NAFLD [27]. Additionally, in male mice, overexpression of *NID2* increased liver fibrosis, which is a key determinant of the progression of simple steatosis to NASH [43]. These findings align with a previous report suggesting a connection between hepatic lipid accumulation and fibrosis in NAFLD [44]. Interestingly, though female mice exhibited increased hepatic lipid accumulation following *NID2* overexpression, no significant differences in fibrosis were noted. These sex-specific differences in fibrosis have also been observed in other models of liver disease and may be influenced by hormonal factors or differences in liver metabolism between males and females [45]. It is known that NAFLD prevalence and severity are higher in men in comparison to women during the reproductive age. However, after menopause, women develop NAFLD at a faster rate, suggesting a protective role of female sex hormones such as estrogen against NAFLD. Animal models also tend to follow a similar trend with higher severity and occurrence of hepatic steatosis, and pro-fibrotic/inflammatory cytokines in males than females, reinstating the differences we observed in our study [45,46].

The development of atherosclerosis is regulated by both systemic metabolic factors and local cellular responses [47]. In line with our hepatic lipid metabolism studies, *NID2* overexpression aggravated aortic atherosclerosis progression in male mice, suggesting a pivotal role of NID2 in atherogenesis. Further, *NID2*-overexpression led to increased lesion size, enhanced lipid accumulation, reduced collagen content, and enlarged necrotic cores in aortic root sections. These data are in compliance with the upregulated expression of *NID2* in atherosclerotic calcified vascular tissues, indicating the deleterious role of NID2 in vascular diseases [15,16]. In contrast, a recent study reported the protective role of NID2 in vascular calcification [18]. The authors observed attenuated NID2 levels in murine calcified aortas and calcified primary rat VSMCs, and showed suppression of vascular calcification in global $Nid2^{-/-}$ mice [18]. Another study from the same research group highlighted NID2's involvement in promoting the contractile phenotype of VSMCs [19]. Both of these studies emphasized the beneficial role of NID2 in regulating the VSMC phenotype. Arteries are composed of different layers with various cell types, including endothelial cells, VSMCs, adventitial fibroblasts, lymphatic endothelial cells, etc. However, the specific role of NID2 in different vascular cell types in the context of vascular pathologies remains to be investigated utilizing cell-specific *NID2*-deficient mice. It is possible that NID2 is playing different roles in different vascular cells. Furthermore, NID2 is recognized as an endogenous ligand for leucine-rich repeat-containing G protein-coupled receptor 4 (LGR4) [18]. Future studies are warranted to discover the other potential receptors of NID2 and investigate atherosclerosis in mice with cell-specific *Lgr4* deletion combined with NID2 overexpression to clarify the role of the NID2-LGR4 axis in atherogenesis. Additionally, reduced hepatic cholesterol efflux capacity in individuals with NAFLD has been linked to the presence of subclinical atherosclerosis [48], hinting that NID2 overexpression in hepatocytes may suppress cholesterol efflux, thereby leading to increased atherosclerosis. Comparable atherosclerosis in female control and *NID2*-overexpressing mice suggests sex-specific responses and implies that factors such as hormonal differences or sex-specific gene regulation modulate the effects of NID2 in atherosclerosis. For instance, estrogen has been shown to exert protective effects against atherosclerosis by modulating lipid metabolism and reducing inflammation [49,50]. Therefore, it is possible that sex hormones may be counteracting pro-atherogenic effects of NID2 in females.

To investigate the molecular mechanisms by which NID2 regulates hepatosteatosis and atherosclerosis, we examined the expression of various proteins and genes involved lipid metabolism. AMPK is a master switch in hepatic metabolism and its activation via phosphorylation (Thr 172) reduces hepatosteatosis by promoting fatty acid oxidation and inhibiting lipid production in the liver [51–53]. Phosphorylated AMPK inactivates ACC (Ser 79 phosphorylation), leading to increased fatty acid oxidation and reduced fatty acid synthesis [30,31]. Our data demonstrated reduced AMPK activation in the livers with *NID2* overexpression, with no changes in the activation status of ACC, hinting an ACC-independent function of AMPK in hepatosteatosis. These findings are consistent with a study by Zordoky et al., which also showed ACC-independent effects of AMPK in myocardial fatty acid oxidation [54]. However, it is unknown how NID2 regulates AMPK phosphorylation. It is possible that NID2, via inhibiting protein kinase C activation, suppresses AMPK activation [18]. Other AMPK-regulated factors such as the liver X receptor and sterol regulatory element-binding protein 1c (SREBP1c) may be mediating pro-steatotic/atherogenic effects of NID2 in mice [55]. We observed no significant differences in hepatic mRNA levels of various lipid uptake, fatty acid synthesis, fatty acid transport, and fatty acid beta oxidation genes, except *Ldlr* between control and *NID2*-AAV-injected mice. *Ldlr* mRNA expression was elevated in mice with *NID2* overexpression, which may represent a compensatory mechanism to clear excess lipids from circulation. Another possibility is that *NID2* overexpression increases proprotein convertase subtilisin/kexin type 9 levels, leading to degradation of LDLR protein and its reduced expression on the surface of hepatocytes, despite elevated mRNA levels [56], potentially contributing to the development of hepatosteatosis in these mice.

A major limitation of the present study is the utilization of *NID2*-AAV under the control of the ubiquitous cytomegalovirus promoter, which drives gene expression in multiple organs in mice. To better understand the cell-specific effects of *NID2* overexpression in NAFLD and atherosclerosis, future investigations with *NID2*-AAV with cell-specific promoter (hepatocytes/vascular cells) are required. Further, in vivo studies using cell-specific *NID2* deficiency are needed to investigate the precise role of endogenous NID2 in the pathophysiology of these diseases. Additionally, further investigations into the sex-specific roles of NID2 are warranted, including the use of ovariectomized female mice or the treatment of sex hormones, such as estradiol (E2), in male mice.

In conclusion, the present study, for the first time, demonstrates the detrimental role of NID2 in hepatosteatosis and atherosclerosis. The presented results suggest that blocking NID2-induced signaling may serve as potential therapeutic approach to suppress both NAFLD and atherosclerosis.

4. Materials and Methods

4.1. Animals and AAV Production

Eight- to ten-week-old male and female *Apoe*$^{-/-}$ mice (The Jackson Laboratory, Bar Harbor, ME, USA, stock # 002052) were used in the present study. One group of *Apoe*$^{-/-}$ mice, designated as control, received an intraperitoneal injection of saline, while another group was administered a single dose of a recombinant AAV expressing human *NID2* gene (AAV8-h*NID2*, referred to as *NID2*-AAV, 6.5 $\times$ 10^{13} viral genomes, IP) under the ubiquitous cytomegalovirus promoter, to induce *NID2* overexpression. The plasmid DNA for the *NID2* vector construct (pAAV-h*NID2*-CMV-amp, # 31829101) was obtained from Applied Biological Materials Inc., Richmond, Canada. The plasmid was packaged into AAV serotype 8 capsid and purified using a density gradient iodixanol solution at the Cincinnati Children's Hospital Medical Center Viral Vector Core [RRID:SCR_022641)-VVL]. Eight- to ten-week-old male wild-type C57BL/6J mice were fed a control diet (Research Diets, Inc., New Brunswick, NJ, USA, D12450J) or a calorie-matched high-fat diet (Research Diets, Inc., New Brunswick, NJ, USA, D12492) for 12 weeks to determine NID2 protein levels using immunoblotting. All mice were housed in a climate-controlled vivarium (12-h light/dark cycle). All animal experiments were conducted according to the National Institutes of Health Guide for the Care and Use of Laboratory Animals, and performed after obtaining approval from the Institutional Animal Care and Use Committee of the University of Tennessee Health Science Center at Memphis, TN, USA (# 22-0319, dated 18 January 2022).

4.2. Atherosclerotic Lesion Analysis

Control and *NID2*-AAV-injected *Apoe*$^{-/-}$ mice were fed a Western diet (Inotiv, Indianapolis, IN, USA, #TD.88137) for 12 weeks to induce hypercholesterolemia and atherosclerosis. In the twelfth week of feeding, whole-body fat and lean mass were measured using the EchoMRI Body Composition Analyzer. Fasting blood glucose (ReliOn Prime Blood Glucose Monitoring System, Bentonville, AR, USA) was determined following a 16 h fast, just before euthanasia. Mice were anesthetized by isoflurane inhalation (3%), and blood (via cardiac puncture), heart, aorta, epididymal adipose tissue, and other tissues were collected for further analysis. Similar regions of the liver from each mouse were processed for histochemistry and molecular analysis. Plasma total cholesterol was determined utilizing the Amplex Red cholesterol assay (Molecular Probes, Eugene, OR, USA, A12216). In situ images of the abdominal area, aortic arch, and heart were captured using a Leica S6E stereomicroscope fitted with a camera.

To assess the atherosclerotic lesion burden in whole aortas, *en face* ORO staining was performed after fixing aortas in 4% paraformaldehyde (PFA). A 2% ORO solution (ThermoFisher Scientific, Ward Hill, MA, USA, A12989.22) was used for staining. Aortas were opened longitudinally, and images were captured to quantify ORO-positive areas. To determine the lipid deposition in the aortic roots, the upper halves of fixed hearts were embedded in optimal cutting temperature (OCT) compound (Fisher Healthcare, Houston, TX, USA, 23-730-571), and serial frozen cross-sections (7 μm) were stained with 2% ORO solution. Images were captured using an Olympus BX43 inverted microscope. Four sections per mouse, spaced 90–100 μm apart, were stained and analyzed, and the mean area of the four sections reported. ORO-positive areas were quantified using Image Pro plus software (Media Cybernetics, Bethesda, MD, USA, version 7.0).

4.3. Hepatic Lipid Accumulation, Triglyceride, and Non-Esterified Fatty Acid Quantitation

To investigate the lipid accumulation in the liver, a similar region of the PFA-fixed and sucrose-dehydrated liver from each mouse was embedded in an OCT compound, and cryo-sectioning was performed. Frozen liver sections (7 μm) were stained with 2% ORO for 10 min at room temperature and counterstained with hematoxylin (Fisher Healthcare, Houston, TX, USA, 22-220-100). For each mouse, at least two sections were stained, and images of five to six random microscopic fields were captured. Image Pro Plus software was used for image analysis.

Liver homogenates were used to extract total lipids using the methanol and chloroform method. Plasma/hepatic triglyceride levels and NEFA levels were quantified following the standard protocols (Wako Pure Chemical Industries, Richmond, VA, USA, 992-02892, 992-02892, 464-01601, 995-34791, and 999-34691), as described previously [57].

4.4. Histochemistry

At least four aortic root sections per mouse, spaced 90–100 μm apart, were stained and analyzed, and the mean area of four sections was reported. Frozen serial cross-sections of aortic roots were washed twice with phosphate-buffered saline (PBS) and stained with H & E (Fisher Healthcare, Houston, TX, USA, 22-220-100 and 22-220-104) as described previously [22,58,59] to evaluate the total lesion and necrotic area. Masson's trichrome staining (Richard Allan Scientific LLC, Kalamazoo, MI, USA, 22-110-648) was performed following the standard protocol to analyze the collagen content.

Frozen or paraffin liver sections were stained with H & E and Sirius red (Fisher Healthcare, Houston, TX, USA, 26357-02) as per the manufacturer's instructions. H & E staining of liver sections was used to visualize the lipid globules, while Sirius red staining was employed to analyze the collagen content (fibrosis). A mean of five to six random microscopic fields per mouse was reported. All image analyses were performed utilizing Image-Pro Plus software.

4.5. Western Blotting

Murine liver and human vascular tissue samples were homogenized in radio-immunoprecipitation assay lysis buffer (RIPA, ThermoScientific, Ward Hill, MA, USA #89900) supplemented with protease and phosphatase inhibitor cocktail (ThermoScientific, Ward Hill, MA, USA #A32959). Equal amounts of protein were separated on SDS-PAGE gels, and resolved bands were transferred onto nitrocellulose membranes (Li-Cor Biosciences, Lincoln, NE, USA). Membranes were blocked (Intercept blocking buffer, Li-Cor Biosciences, Lincoln, NE, USA, #927-60001) and incubated overnight at 4 °C with indicated primary antibodies. The next day, membranes were washed and probed with IRDye-conjugated secondary antibodies (Li-Cor Biosciences, Lincoln, NE, USA). After washing, membranes were scanned with an Odyssey DLx Infrared Imaging System (Li-Cor Biosciences, Lincoln, NE, USA), and band intensities were determined using the NIH ImageJ software (version 1.53a). The following primary antibodies were used: NID2 (Proteintech, Rosemont, IL, USA #13530-1-AP), total ACC (Cell Signaling Technology, Danvers, MA, USA, #3662S), pACC^{Ser79} (Cell Signaling Technology, Danvers, MA, USA, #11818S), total AMPKα (Cell Signaling Technology, Danvers, MA, USA, #2793S), pAMPKα^{Thr172} (Cell Signaling Technology, Danvers, MA, USA, #2535S), IL-6 (Cell Signaling Technology, Danvers, MA, USA, #12912S), TNFα (Cell Signaling Technology, Danvers, MA, USA, #11948T), β-Tubulin (Cell Signaling Technology, Danvers, MA, USA, #86298S), and GAPDH (Santa Cruz Biotechnology, Dallas, TX, USA #sc-365062). All the antibodies except GAPDH and β-Tubulin were used at a 1:1000 dilution. GAPDH and β-Tubulin were utilized at a 1:2000 dilution.

4.6. Quantitative Reverse-Transcriptase PCR

Liver tissue samples were homogenized in TRIzol reagent (ThermoFisher Scientific, Ward Hill, MA, USA, #15596018), and total RNA was extracted according to the manufacturer's instructions. Complementary DNA was synthesized using the RevertAid RT Reverse Transcription Kit (ThermoFisher Scientific, Ward Hill, MA, USA, #K1691). The qRT-PCR was performed using PowerUp SYBR Green Master Mix (ThermoFisher Scientific, Ward Hill, MA, USA, #A25742) in a QuantStudio 3 Real-Time PCR System (Applied Biosystems, Waltham, MA, USA). Relative gene expression was calculated using the $2^{-\Delta\Delta Ct}$ method and *Gapdh* as a housekeeping gene. Primer sequences used for qRT-PCR are listed in Supplementary Table S1.

4.7. Statistical Analysis

Sample sizes (n) for each experiment are mentioned in the figure legends. Statistical analyses were conducted using GraphPad Prism 10 (La Jolla, CA, USA). The normality of the data was assessed by the Shapiro–Wilk test. Comparisons between the two groups were performed using a two-tailed Student's t-test for parametric data or a Mann–Whitney U test for non-parametric data. For parametric tests, the same standard deviation was assumed across groups. A p-value < 0.05 was considered statistically significant.

Supplementary Materials: The following supporting information can be downloaded at: https://www.mdpi.com/article/10.3390/ijms252312782/s1.

Author Contributions: All authors contributed data and analysis to the manuscript. Conceptualization: I.K. and B.S.; methodology: I.K., B.K.S. and B.S.; validation: I.K.; formal analysis: I.K., A.P. and R.V.A.; investigation: I.K., A.P., R.V.A., B.S., M.O.-B. and M.A.G.; resources: F.P., U.P.S., J.J. and B.S.; data curation: I.K. and B.S.; visualization: I.K. and B.S.; writing—original draft preparation: I.K.; writing—review and editing: B.S.; supervision: B.S.; project administration: B.S.; funding acquisition: B.S. All authors have read and agreed to the published version of the manuscript.

Funding: This work was supported by the National Institutes of Health grants (K99HL146954 and R00HL146954) and the UTHSC College of Pharmacy Research Seed Grant awarded to B.S.

Institutional Review Board Statement: The experiments were performed after obtaining approval from the Institutional Animal Care and Use Committee of the University of Tennessee Health Science Center at Memphis, TN, USA (22-0319).

Informed Consent Statement: Not applicable.

Data Availability Statement: The data presented in this study are available upon reasonable request from the corresponding author.

Conflicts of Interest: The authors have declared that no conflicts of interest exist.

References

1. Han, S.K.; Baik, S.K.; Kim, M.Y. Non-alcoholic fatty liver disease: Definition and subtypes. *Clin. Mol. Hepatol.* **2023**, *29*, S5–S16. [CrossRef] [PubMed]
2. Polyzos, S.A.; Mantzoros, C.S. Making progress in nonalcoholic fatty liver disease (NAFLD) as we are transitioning from the era of NAFLD to dys-metabolism associated fatty liver disease (DAFLD). *Metabolism* **2020**, *111S*, 154318. [CrossRef] [PubMed]
3. Riazi, K.; Azhari, H.; Charette, J.H.; Underwood, F.E.; King, J.A.; Afshar, E.E.; Swain, M.G.; Congly, S.E.; Kaplan, G.G.; Shaheen, A.A. The prevalence and incidence of NAFLD worldwide: A systematic review and meta-analysis. *Lancet Gastroenterol. Hepatol.* **2022**, *7*, 851–861. [CrossRef]

4. Loomba, R.; Ratziu, V.; Harrison, S.A.; NASH Clinical Trial Design International Working Group. Expert Panel Review to Compare FDA and EMA Guidance on Drug Development and Endpoints in Nonalcoholic Steatohepatitis. *Gastroenterology* **2022**, *162*, 680–688. [CrossRef] [PubMed]
5. Harrison, S.A.; Taub, R.; Neff, G.W.; Lucas, K.J.; Labriola, D.; Moussa, S.E.; Alkhouri, N.; Bashir, M.R. Resmetirom for nonalcoholic fatty liver disease: A randomized, double-blind, placebo-controlled phase 3 trial. *Nat. Med.* **2023**, *29*, 2919–2928. [CrossRef]
6. Harrison, S.A.; Bedossa, P.; Guy, C.D.; Schattenberg, J.M.; Loomba, R.; Taub, R.; Labriola, D.; Moussa, S.E.; Neff, G.W.; Rinella, M.E.; et al. A Phase 3, Randomized, Controlled Trial of Resmetirom in NASH with Liver Fibrosis. *N. Engl. J. Med.* **2024**, *390*, 497–509. [CrossRef]
7. Deprince, A.; Haas, J.T.; Staels, B. Dysregulated lipid metabolism links NAFLD to cardiovascular disease. *Mol. Metab.* **2020**, *42*, 101092. [CrossRef]
8. Finney, A.C.; Das, S.; Kumar, D.; McKinney, M.P.; Cai, B.; Yurdagul, A., Jr.; Rom, O. The interplay between nonalcoholic fatty liver disease and atherosclerotic cardiovascular disease. *Front. Cardiovasc. Med.* **2023**, *10*, 1116861. [CrossRef] [PubMed]
9. Kohfeldt, E.; Sasaki, T.; Gohring, W.; Timpl, R. Nidogen-2: A new basement membrane protein with diverse binding properties. *J. Mol. Biol.* **1998**, *282*, 99–109. [CrossRef]
10. Srisuttee, R.; Arayataweegool, A.; Mahattanasakul, P.; Tangjaturonrasme, N.; Kerekhanjanarong, V.; Keelawat, S.; Mutirangura, A.; Kitkumthorn, N. Evaluation of NID2 promoter methylation for screening of Oral squamous cell carcinoma. *BMC Cancer* **2020**, *20*, 218. [CrossRef]
11. Torky, H.A.; Sherif, A.; Abo-Louz, A.; Ali, M.; Ahmed, A.; Ali, A. Evaluation of Serum Nidogen-2 as a Screening and Diagnostic Tool for Ovarian Cancer. *Gynecol. Obstet. Investig.* **2018**, *83*, 461–465. [CrossRef] [PubMed]
12. Yu, Z.H.; Wang, Y.M.; Jiang, Y.Z.; Ma, S.J.; Zhong, Q.; Wan, Y.Y.; Wang, X.W. NID2 can serve as a potential prognosis prediction biomarker and promotes the invasion and migration of gastric cancer. *Pathol. Res. Pract.* **2019**, *215*, 152553. [CrossRef] [PubMed]
13. Wang, J.; Zhao, Y.; Xu, H.; Ma, J.; Liang, F.; Zou, Q.; Lin, F. Silencing NID2 by DNA Hypermethylation Promotes Lung Cancer. *Pathol. Oncol. Res.* **2020**, *26*, 801–811. [CrossRef] [PubMed]
14. Pereira, B.A.; Ritchie, S.; Chambers, C.R.; Gordon, K.A.; Magenau, A.; Murphy, K.J.; Nobis, M.; Tyma, V.M.; Liew, Y.F.; Lucas, M.C.; et al. Temporally resolved proteomics identifies nidogen-2 as a cotarget in pancreatic cancer that modulates fibrosis and therapy response. *Sci. Adv.* **2024**, *10*, eadl1197. [CrossRef] [PubMed]
15. Lorentzen, L.G.; Yeung, K.; Eldrup, N.; Eiberg, J.P.; Sillesen, H.H.; Davies, M.J. Proteomic analysis of the extracellular matrix of human atherosclerotic plaques shows marked changes between plaque types. *Matrix Biol. Plus* **2024**, *21*, 100141. [CrossRef]
16. Theofilatos, K.; Stojkovic, S.; Hasman, M.; van der Laan, S.W.; Baig, F.; Barallobre-Barreiro, J.; Schmidt, L.E.; Yin, S.; Yin, X.; Burnap, S.; et al. Proteomic Atlas of Atherosclerosis: The Contribution of Proteoglycans to Sex Differences, Plaque Phenotypes, and Outcomes. *Circ. Res.* **2023**, *133*, 542–558. [CrossRef]
17. Lou, Y.; Li, P.H.; Liu, X.Q.; Wang, T.X.; Liu, Y.L.; Chen, C.C.; Ma, K.L. ITGAM-mediated macrophages contribute to basement membrane damage in diabetic nephropathy and atherosclerosis. *BMC Nephrol.* **2024**, *25*, 72. [CrossRef]
18. Chen, Y.; Mao, C.; Gu, R.; Zhao, R.; Li, W.; Ma, Z.; Jia, Y.; Yu, F.; Luo, J.; Fu, Y.; et al. Nidogen-2 is a Novel Endogenous Ligand of LGR4 to Inhibit Vascular Calcification. *Circ. Res.* **2022**, *131*, 1037–1054. [CrossRef]
19. Mao, C.; Ma, Z.; Jia, Y.; Li, W.; Xie, N.; Zhao, G.; Ma, B.; Yu, F.; Sun, J.; Zhou, Y.; et al. Nidogen-2 Maintains the Contractile Phenotype of Vascular Smooth Muscle Cells and Prevents Neointima Formation via Bridging Jagged1-Notch3 Signaling. *Circulation* **2021**, *144*, 1244–1261. [CrossRef]
20. Honda, O.; Sugiyama, S.; Kugiyama, K.; Fukushima, H.; Nakamura, S.; Koide, S.; Kojima, S.; Hirai, N.; Kawano, H.; Soejima, H.; et al. Echolucent carotid plaques predict future coronary events in patients with coronary artery disease. *J. Am. Coll. Cardiol.* **2004**, *43*, 1177–1184. [CrossRef]
21. Mathiesen, E.B.; Bonaa, K.H.; Joakimsen, O. Echolucent plaques are associated with high risk of ischemic cerebrovascular events in carotid stenosis: The tromso study. *Circulation* **2001**, *103*, 2171–2175. [CrossRef] [PubMed]
22. Singla, B.; Lin, H.P.; Chen, A.; Ahn, W.; Ghoshal, P.; Cherian-Shaw, M.; White, J.; Stansfield, B.K.; Csanyi, G. Role of R-spondin 2 in arterial lymphangiogenesis and atherosclerosis. *Cardiovasc. Res.* **2021**, *117*, 1489–1509. [CrossRef] [PubMed]
23. Liu, Y.; Zhao, Y.; Shukha, Y.; Lu, H.; Wang, L.; Liu, Z.; Liu, C.; Zhao, Y.; Wang, H.; Zhao, G.; et al. Dysregulated oxalate metabolism is a driver and therapeutic target in atherosclerosis. *Cell. Rep.* **2021**, *36*, 109420. [CrossRef] [PubMed]
24. Flessa, C.M.; Nasiri-Ansari, N.; Kyrou, I.; Leca, B.M.; Lianou, M.; Chatzigeorgiou, A.; Kaltsas, G.; Kassi, E.; Randeva, H.S. Genetic and Diet-Induced Animal Models for Non-Alcoholic Fatty Liver Disease (NAFLD) Research. *Int. J. Mol. Sci.* **2022**, *23*, 15791. [CrossRef] [PubMed]
25. Getz, G.S.; Reardon, C.A. Animal models of atherosclerosis. *Arterioscler. Thromb. Vasc. Biol.* **2012**, *32*, 1104–1115. [CrossRef] [PubMed]
26. Kawano, Y.; Cohen, D.E. Mechanisms of hepatic triglyceride accumulation in non-alcoholic fatty liver disease. *J. Gastroenterol.* **2013**, *48*, 434–441. [CrossRef]
27. Lee, E.; Korf, H.; Vidal-Puig, A. An adipocentric perspective on the development and progression of non-alcoholic fatty liver disease. *J. Hepatol.* **2023**, *78*, 1048–1062. [CrossRef]
28. Holmer, M.; Hagstrom, H.; Chen, P.; Danielsson, O.; Aouadi, M.; Ryden, M.; Stal, P. Associations between subcutaneous adipocyte hypertrophy and nonalcoholic fatty liver disease. *Sci. Rep.* **2022**, *12*, 20519. [CrossRef]

29. Day, E.A.; Ford, R.J.; Steinberg, G.R. AMPK as a Therapeutic Target for Treating Metabolic Diseases. *Trends Endocrinol. Metab.* **2017**, *28*, 545–560. [CrossRef]
30. Viollet, B.; Foretz, M.; Guigas, B.; Horman, S.; Dentin, R.; Bertrand, L.; Hue, L.; Andreelli, F. Activation of AMP-activated protein kinase in the liver: A new strategy for the management of metabolic hepatic disorders. *J. Physiol.* **2006**, *574*, 41–53. [CrossRef]
31. Foretz, M.; Even, P.C.; Viollet, B. AMPK Activation Reduces Hepatic Lipid Content by Increasing Fat Oxidation In Vivo. *Int. J. Mol. Sci.* **2018**, *19*, 2826. [CrossRef] [PubMed]
32. Song, C.; Long, X.; He, J.; Huang, Y. Recent evaluation about inflammatory mechanisms in nonalcoholic fatty liver disease. *Front. Pharmacol.* **2023**, *14*, 1081334. [CrossRef] [PubMed]
33. Horton, J.D.; Shimomura, I.; Brown, M.S.; Hammer, R.E.; Goldstein, J.L.; Shimano, H. Activation of cholesterol synthesis in preference to fatty acid synthesis in liver and adipose tissue of transgenic mice overproducing sterol regulatory element-binding protein-2. *J. Clin. Investig.* **1998**, *101*, 2331–2339. [CrossRef] [PubMed]
34. Wojcik-Cichy, K.; Koslinska-Berkan, E.; Piekarska, A. The influence of NAFLD on the risk of atherosclerosis and cardiovascular diseases. *Clin. Exp. Hepatol.* **2018**, *4*, 1–6. [CrossRef] [PubMed]
35. Tsao, C.W.; Aday, A.W.; Almarzooq, Z.I.; Anderson, C.A.M.; Arora, P.; Avery, C.L.; Baker-Smith, C.M.; Beaton, A.Z.; Boehme, A.K.; Buxton, A.E.; et al. Heart Disease and Stroke Statistics-2023 Update: A Report From the American Heart Association. *Circulation* **2023**, *147*, e93–e621. [CrossRef] [PubMed]
36. Kimura, N.; Toyoshima, T.; Kojima, T.; Shimane, M. Entactin-2: A new member of basement membrane protein with high homology to entactin/nidogen. *Exp. Cell. Res.* **1998**, *241*, 36–45. [CrossRef]
37. Chai, A.W.Y.; Cheung, A.K.L.; Dai, W.; Ko, J.M.Y.; Lee, N.P.Y.; Chan, K.T.; Law, S.Y.; Lung, M.L. Elevated levels of serum nidogen-2 in esophageal squamous cell carcinoma. *Cancer Biomark.* **2018**, *21*, 583–590. [CrossRef]
38. Wang, X.; Ren, J.; Fang, F.; Wang, E.; Li, J.; He, W.; Zhang, Z.; Shen, Y.; Liu, X. Matrix vesicles from osteoblasts promote atherosclerotic calcification. *Matrix Biol.* **2024**, *134*, 79–92. [CrossRef]
39. Basaranoglu, M.; Neuschwander-Tetri, B.A. Nonalcoholic Fatty Liver Disease: Clinical Features and Pathogenesis. *Gastroenterol. Hepatol.* **2006**, *2*, 282–291.
40. Targher, G.; Bertolini, L.; Poli, F.; Rodella, S.; Scala, L.; Tessari, R.; Zenari, L.; Falezza, G. Nonalcoholic fatty liver disease and risk of future cardiovascular events among type 2 diabetic patients. *Diabetes* **2005**, *54*, 3541–3546. [CrossRef]
41. Cohen, J.C.; Horton, J.D.; Hobbs, H.H. Human fatty liver disease: Old questions and new insights. *Science* **2011**, *332*, 1519–1523. [CrossRef] [PubMed]
42. Samuel, V.T.; Shulman, G.I. Mechanisms for insulin resistance: Common threads and missing links. *Cell* **2012**, *148*, 852–871. [CrossRef] [PubMed]
43. Taylor, R.S.; Taylor, R.J.; Bayliss, S.; Hagstrom, H.; Nasr, P.; Schattenberg, J.M.; Ishigami, M.; Toyoda, H.; Wai-Sun Wong, V.; Peleg, N.; et al. Association Between Fibrosis Stage and Outcomes of Patients With Nonalcoholic Fatty Liver Disease: A Systematic Review and Meta-Analysis. *Gastroenterology* **2020**, *158*, 1611–1625. [CrossRef]
44. Anstee, Q.M.; Targher, G.; Day, C.P. Progression of NAFLD to diabetes mellitus, cardiovascular disease or cirrhosis. *Nat. Rev. Gastroenterol. Hepatol.* **2013**, *10*, 330–344. [CrossRef]
45. Lonardo, A.; Nascimbeni, F.; Ballestri, S.; Fairweather, D.; Win, S.; Than, T.A.; Abdelmalek, M.F.; Suzuki, A. Sex Differences in Nonalcoholic Fatty Liver Disease: State of the Art and Identification of Research Gaps. *Hepatology* **2019**, *70*, 1457–1469. [CrossRef]
46. Norheim, F.; Hui, S.T.; Kulahcioglu, E.; Mehrabian, M.; Cantor, R.M.; Pan, C.; Parks, B.W.; Lusis, A.J. Genetic and hormonal control of hepatic steatosis in female and male mice. *J. Lipid. Res.* **2017**, *58*, 178–187. [CrossRef]
47. Yurdagul, A., Jr.; Finney, A.C.; Woolard, M.D.; Orr, A.W. The arterial microenvironment: The where and why of atherosclerosis. *Biochem. J.* **2016**, *473*, 1281–1295. [CrossRef]
48. Fadaei, R.; Poustchi, H.; Meshkani, R.; Moradi, N.; Golmohammadi, T.; Merat, S. Impaired HDL cholesterol efflux capacity in patients with non-alcoholic fatty liver disease is associated with subclinical atherosclerosis. *Sci. Rep.* **2018**, *8*, 11691. [CrossRef] [PubMed]
49. Mendelsohn, M.E.; Karas, R.H. The protective effects of estrogen on the cardiovascular system. *N. Engl. J. Med.* **1999**, *340*, 1801–1811. [CrossRef] [PubMed]
50. Moolman, J.A. Unravelling the cardioprotective mechanism of action of estrogens. *Cardiovasc. Res.* **2006**, *69*, 777–780. [CrossRef]
51. Sharma, A.; Anand, S.K.; Singh, N.; Dwarkanath, A.; Dwivedi, U.N.; Kakkar, P. Berbamine induced activation of the SIRT1/LKB1/AMPK signaling axis attenuates the development of hepatic steatosis in high-fat diet-induced NAFLD rats. *Food Funct.* **2021**, *12*, 892–909. [CrossRef]
52. Meng, Z.; Liu, Q.; Sun, F.; Qiao, L. Hepatitis C virus nonstructural protein 5A perturbs lipid metabolism by modulating AMPK/SREBP-1c signaling. *Lipids. Health Dis.* **2019**, *18*, 191. [CrossRef] [PubMed]
53. Smith, B.K.; Marcinko, K.; Desjardins, E.M.; Lally, J.S.; Ford, R.J.; Steinberg, G.R. Treatment of nonalcoholic fatty liver disease: Role of AMPK. *Am. J. Physiol. Endocrinol. Metab.* **2016**, *311*, E730–E740. [CrossRef] [PubMed]
54. Zordoky, B.N.; Nagendran, J.; Pulinilkunnil, T.; Kienesberger, P.C.; Masson, G.; Waller, T.J.; Kemp, B.E.; Steinberg, G.R.; Dyck, J.R. AMPK-dependent inhibitory phosphorylation of ACC is not essential for maintaining myocardial fatty acid oxidation. *Circ. Res.* **2014**, *115*, 518–524. [CrossRef] [PubMed]
55. Yun, Y.R.; Kim, J.H.; Kim, J.H.; Jung, M.H. Protective effects of gomisin N against hepatic steatosis through AMPK activation. *Biochem. Biophys. Res. Commun.* **2017**, *482*, 1095–1101. [CrossRef]

56. Lagace, T.A. PCSK9 and LDLR degradation: Regulatory mechanisms in circulation and in cells. *Curr. Opin. Lipidol.* **2014**, *25*, 387–393. [CrossRef]
57. Kim, S.; Choi, S.; Dutta, M.; Asubonteng, J.O.; Polunas, M.; Goedken, M.; Gonzalez, F.J.; Cui, J.Y.; Gyamfi, M.A. Pregnane X receptor exacerbates nonalcoholic fatty liver disease accompanied by obesity- and inflammation-prone gut microbiome signature. *Biochem. Pharmacol.* **2021**, *193*, 114698. [CrossRef]
58. Singla, B.; Aithbathula, R.V.; Pervaiz, N.; Kathuria, I.; Swanson, M.; Ekuban, F.A.; Ahn, W.; Park, F.; Gyamfi, M.; Cherian-Shaw, M.; et al. CD47 Activation by Thrombospondin-1 in Lymphatic Endothelial Cells Suppresses Lymphangiogenesis and Promotes Atherosclerosis. *Arterioscler. Thromb. Vasc. Biol.* **2023**, *43*, 1234–1250. [CrossRef]
59. Singla, B.; Lin, H.P.; Ahn, W.; Xu, J.; Ma, Q.; Sghayyer, M.; Dong, K.; Cherian-Shaw, M.; Zhou, J.; Huo, Y.; et al. Loss of myeloid cell-specific SIRPalpha, but not CD47, attenuates inflammation and suppresses atherosclerosis. *Cardiovasc. Res.* **2022**, *118*, 3097–3111. [CrossRef]

International Journal of *Molecular Sciences*

MDPI

Article

MiRNA-34a, miRNA-145, and miRNA-222 Expression, Matrix Metalloproteinases, TNF-α and VEGF in Patients with Different Phenotypes of Coronary Artery Disease

Alfiya Oskarovna Iusupova [1,*], Nikolay Nikolaevich Pakhtusov [1], Olga Alexandrovna Slepova [1], Natalia Vladimirovna Khabarova [1], Elena Vitalievna Privalova [1], Irina Vladimirovna Bure [2,3], Marina Vyacheslavovna Nemtsova [2,4] and Yuri Nikitich Belenkov [1]

1 Department of Hospital Therapy No 1, I.M. Sechenov First Moscow State Medical University (Sechenov University), 119048 Moscow, Russia; pakhtusovnn@gmail.com (N.N.P.); slepova_o_a@staff.sechenov.ru (O.A.S.); khabarova_n_v@staff.sechenov.ru (N.V.K.); privalova_e_v@staff.sechenov.ru (E.V.P.); belenkov_yu_n@staff.sechenov.ru (Y.N.B.)

2 Laboratory of Medical Genetics, I.M. Sechenov First Moscow State Medical University (Sechenov University), 119048 Moscow, Russia; bureira@mail.ru (I.V.B.); nemtsova_m_v@mail.ru (M.V.N.)

3 Research Institute of Molecular and Personalized Medicine, Russian Medical Academy of Continuous Professional Education, I.M. Sechenov First Moscow State Medical University (Sechenov University), 119048 Moscow, Russia

4 Laboratory of Epigenetics, Research Centre for Medical Genetics, 115522 Moscow, Russia

* Correspondence: yusalya28@gmail.com

Abstract: The development of different phenotypes of coronary artery (CA) lesions is regulated via many various factors, such as pro-inflammatory agents, zinc-dependent endopeptidases, growth factors and circulating microRNAs (miRs). To evaluate the expression levels of miR-34a, miR-145 and miR-222, tumor necrosis factor α (TNF-α), matrix metalloproteinases (MMP-1, -9, -13 and -14) and vascular endothelial growth factor (VEGF) in patients with different phenotypes of coronary artery disease (CAD): ischemia/angina with non-obstructive coronary arteries (INOCA/ANOCA) and obstructive CAD (oCAD) compared with a control group. This cross-sectional observational study included 157 subjects with a verified CAD diagnosis (51 patients with INOCA, 76 patients with oCAD and 30 healthy volunteers). The expression of miR-34a, miR-145 and miR-222 (RT-PCR) and the levels of VEGF, TNF-α, MMP-1, MMP-9, MMP-13 and MMP-14 (ELISA) were estimated in plasma samples. A higher concentration of MMP-9 was found in oCAD-group samples compared to the INOCA/ANOCA group. The INOCA/ANOCA group was characterized by higher levels of TNF-α. Based on multivariate regression analysis, a mathematical model predicting the type of CA lesion was constructed. MiR-145 was the independent predictor of INOCA/ANOCA (p = 0.006). Changes in concentrations of MMP-9 and MMP-14 were found in both investigated CAD groups, with MMP-9 levels being significantly higher in obstructive CAD samples than in INOCA/ANOCA, which confirms the role of inflammation in the development of atherosclerosis. A multivariate regression analysis allowed us to achieve a model that can predict the phenotype of stable CAD, and MiR-145 can be assumed as an independent predictor of INOCA/ANOCA.

Keywords: microRNA (miR-34a: miR-145: miR-222); matrix metalloproteinases (MMP-1: MMP-9: MMP-13: MMP-14); tumor necrosis factor α (TNF-α); vascular endothelial growth factor (VEGF); ischemia/angina with non-obstructive coronary arteries (INOCA/ANOCA); coronary artery disease (CAD)

1. Introduction

The prevalence of metabolic risk factors and the aging of the population in developed countries lead to the persistence of high mortality rates from non-communicable diseases and from coronary artery disease (CAD) in the world [1]. According to the World Health Organization (WHO) in 2021, the mortality rate from CAD reached 17.9 million people [2]. Among patients with CAD, there are phenotypes with ischemia/angina and non-obstructive coronary arteries (INOCA/ANOCA), the prevalence of which, in the population with CAD, according to some studies, reaches 13% [3]. At the same time, INOCA/ANOCA is significantly more common in women (61%, and, in accordance with other data—65%) than in men (32%) [4–7]. The development of different types of CA lesions is regulated via many various factors, among which pro-inflammatory agents play a significant role. According to a study by Karakayali M. et al., the systemic immuno-inflammatory index (SII, platelet × neutrophil/lymphocyte ratio) is independently associated with the presence of INOCA [8]. It is known that, in the case of INOCA, an increase in the systemic inflammation response index (SIRI) plays a potentially important role in the diagnosis of the slow coronary flow phenomenon [9]. Additionally, numerous factors—including pro-inflammatory cytokines (IL and TNF-α), reactive oxygen species (ROS), an imbalance between vasodilation (NO) and vasoconstriction mediators, several zinc-dependent endopeptidases (matrix metalloproteinases, MMP) and growth factors (such as VEGF)—influence the progression of CA atherosclerosis. This effect was particularly demonstrated in the study by Beatty et al., which showed that TNF-α induces the activation of macrophages, T-helper 1 lymphocytes and endothelial cells in atherosclerosis. Activated endothelial cells produce receptors and adhesion molecules that promote abnormal leukocyte migration into the vascular wall, leading to the dysregulated secretion of pro-inflammatory cytokines. The authors conclude that TNF-α and IL-6 play significant roles as risk factors for the development of CAD [10].

MMPs are zinc-dependent endopeptidases, which consist of pro-peptide, the C-terminal domain and the catalytic domain [11]. MMPs are synthesized in the latent form and regulated via a number of proinflammatory factors. MMPs are involved in the processes of extracellular matrix degradation [12].

The classification of MMPs is based on substrate specificity and sequence similarity. Among the groups of MMPs, there are collagenases, gelatinases, stromelysins, matrilysins, membrane-type MMPs and others [13,14]. It is known that foam and smooth muscle cells (SMCs) produce MMPs, which play a significant value in the formation and growth of atherosclerotic plaques [15]. At the same time, MMPs produced by macrophages are implicated in the process of fibrous-cap thinning and plaque destabilization [16]. Thus, the increased expression of activated MMP-13 is related to increased collagenolysis in vivo, mainly in atheromatous plaques, and a decrease in the accumulation of SMC at different stages of atherogenesis, in particular, at the preclinical stage [17]. The investigation by Lehrke M. et al. demonstrated that the level of circulating MMP-1 can be used as a predictive marker of the presence of atherosclerotic plaques [18].

The study of the significance of circulating microRNAs (miRs) in the epigenetic regulation of the development and progression of atherosclerosis is also of considerable interest. MiRs are short non-coding RNA molecules that modify gene expression through the inhibition of translation or enhancing mRNA destruction. Recent research highlights the significance of miRNAs as promising diagnostic biomarkers for assessing the severity of CA stenosis. In particular, the expression of miR-34a increases in the heart during myocardial hypertrophy caused by stretching, adrenergic stimulation and hypoxia, which has been shown to contribute to the disruption of angiogenesis by uncoupling hypoxia-inducible factor 1-α–VEGF (HIF-1α-VEGF) signaling [19]. In addition, it is known that miR-34a, miR-92a, miR-181c and miR-210 participate in the regulation of endothelial function of the vascular wall by inducing or reducing the level of oxidative stress markers [20,21].

The expression of miR-145 decreases in acute coronary syndrome (ACS), which makes it possible to consider this miR as a potential diagnostic biomarker. A negative correlation of miR-145 with markers of endothelial damage (von Willebrand factor (vWF) and heart-type fatty acid-binding protein (H-FABP)) and pro-inflammatory cytokines (IL-6 and TNF-α) was also found [22]. In turn, miR-221 and miR-222 participate in the processes of control of endothelial inflammation, angiogenesis and the apoptosis of endothelial cells [23].

According to the literature data, there is isolated evidence on the expression of miR-34a, miR-145 and miR-222 in patients with CAD, including those with INOCA/ANOCA. It should be noted that, in patients with CAD (obstructive and non-obstructive phenotypes), no investigation was conducted on the possible association of the expression of these miRs with pro-inflammatory cytokines (TNF-α), MMPs and growth factors (VEGF). The study of miR expression levels in such patients can clarify some aspects of the atherogenesis in CA and, in consequence, may be important for determining their potential as possible diagnostic biomarkers and for the development of new therapies with antagomiRs.

2. Results

2.1. Basic Clinical Characteristics

Plasma samples were collected from patients admitted to the cardiology department presenting with complaints of chest pain and dyspnea. All participants underwent stress tests, including stress echocardiography, myocardial scintigraphy, and cardiac MRI with stress, to elucidate the diagnosis of coronary artery disease (CAD). In patients with identified myocardial ischemia, coronary artery imaging (coronary angiography or MSCT) was additionally conducted to assess the necessity for revascularization. The study comprised 127 patients categorized into two groups based on the extent of coronary artery obstruction: the first group included 51 patients with hemodynamically insignificant stenosis (INOCA/ANOCA, stenosis less than 50%), while the second group included 76 patients with coronary artery obstruction (obstructive CAD, stenosis exceeding 50%). The control group consisted of 30 healthy volunteers devoid of risk factors for cardiovascular diseases. The design of the study is presented in Figure 1.

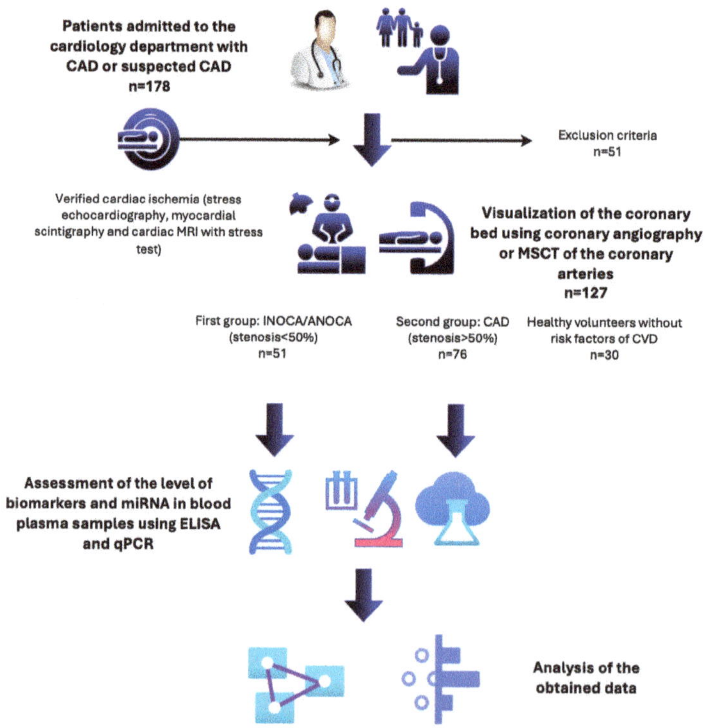

Figure 1. The design of the study. CAD—coronary artery disease; INOCA/ANOCA—ischemia/angina with non-obstructive coronary arteries; qPCR—quantitative polymerase chain reaction; MRI—magnetic resonance imaging; MSCT—multi-detector computed tomography.

The general clinical and demographic characteristics of the groups are summarized in Table 1 [24]. The groups included in the study were comparable according to the main clinical and demographic indicators (age and body mass index (BMI)). In the INOCA/ANOCA group, the majority were women (60.8% women vs. 39.2% men).

Table 1. Basic clinical characteristics.

	All CAD (n = 127)	INOCA/ANOCA (n = 51)	Obstructive CAD (n = 76)	Control (n = 30)	*p*-Value
Men (%)	71 (57.4)	20 (39.2)	51 (67.1)	10 (33.3)	0.001 * $p_{INOCA/ANOCA–obstructive\ CAD} = 0.004$ $p_{obstructive\ CAD–Control} = 0.003$
Women (%)	56 (42.6)	31 (60.8)	25 (32.9)	20 (66.7)	
Age (year)	64 [57; 71]	64 [59; 70.5]	63 [56; 71]	28.5 [26; 39.2]	<0.001 * $p_{control–INOCA/ANOCA} < 0.001$ $p_{control–obstructive\ CAD} < 0.001$
BMI (kg/m^2)	27.4 [25; 30.2]	26.20 [25.67; 30.40]	27.4 [24.77; 29.75]	21.95 [20.75; 25.23]	<0.001 * $p_{control–INOCA/ANOCA} < 0.001$ $p_{control–obstructive\ CAD} < 0.001$
Smoking (%)	9 (7.8)	3 (7.7)	6 (7.9)	-	0.953
Hemoglobin (g/L)	144 [135; 155]	142 [134; 151]	144 [133; 152]	136 [129; 152]	0.459
Glucose (mmol/L)	5.45 ± 0.54	5.53 [5.25; 5.81]	5.43 [5.31; 5.54]	4.9 [4.67; 5.35]	0.005 * $p_{INOCA/ANOCA–Control} = 0.011$ $p_{obstructive\ CAD–Control} = 0.007$
Creatinine (µmol/L)	89 [77.5; 99.15]	80.45 [72.08; 91.67]	91.5 [81; 101.32]	82 [77.7; 87]	0.009 * $p_{INOCA/ANOCA–obstructive\ CAD} = 0.023$
Total cholesterol (mmol/L)	4.05 [3.45; 5.21]	4.45 [3.49; 5.36]	3.79 [3.25; 4.36]	4.94 [4.39; 5.52]	<0.001 * $p_{INOCA/ANOCA–obstructive\ CAD} = 0.015$ $p_{obstructive\ CAD–Control} < 0.001$
LDL (mmol/L)	2.35 [1.81; 2.99]	2.72 [2.03; 3.2]	2.16 [1.58; 2.55]	2.54 [2.28; 3.21]	0.006 * $p_{obstructive\ CAD–INOCA/ANOCA} = 0.016$ $p_{control\ –\ obstructive\ CAD} = 0.044$
HDL (mmol/L)	1.24 ± 0.47	1.31 [1.03; 1.46]	1.08 [1.08; 1.32]	1.62 [1.35; 1.9]	<0.001 * $p_{control–INOCA/ANOCA} = 0.021$ $p_{control–obstructive\ CAD} < 0.001$

* Statistically significant—$p < 0.05$; n—number of patients in the group; CAD—coronary artery disease; INOCA/ANOCA—ischemia/angina with non-obstructive coronary arteries; BMI—body mass index; LDL—low-density lipoproteins; HDL—high-density lipoproteins.

In the group with hemodynamically significant CA stenosis, the levels of total cholesterol and LDL were lower than in the INOCA/ANOCA group. We assume that these results can be explained by better control of lipid spectrum parameters due to the administration of higher doses of statins.

The therapy that patients received at the time of hospitalization is summarized in Table 2.

Table 2. CAD patients' therapy characteristics.

	INOCA/ANOCA	Obstructive CAD	p-Value
ACE inhibitors	18 (35.3)	47 (61.8)	0.027 *
ARB II	17(33.3)	20 (26.7)	0.123
Beta blockers	26 (86.7)	53 (81.5)	0.535
Calcium channel blockers	16 (53.3)	24 (36.9)	0.33
Antiaggregants	26 (66.7)	62 (81.5)	0.202
Anticoagulants	4 (10.2)	7 (9.2)	0.738
Antiarrhythmic drugs	3 (7.7)	8 (10.5)	1.000
HMG-CoA reductase inhibitors	29 (74.4)	63 (82.9)	0.539

INOCA/ANOCA—ischemia/angina with non-obstructive coronary arteries; ACE inhibitors—angiotensin-converting enzyme inhibitors; ARB II—angiotensin II receptor blockers; *—statistically signficant $p < 0.05$

2.2. Concentration of MMPs, TNF-α and VEGF in Plasma

Statistically significant differences were revealed when the levels of MMPs-9 and -14 and TNF-α were compared in the study groups and the control group. The level of VEGF was significantly higher only in the INOCA/ANOCA group compared to the control group. Also, we found differences between the different phenotypes of CAD in the case of TNF-α and MMP-9.

The highest level of MMP-9 was observed in the group with significant stenoses of CA. In addition, in this group, concentrations of VEGF and TNF-α were lower when compared with INOCA/ANOCA. The differences in MMP-1 and MMP-13 levels in both groups were statistically insignificant (Table 3) [24].

Table 3. The concentration of VEGF, TNF-α and MMPs in plasma.

Proteins	Groups	Concentration (Me [Q1–Q3])	p-Value
VEGF, ng/mL	INOCA/ANOCA Obstructive CAD Control	41.66 [36.23–47.58] 36.4 [13.12–66.05] 35.03 [10.50–41.62]	0.043 * $p_{INOCA/ANOCA–control} = 0.036$
TNF-α, ng/mL	INOCA/ANOCA Obstructive CAD Control	28.33 [13.97–29.74] 13.85 [10.76–25.30] 28.23 [14.17–28.73]	<0.004 * $p_{control–obstructive\ CAD} = 0.037$ $p_{INOCA/ANOCA–\ obstructive\ CAD} = 0.03$
MMP-1, ng/mL	INOCA/ANOCA Obstructive CAD Control	0.21 [0.17–0.29] 0.23 [0.21–0.23] 0.24 [0.22–0.32]	0.161
MMP-9 ng/mL	INOCA/ANOCA Obstructive CAD Control	3.58 [1.98–6.18] 7.2 [4.25–10.68] 5.45 [4.02–6.81]	<0.001 * $p_{obstructive\ CAD–INOCA/ANOCA} < 0.001$
MMP-13, ng/mL	INOCA/ANOCA Obstructive CAD Control	123.95 [68.85–285.43] 91.57 [49.77–339.51] 67.5 [47.79–111.30]	0.055
MMP-14, ng/mL	INOCA/ANOCA Obstructive CAD Control	0.71 [0.29–1.04] 0.45 [0.26–0.78] 1.00 [0.75–1.31]	<0.001 * $p_{obstructive\ CAD–control} < 0.001$ $p_{control–INOCA} = 0.02$

* Statistically significant—$p < 0.05$; CAD—coronary artery disease; INOCA/ANOCA—ischemia/angina with non-obstructive coronary arteries; VEGF—vascular endothelial growth factor; TNF-α—tumor necrosis factor-α; MMP—matrix metalloproteinase.

2.3. MiRNA Expression in Plasma

In patients with different phenotypes, CAD expression of miR-34a ($p < 0.001$) and miR-222 ($p < 0.001$) was higher than in the control group. Analyzing the expression of miR-145 can establish that significant differences from the control are present only in the INOCA group ($p = 0.039$) (Figure 2) [24].

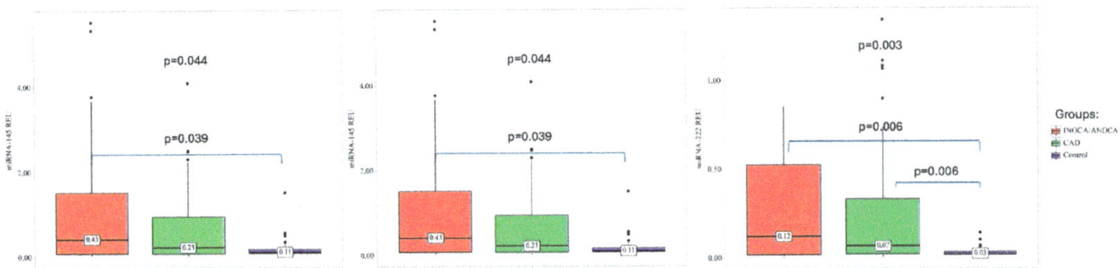

Figure 2. MiRNAs expression in plasma of CAD patients and healthy volunteers (control). All values are presented as the median and CI. Statistically significant—$p < 0.05$; CAD—coronary artery disease, INOCA/ANOCA—ischemia/angina with non-obstructive coronary arteries.

2.4. Correlations of VEGF, TNF-α and MMPs with Circulating miRNAs

According to the correlation analysis, in the INOCA/ANOCA group, notable associations were recorded between VEGF and MMP-1 ($p = 0.668$; $p < 0.001$), as well as MMP-14 ($p = 0.629$; $p < 0.001$). In the obstructive CAD group, a moderate association was observed between VEGF and MMP-9 ($\rho = 0.400$; $p < 0.001$) and a strong association between MMP-1 ($\rho = 0.825$; $p < 0.001$) and MMP-14 ($\rho = 0.736$; $p < 0.001$).

In the INOCA/ANOCA group, there were observed moderate correlations of miR-145 with VEGF ($\rho = 0.442$; $p = 0.013$) and TNF-α (negative relationship, $\rho = -0.386$; $p = 0.032$) and a strong negative linkage with MMP-13 ($\rho = -0.729$; $p < 0.001$). A moderate positive association of miR-222 with VEGF ($\rho = 0.414$; $p = 0.021$), a significant correlation with MMP-1 ($\rho = 0.652$; $p < 0.001$) and a strong correlation with MMP-14 ($\rho = 0.701$; $p < 0.001$) were also found.

In the obstructive CAD group, a significant correlation of miR-145 with VEGF ($\rho = 0.584$; $p < 0.001$) and a strong negative association with MMP-13 ($\rho = -0.380$; $p = 0.002$) were observed. In addition, a moderate association of miRNA-222 with TNF-α ($\rho = 0.363$; $p = 0.004$) and a significant correlation with VEGF ($\rho = 0.595$; $p < 0.001$), as well as a strong linkage with MMP-1 ($\rho = 0.726$; $p < 0.001$) and with MMP-14 ($\rho = 0.727$; $p < 0.001$) were demonstrated.

Univariate logistic regression determined expression of miR-145 as significant predictor of INOCA/ANOCA (Table 4).

Table 4. Univariate logistic regression analysis for different phenotypes of CAD.

Factor/Predictor	B	Exp (B) [95%CI]	*p*	Pseudo R-squ
Gender (male/female)	−1.409	0.244 [0.094, 0.636]	$p = 0.004$ *	0.080
Smoking (n)	0.063	1.064 [0.244, 4.641]	$p = 0.933$	0.000
Hypertension (n)	0.138	1.147 [0.210, 6.28]	$p = 0.874$	0.000
Dyslipidemia (n)	0.323	1.381 [0.138, 13.85]	$p = 0.784$	0.001
Angina pain (n)	0.642	1.899 [0.629, 5.736]	$p = 0.255$	0.012
Fasting glucose (mmol/L)	0.018	1.018 [1.004, 1.033]	$p = 0.014$ *	0.053
Myocardial infarction (n)	−1.488	0.226 [0.077, 0.662]	$p = 0.007$ *	0.073
ACE inhibitors	−1.082	0.339 [0.138, 0.831]	$p = 0.018$ *	0.049
ARB II	0.799	2.222 [0.876, 5.637]	$p = 0.093$	0.024
Beta blockers	0.386	1.471 [0.432, 5.01]	$p = 0.536$	0.003
Calcium channel blocker	0.669	1.952 [0.813, 4.691]	$p = 0.135$	0.019
Antiaggregants	−1.157	0.314 [0.066, 1.505]	$p = 0.148$	0.018
Statins	−0.776	0.460 [0.028, 7.619]	$p = 0.588$	0.002

Table 4. *Cont.*

Factor/Predictor	B	Exp (B) [95%CI]	p	Pseudo R-squ
Age (years)	0.004	1.004 [0.953, 1.058]	$p = 0.871$	0.000
BMI (kg/m^2)	0.007	1.006 [0.903, 1.122]	$p = 0.905$	0.000
VEGF (ng/mL)	0.000	1.000 [0.998, 1.001]	$p = 0.691$	0.001
TNF-α (ng/mL)	−0.002	0.998 [0.992, 1.004]	$p = 0.433$	0.006
MMP-1 (ng/mL)	−0.046	0.955 [0.587, 1.553]	$p = 0.853$	0.000
MMP-9 (ng/mL)	−0.044	0.957 [0.906, 1.011]	$p = 0.118$	0.029
MMP-13 (ng/mL)	0.000	1.000 [1.000, 1.0]	$p = 0.972$	0.000
MMP-14 (ng/mL)	−0.025	0.975 [0.890, 1.07]	$p = 0.600$	0.003
miR-34a REU	−0.050	0.951 [0.869, 1.041]	$p = 0.274$	0.010
miR-145 REU	0.444	1.558 [1.066, 2.277]	$p = 0.022$ *	0.042
miR-222 REU	0.458	1.581 [0.422, 5.93]	$p = 0.497$	0.003

* Statistically significant—$p < 0.05$; CAD—coronary artery disease; BMI—body mass index; ACE inhibitors—angiotensin-converting enzyme inhibitors; ARB II—angiotensin II receptor blockers; VEGF—vascular endothelial growth factor; TNF-α—tumor necrosis factor-α; MMP—matrix metalloproteinase.

The mathematical model was created based on multivariate regression analysis. Based on the obtained data, it can be assumed that miRNA-145 may be an independent predictor of INOCA/ANOCA (Table 5).

Table 5. Multivariate logistic regression analysis for CAD and INOCA/ANOCA groups.

Variables	Coef (B)	Exp (B)	p
miR-145 REU	0.921	2.512 [1.294, 4.875]	$p = 0.006$ *
Gender (male/female)	−1.116	0.328 [0.121, 0.889]	$p = 0.029$ *

* Statistically significant—$p < 0.05$.

The probability of INOCA/ANOCA can be proposed according to the results of an ROC analysis ((cut-off = 0.48) with sensitivity of 77.8% [50.0; 100.0]%, specificity of 78.9% [62.5; 93.3]% and ROC-AUC = 77.8% [60.2; 93.8]%) (Figure 3).

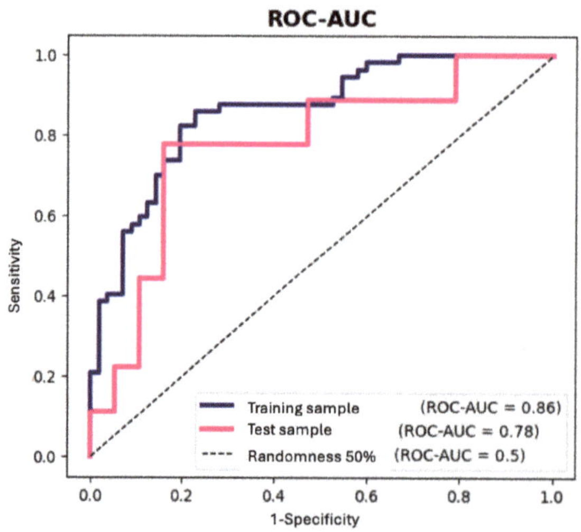

Figure 3. Diagnostic value analysis of the model by ROC curve.

3. Discussion

The development and progression of CA atherosclerosis in stable CAD is influenced by many independent factors that play a crucial role in the formation of different variants of CA lesions. One of these factors is angiogenesis, in the regulation of which VEGF is actively involved. Several members of VEGF family participate in the processes of atherogenesis. In previous studies, it has been demonstrated that VEGF can influence the growth and instability of atherosclerotic plaque through angiogenesis-independent processes [25,26].

It is known that, in metabolic syndrome, the activity of angiogenesis processes in CA may be reduced, despite the increased expression of VEGF, which is associated with an altered VEGF signaling pathway—VEGF/VEGFR signaling [27]. VEGF is not only involved in angiogenesis, stimulating the proliferation and growth of endothelial cells, but also affects pro-inflammatory cytokines and cells: it increases the levels of TNF-α and IL-1 in monocytes and reduces IL-6. Similar results were obtained in our study from plasma samples with obstructive CAD [28].

TNF-α is predominantly produced by activated macrophages and many other types of cells. Recent studies have demonstrated that TNF-α and VEGFA gene expression was significantly lower in patients with INOCA compared to patients with obstructive CAD [29].

In addition, the expression of MMP-1, MMP-3 and MMP-13 can be enhanced through VEGF [30]. The risk of CAD and various severities of the disease may have a relationship with changes in MMP levels. Our study revealed significant differences between levels of MMP-9 and MMP-14 in samples with different phenotypes of CAD compared to the control group. Direct correlations of VEGF with MMP-1, MMP-9 and MMP-14 were found in obstructive CA lesions, and only MMP-1 and MMP-14 with non-obstructive ones.

According to Buchler A., et al. and Quillard T., et al., the increased expression of activated MMP-13 is associated with increased collagenolysis in vivo, which accelerates vascular remodeling processes in atherosclerotic lesions [17,31]. In the study of Gaubatz J. W. et al. a positive relationship between plasma levels of MMP-1 and the calcification of the carotid arteries was revealed [32]. At the same time, in the study of Polonskaya Y.V. et al. the levels of MMP-1 and MMP-9 were increased in calcified plaques, but according to logistic regression analysis, the relative risk of CA plaque calcification was associated only with MMP-9 [33].

MMP-9 is also associated with plaque instability, while MMP-13 is involved in the initial and later stages of atherogenesis [34]. MMP-13 promotes the degradation of the extracellular matrix, thus leading to plaque destabilization [31,35].

Currently, the role of MMP-14 in the development of CAD has been proven in many studies. Thus, high levels of MMP-14 were independently correlated with CVD [36]. An increased expression of MMP-14 was detected by Johnson J.L. et al. in the foam cells of unstable atherosclerotic plaques [37].

In our study, the absence of significant differences between the groups in MMP-1 and MMP-13 levels may be due to the fact that MMP activity was determined only in stable CAD, and the inclusion of a group with ACS may help reveal these differences.

It has been established that miRs are involved in the regulation of various processes, among which the most important in atherogenesis are endothelial damage, inflammation development, the activation of macrophages, the formation of foam cells in the vascular wall, the proliferation, migration and apoptosis of SMCs and, as a consequence, vascular remodeling [16,38]. Epigenetic regulation, in particular microRNAs, changes with age, and some microRNAs undergo an age-dependent decrease, while the expression of others, on the contrary, increases during life. The younger age and demographic characteristics of the control group are due to the fact that we recruited healthy volunteers without risk factors for cardiovascular diseases (for example, those without obesity and overweight, those without acute and chronic diseases and non-smokers).

In the present study, the level of expression of miR-145 in the groups significantly differed and reached the highest values in patients with INOCA/ANOCA. It should be noted that a negative high-strength correlation was found between miR-145 and MMP-13. According to available scientific data, miR-145-5p can act as a "cardioprotective" molecule in patients with myocardial ischemia and, through the negative regulation of CD40, is involved in reducing the activity of the inflammatory response and apoptosis caused by hypoxia [39]. The overexpression of miR-145 can eliminate endothelial damage and reduce the activity of abnormal inflammation, which makes it possible to consider this miR as a potential candidate for targeted ACS therapy [22].

Different phenotypes of CAD can be united by the presence of endothelial dysfunction. It can be hypothesized that INOCA/ANOCA represents an initial stage in the progression of classical CAD. The anti-atherogenic miRNA-145 may function as part of a compensatory mechanism protecting vascular walls against stenotic atherosclerosis.

In the study by Wu S. et al., a negative relationship between miR-145 expression and levels of vWF, H-FABP, IL-6 and TNF-α was demonstrated. Thus, the authors concluded that the reduced expression of miR-145 in serum can serve as a potential diagnostic biomarker of ACS [22]. In our study, similar results were obtained in the INOCA/ANOCA group: a moderate negative correlation between miR-145 and TNF-α was revealed. According to the work of Zhang X. et al., miR-145-5p expression was reduced in blood samples and arterial walls of patients with stenotic atherosclerosis of the CA [40]. Kumar A. et al. found that lower levels of miR-145 and miR-155, along with endothelial dysfunction, were associated with the severity of CKD and with a higher risk of CVD development [41]. Thus, our data support the assumption that a lower level of miR-145 expression in obstructive CAD, in contrast to INOCA, may be associated with a more severe atherosclerotic lesion of CA.

As for the analysis of miR-34a, the minimal level of expression of this miR was observed in the control group, represented by healthy volunteers without CVD risk factors, while in obstructive and non-obstructive CA lesions, the expression was significantly higher. Similar results were obtained by Gatsiou A. et al.: high miR-34a levels were independently associated with the presence of CAD, while the simultaneous overexpression of miR-34-a/c or all three miR-34a/b/c was associated with increased stiffness of the aorta [42].

MiR-34a promotes the downregulation of SIRT1 and VEGF protein expression, causing a disruption of angiogenesis processes and inducing cell death [19]. A study of the role of miR-21, -34a, -146a, -146b-5p and -210 demonstrated a significant increase in their expression in atherosclerotic plaques in contrast to intact arteries [43]. All of these data confirm a significant upregulation in miR-34a expression levels in the plasma of patients with CAD compared to the control group [44].

Similar results were obtained from studying miR-222, the expression of which was significantly higher in both study groups when compared with the control. According to available scientific data, miR-222 also takes part in atherogenesis. MiR-221/222 and miR-155 suppress the inflammatory response induced via angiotensin II in endothelial cells, affecting transcription factor Ets-1 and the genes vascular cell adhesion molecule 1 (VCAM-1) and monocyte chemoattractant protein-1 (MCP1) [45]. The overexpression of miR-19b-3p, miR-221-3p and miR-222-3p induced via inflammatory cytokines TNF-α and IFNγ resulted in intracellular ROS accumulation, leading to cell apoptosis [46]. In obstructive CAD, a moderate association between miR-222 and TNF-α expression was found, as well as a high-strength correlation with MMP-1 and MMP-14 [47]. Karere G.M. et al. identified vascular miRs expressed in baboons and humans and potential novel miRs associated with atherosclerosis. The expression of miR-144-3p, miR-146a-5p, miR-21 and miR-221/222-3p was increased in fibrous plaques, while miR-195-5p was decreased. These results indicate that some miRs are not only specific to a particular type of lesion but also exhibit different levels of expression at various stages of the disease. This indicates their potential importance in the initiation and development of atherosclerosis [48].

In our study, according to the results of multivariate regression analysis, miR-145 was identified as an independent predictor of the non-obstructive phenotype of stable CAD.

In accordance with the results of the ROC analysis, it was concluded that various miRs can be considered potential diagnostic noninvasive markers of CAD. Multivariate logistic regression analysis revealed that levels of circulating miR-145 and miR-155 were associated with CAD and may be powerful markers for detecting CAD [49]. O'Sullivan J. et. al. concluded that four miRNAs (miR-15a-5p, miR-146a-5p, miR-16-5p and miR-93-5p) were predictors of stable CAD development [50]. Zhang L. et. al. suggested other miRs (miR-29a-3p, miR-574-3p and miR-574-5p with AUCs 0.83, 0.792 and 0.789, respectively) as potential markers for the noninvasive diagnosis of CAD [51].

Recent data suggest that plasma levels of miR-23b and miR-143 may be useful as non-invasive biomarkers for in-stent restenosis [52]. Gholipour A. et al. established the potential value of miR-6721-5p as a biomarker for CAD [53].

Our results can be useful in the comprehension of potential roles of miRs, and we plan to continue our research on the mechanisms of the epigenetic regulation of the pathogenesis of different phenotypes of CAD. An investigation of the pathogenesis of atherosclerotic CA lesions may be important for determining the potential role of miRs as possible diagnostic biomarkers and in the development of new treatment methods using antagomiRs. It is necessary to continue careful study and fundamental research in order to solve this complicated problem.

4. Materials and Methods

4.1. Patient Population

This article represents a continuation of our efforts within a grant project [24]. Over the course of the year, we recruited an additional cohort of patients and augmented the number of samples in all groups, except for the control group. As of the current writing, 127 individuals who met the inclusion criteria and provided informed consent from 2020 to 2024 have been enrolled in the ongoing cross-sectional observational study. The study was conducted in accordance with the principles of the Declaration of Helsinki, and it received approval from the Ethics Committee of Sechenov University (Protocol No. 01-21, dated 22 January 2021).

The participants in the study consisted of men and women aged 45 to 75 years who had been diagnosed with CAD. The diagnosis of myocardial ischemia in hospitalized patients with stable angina or its equivalents was performed using instrumental methods, including stress echocardiography (EchoCG) and single-photon emission computed tomography (SPECT), conducted in conjunction with stress tests. Based on the outcomes of coronary angiography (CAG) or multispiral computed tomography (CT), the patients were categorized into two groups: the first group (non-obstructive coronary artery disease, characterized by stenosis < 50% or unchanged arteries) increased from 20 to 51 individuals, while the second group (obstructive coronary artery disease with hemodynamically significant stenosis) expanded from 44 to 76 individuals. The control group, consisting of 30 healthy volunteers without cardiovascular diseases and risk factors, remained unchanged.

The exclusion criteria were as follows: diabetes mellitus, acute coronary syndrome, myocardial infarction or stroke within the preceding three months, chronic heart failure of functional class III-IV (as per the NYHA classification), autoimmune and oncological diseases, decompensated liver diseases, portal hypertension, uncontrolled bronchial asthma, chronic obstructive pulmonary disease, acute gastric or duodenal ulcers, acute chronic pancreatitis, malignant neoplasms, thyroid pathologies, Cushing's syndrome, acute or terminal renal failure (GFR < 15 mL/min/1.73 m^2), mental disorders, alcoholism, drug addiction, substance abuse, pregnancy and breastfeeding.

4.2. Collection of Blood Samples and ELISA

Blood plasma samples were collected in tubes with EDTA K3 as an anticoagulant, centrifuged for 20 min at 1000× g (1000 RCF) and further frozen in cryotubes at −80 °C. To estimate the MMPs' levels, a VEGF and TNF-α enzyme immunoassay (ELISA) was performed using the ELISA analyzer of Adaltis Personal Lab (Rome, Italy) and Wuhan Fine

Biotech Co., Ltd. kits (Wuhan, China) (catalog numbers: EH0232, EH0238, EH0234, EH0369, EH0302 and EH0327). The coefficient of variation (CV) for the sets was 10% and 12%, respectively. All patients had undergone standard biochemical tests, including indicators of the lipid spectrum, glucose and uric acid.

4.3. RNA Extraction and Reverse-Transcription–Polymerase Chain Reaction (RT-PCR) Assay

Total RNA was extracted from blood samples using Qiazol reagent (Qiagen, Hilden, Germany), following the protocol of the manufacturer with small modifications. The concentration and purity of the obtained RNA was estimated on the NanoDrop 2000 microvolume spectrophotometer (Thermo Fisher Scientific, New York, NY, USA). The process of extraction was repeated for each sample until a sufficient amount of RNA was obtained.

cDNA was synthesized from 300 ng of total RNA using MiScript II RT Kit (Qiagen) under the recommended protocol. Real-time PCR was performed on the CFX96 Real-Time PCR Detection System (Bio-Rad, Hercules, CA, USA) in three repetitions for each transcript and control, using the MiScript SYBR Green PCR Kit (Qiagen) according to the manufacturer's recommended protocol. Primers for all three investigated miRNAs were designed according to the instructions (Table 6) [54]. The presynthesized MiScript Primer Assay (Ce_miR-39_1, identification code MS00019789, Qiagen, Germany) was used for the exogenous control, cel-miR-39-3p. Data of the ncRNAs' expression were normalized and analyzed using the $2^{-\Delta\Delta Ct}$ method. The results are presented as REU (relative units of expression).

Table 6. Primer sequences for RT-PCR.

miRNA	Primer Sequence
miR-34a	5′-TGGCAGTGTCTTAGCTGGTTGT-3′
miR-145	5′-TCCAGTTTTCCCAGGAATCCCT-3′
miR-222	5′-CTCAGTAGCCAGTGTAGATCCT-3′

4.4. Statistical Analysis

The data presented in this paper are provided in the figures and tables. The statistical analysis of the results was performed using the program StatTech v.v. 3.1.10 (StatTech, Kazan, Russia) and the free Python computing software environment (v.3.11).

4.4.1. Clinical Data Analyses

Demographic, clinical and laboratory data were compared via either a Kruskal–Wallis test, Dunn test and Fisher's exact test for categorical variables. The two groups were compared quantitatively with an abnormal distribution using the Mann–Whitney U-test.

4.4.2. Multiple Logistic Regression

Multiple logistic regression (MLR) was used to build a model for predicting the presence/absence of a characteristic. The choice of the method was based on the dichotomy of the dependent variable and the fact that independent variables characterize both categorical and quantitative characteristics. The independent variables were selected through step-by-step reverse selection using Wald statistics as an exclusion criterion. The statistical significance of the obtained model was determined using the criterion χ^2. To balance the training data set for a more stable predictive model, the SMOTE (Synthetic Minority Over-sampling Technique) method was employed. To estimate the quality of the constructed model, the following criteria were used: ROC-AUC, accuracy, sensitivity, specificity, and DCA analysis (decision curve analysis). Metrics were calculated together with the 95% CI. The 95% CI was calculated using the bootstrap method with a sample of 1000 instances. The threshold value was chosen in accordance with the maximization of sensitivity and specificity.

4.5. Study Limitations

This study involved potential limitations. According to the European clinical guidelines for chronic coronary syndromes (2024), the incidence of INOCA/ANOCA is higher in women. So, this fact limited our sample size and the ability to obtain fully comparable study groups. The control group included healthy volunteers without any risk factors for cardiovascular diseases (for example, those without acute and chronic diseases, obesity, overweight and non-smokers) who were younger than the main groups of patients with different phenotypes of CAD.

5. Conclusions

The aim of this study was to evaluate the expression levels of miR-34a, miR-145 and miR-222, TNF-α, MMP-1, -9, -13 and -14, and VEGF in order to search for possible diagnostic markers of different phenotypes of CAD. Changes in MMP levels may be associated with an increased risk of the development of CAD and varying severity of the disease. In our study, MMP-9 levels were significantly different between the groups with obstructive CAD and INOCA/ANOCA. Direct correlations of VEGF with MMP-1, MMP-9 and MMP-14 were found in obstructive CAD, versus only MMP-1 and MMP-14 in INOCA/ANOCA.

MiRs can be considered potential diagnostic markers of stable CAD. The multivariate regression analysis allowed us to achieve a model that can predict the phenotype of coronary artery lesions with high sensitivity and specificity among patients with stable CAD. Thus, we can assume that miR-145 can be potentially used as a predictor of INOCA/ANOCA.

Author Contributions: Conceptualization, Y.N.B. and A.O.I.; methodology, I.V.B.; software, N.N.P.; validation, M.V.N. and I.V.B.; formal analysis, N.N.P.; investigation, N.N.P., O.A.S. and I.V.B.; resources, M.V.N. and I.V.B.; data curation, N.N.P.; writing—original draft preparation, A.O.I., N.N.P., O.A.S. and N.V.K.; writing—review and editing, M.V.N. and E.V.P.; visualization, N.N.P.; supervision, A.O.I.; project administration, Y.N.B.; funding acquisition, Y.N.B. All authors have read and agreed to the published version of the manuscript.

Funding: The study was financially supported by the Russian Science Foundation in the form of scientific project No. 22-15-00424, a scientific grant, «The role of activation of the WNT signaling cascade, the processes of its epigenetic regulation and immune-mediated inflammation in the progression of atherosclerosis and the possibility of influencing it by therapeutic neoangiogenesis in patients with stable coronary heart disease».

Institutional Review Board Statement: The study was conducted in accordance with the Declaration of Helsinki and approved by the Ethics Committee of the Sechenov University (Number: 01–21, 22 January 2021).

Informed Consent Statement: Informed consent was obtained from all subjects involved in the study.

Data Availability Statement: The data presented in this study are available upon request from the corresponding author. The data are not publicly available because some data sets will be used for further research.

Conflicts of Interest: The authors declare no conflicts of interest.

References

1. Ralapanawa, U.; Sivakanesan, R. Epidemiology and the Magnitude of Coronary Artery Disease and Acute Coronary Syndrome: A Narrative Review. *J. Epidemiol. Glob. Health* **2021**, *11*, 169–177. [CrossRef] [PubMed]
2. Silva, S.; Fatumo, S.; Nitsch, D. Mendelian Randomization Studies on Coronary Artery Disease: A Systematic Review and Meta-Analysis. *Syst. Rev.* **2024**, *13*, 29. [CrossRef] [PubMed]
3. Reynolds, H.R.; Diaz, A.; Cyr, D.D.; Shaw, L.J.; Mancini, G.B.J.; Leipsic, J.; Budoff, M.J.; Min, J.K.; Hague, C.J.; Berman, D.S.; et al. Ischemia With Nonobstructive Coronary Arteries: Insights From the ISCHEMIA Trial. *JACC Cardiovasc. Imaging* **2023**, *16*, 63–74. [CrossRef] [PubMed]
4. Pepine, C.J.; Ferdinand, K.C.; Shaw, L.J.; Light-McGroary, K.A.; Shah, R.U.; Gulati, M.; Duvernoy, C.; Walsh, M.N.; Bairey Merz, C.N. Emergence of Nonobstructive Coronary Artery Disease: A Woman's Problem and Need for Change in Definition on Angiography. *J. Am. Coll. Cardiol.* **2015**, *66*, 1918–1933. [CrossRef]

5. Mileva, N.; Nagumo, S.; Mizukami, T.; Sonck, J.; Berry, C.; Gallinoro, E.; Monizzi, G.; Candreva, A.; Munhoz, D.; Vassilev, D.; et al. Prevalence of Coronary Microvascular Disease and Coronary Vasospasm in Patients with Nonobstructive Coronary Artery Disease: Systematic Review and Meta-Analysis. *J. Am. Heart Assoc.* **2022**, *11*, e023207. [CrossRef]
6. Chang, A.; Kang, N.; Chung, J.; Gupta, A.R.; Parwani, P. Evaluation of Ischemia with No Obstructive Coronary Arteries (INOCA) and Contemporary Applications of Cardiac Magnetic Resonance (CMR). *Medicina* **2023**, *59*, 1570. [CrossRef]
7. Jespersen, L.; Hvelplund, A.; Abildstrøm, S.Z.; Pedersen, F.; Galatius, S.; Madsen, J.K.; Jørgensen, E.; Kelbæk, H.; Prescott, E. Stable Angina Pectoris with No Obstructive Coronary Artery Disease Is Associated with Increased Risks of Major Adverse Cardiovascular Events. *Eur. Heart J.* **2012**, *33*, 734–744. [CrossRef]
8. Karakayali, M.; Altunova, M.; Yakisan, T.; Aslan, S.; Omar, T.; Artac, I.; Ilis, D.; Arslan, A.; Cagin, Z.; Karabag, Y.; et al. The Relationship between the Systemic Immune-Inflammation Index and Ischemia with Non-Obstructive Coronary Arteries in Patients Undergoing Coronary Angiography. *Arq. Bras. Cardiol.* **2024**, *121*, e20230540. [CrossRef]
9. Chen, Y.-D.; Wen, Z.-G.; Long, J.-J.; Wang, Y. Association Between Systemic Inflammation Response Index and Slow Coronary Flow Phenomenon in Patients with Ischemia and No Obstructive Coronary Arteries. *Int. J. Gen. Med.* **2024**, *17*, 4045–4053. [CrossRef]
10. Beatty, C.; Richardson, K.P.; Tran, P.M.H.; Satter, K.B.; Hopkins, D.; Gardiner, M.; Sharma, A.; Purohit, S. Multiplex Analysis of Inflammatory Proteins Associated with Risk of Coronary Artery Disease in Type-1 Diabetes Patients. *Clin. Cardiol.* **2024**, *47*, e24143. [CrossRef]
11. Hu, Q.; Ecker, M. Overview of MMP-13 as a Promising Target for the Treatment of Osteoarthritis. *Int. J. Mol. Sci.* **2021**, *22*, 1742. [CrossRef] [PubMed]
12. Ramírez-Carracedo, R.; Hernández, I.; Moreno-Gómez-Toledano, R.; Díez-Mata, J.; Tesoro, L.; González-Cucharero, C.; Jiménez-Guirado, B.; Alcharani, N.; Botana, L.; Saura, M.; et al. NOS3 Prevents MMP-9, and MMP-13 Induced Extracellular Matrix Proteolytic Degradation through Specific MicroRNA-Targeted Expression of Extracellular Matrix Metalloproteinase Inducer in Hypertension-Related Atherosclerosis. *J. Hypertens.* **2024**, *42*, 685–693. [CrossRef] [PubMed]
13. Parks, W.C.; Shapiro, S.D. Matrix Metalloproteinases in Lung Biology. *Respir. Res.* **2001**, *2*, 10–19. [CrossRef] [PubMed]
14. Hey, S.; Linder, S. Matrix Metalloproteinases at a Glance. *J. Cell Sci.* **2024**, *137*, jcs261898. [CrossRef]
15. Ramirez-Carracedo, R.; Tesoro, L.; Hernandez, I.; Diez-Mata, J.; Filice, M.; Toro, R.; Rodriguez-Piñero, M.; Zamorano, J.L.; Saura, M.; Zaragoza, C. Non-Invasive Detection of Extracellular Matrix Metalloproteinase Inducer EMMPRIN, a New Therapeutic Target against Atherosclerosis, Inhibited by Endothelial Nitric Oxide. *Int. J. Mol. Sci.* **2018**, *19*, 3248. [CrossRef]
16. Maitrias, P.; Metzinger-Le Meuth, V.; Nader, J.; Reix, T.; Caus, T.; Metzinger, L. The Involvement of MiRNA in Carotid-Related Stroke. *Arterioscler. Thromb. Vasc. Biol.* **2017**, *37*, 1608–1617. [CrossRef]
17. Buchler, A.; Munch, M.; Farber, G.; Zhao, X.; Al-Haddad, R.; Farber, E.; Rotstein, B.H. Selective Imaging of Matrix Metalloproteinase-13 to Detect Extracellular Matrix Remodeling in Atherosclerotic Lesions. *Mol. Imaging Biol.* **2022**, *24*, 93–103. [CrossRef]
18. Lehrke, M.; Greif, M.; Broedl, U.C.; Lebherz, C.; Laubender, R.P.; Becker, A.; von Ziegler, F.; Tittus, J.; Reiser, M.; Becker, C.; et al. MMP-1 Serum Levels Predict Coronary Atherosclerosis in Humans. *Cardiovasc. Diabetol.* **2009**, *8*, 50. [CrossRef]
19. Reddy, S.; Hu, D.-Q.; Zhao, M.; Ichimura, S.; Barnes, E.A.; Cornfield, D.N.; Alejandre Alcázar, M.A.; Spiekerkoetter, E.; Fajardo, G.; Bernstein, D. MicroRNA-34a-Dependent Attenuation of Angiogenesis in Right Ventricular Failure. *J. Am. Heart Assoc.* **2024**, *13*, e029427. [CrossRef]
20. Li, Q.; Kim, Y.-R.; Vikram, A.; Kumar, S.; Kassan, M.; Gabani, M.; Lee, S.K.; Jacobs, J.S.; Irani, K. P66Shc-Induced MicroRNA-34a Causes Diabetic Endothelial Dysfunction by Downregulating Sirtuin1. *Arterioscler. Thromb. Vasc. Biol.* **2016**, *36*, 2394–2403. [CrossRef]
21. Wu, J.; Liang, W.; Tian, Y.; Ma, F.; Huang, W.; Jia, Y.; Jiang, Z.; Wu, H. Inhibition of P53/MiR-34a Improves Diabetic Endothelial Dysfunction via Activation of SIRT1. *J. Cell Mol. Med.* **2019**, *23*, 3538–3548. [CrossRef] [PubMed]
22. Wu, S.; Sun, H.; Sun, B. MicroRNA-145 Is Involved in Endothelial Cell Dysfunction and Acts as a Promising Biomarker of Acute Coronary Syndrome. *Eur. J. Med. Res.* **2020**, *25*, 2. [CrossRef] [PubMed]
23. Qin, B.; Cao, Y.; Yang, H.; Xiao, B.; Lu, Z. MicroRNA-221/222 Regulate Ox-LDL-Induced Endothelial Apoptosis via Ets-1/P21 Inhibition. *Mol. Cell Biochem.* **2015**, *405*, 115–124. [CrossRef] [PubMed]
24. Iusupova, A.O.; Pakhtusov, N.N.; Slepova, O.A.; Belenkov, Y.N.; Privalova, E.V.; Bure, I.V.; Vetchinkina, E.A.; Nemtsova, M.V. MiRNA-21a, MiRNA-145, and MiRNA-221 Expression and Their Correlations with WNT Proteins in Patients with Obstructive and Non-Obstructive Coronary Artery Disease. *Int. J. Mol. Sci.* **2023**, *24*, 7613. [CrossRef] [PubMed]
25. Couffinhal, T.; Kearney, M.; Witzenbichler, B.; Chen, D.; Murohara, T.; Losordo, D.W.; Symes, J.; Isner, J.M. Vascular Endothelial Growth Factor/Vascular Permeability Factor (VEGF/VPF) in Normal and Atherosclerotic Human Arteries. *Am. J. Pathol.* **1997**, *150*, 1673–1685.
26. Mao, Y.; Liu, X.Q.; Song, Y.; Zhai, C.G.; Xu, X.L.; Zhang, L.; Zhang, Y. Fibroblast Growth Factor-2/Platelet-Derived Growth Factor Enhances Atherosclerotic Plaque Stability. *J. Cell Mol. Med.* **2020**, *24*, 1128–1140. [CrossRef]
27. Bartkowiak, K.; Bartkowiak, M.; Jankowska-Steifer, E.; Ratajska, A.; Kujawa, M.; Aniołek, O.; Niderla-Bielińska, J. Metabolic Syndrome and Cardiac Vessel Remodeling Associated with Vessel Rarefaction: A Possible Underlying Mechanism May Result from a Poor Angiogenic Response to Altered VEGF Signaling Pathways. *J. Vasc. Res.* **2024**, *61*, 151–159. [CrossRef]

28. Zhao, Q.; Egashira, K.; Inoue, S.; Usui, M.; Kitamoto, S.; Ni, W.; Ishibashi, M.; Hiasa Ki, K.; Ichiki, T.; Shibuya, M.; et al. Vascular Endothelial Growth Factor Is Necessary in the Development of Arteriosclerosis by Recruiting/Activating Monocytes in a Rat Model of Long-Term Inhibition of Nitric Oxide Synthesis. *Circulation* **2002**, *105*, 1110–1115. [CrossRef]
29. Bonanni, A.; d'Aiello, A.; Pedicino, D.; Di Sario, M.; Vinci, R.; Ponzo, M.; Ciampi, P.; Lo Curto, D.; Conte, C.; Cribari, F.; et al. Molecular Hallmarks of Ischemia with Non-Obstructive Coronary Arteries: The "INOCA versus Obstructive CCS" Challenge. *J. Clin. Med.* **2022**, *11*, 1711. [CrossRef]
30. Pufe, T.; Harde, V.; Petersen, W.; Goldring, M.B.; Tillmann, B.; Mentlein, R. Vascular Endothelial Growth Factor (VEGF) Induces Matrix Metalloproteinase Expression in Immortalized Chondrocytes. *J. Pathol.* **2004**, *202*, 367–374. [CrossRef]
31. Quillard, T.; Tesmenitsky, Y.; Croce, K.; Travers, R.; Shvartz, E.; Koskinas, K.C.; Sukhova, G.K.; Aikawa, E.; Aikawa, M.; Libby, P. Selective Inhibition of Matrix Metalloproteinase-13 Increases Collagen Content of Established Mouse Atherosclerosis. *Arterioscler. Thromb. Vasc. Biol.* **2011**, *31*, 2464–2472. [CrossRef] [PubMed]
32. Gaubatz, J.W.; Ballantyne, C.M.; Wasserman, B.A.; He, M.; Chambless, L.E.; Boerwinkle, E.; Hoogeveen, R.C. Association of Circulating Matrix Metalloproteinases with Carotid Artery Characteristics: The Atherosclerosis Risk in Communities Carotid MRI Study. *Arterioscler. Thromb. Vasc. Biol.* **2010**, *30*, 1034–1042. [CrossRef] [PubMed]
33. Polonskaya, Y.V.; Kashtanova, E.V.; Murashov, I.S.; Striukova, E.V.; Kurguzov, A.V.; Stakhneva, E.M.; Shramko, V.S.; Maslatsov, N.A.; Chernyavsky, A.M.; Ragino, Y.I. Association of Matrix Metalloproteinases with Coronary Artery Calcification in Patients with CHD. *J. Pers. Med.* **2021**, *11*, 506. [CrossRef] [PubMed]
34. Tarín, C.; Gomez, M.; Calvo, E.; López, J.A.; Zaragoza, C. Endothelial Nitric Oxide Deficiency Reduces MMP-13-Mediated Cleavage of ICAM-1 in Vascular Endothelium: A Role in Atherosclerosis. *Arterioscler. Thromb. Vasc. Biol.* **2009**, *29*, 27–32. [CrossRef] [PubMed]
35. Deguchi, J.-O.; Aikawa, E.; Libby, P.; Vachon, J.R.; Inada, M.; Krane, S.M.; Whittaker, P.; Aikawa, M. Matrix Metalloproteinase-13/Collagenase-3 Deletion Promotes Collagen Accumulation and Organization in Mouse Atherosclerotic Plaques. *Circulation* **2005**, *112*, 2708–2715. [CrossRef]
36. Melin, E.O.; Dereke, J.; Hillman, M. Galectin-3, Metalloproteinase-2 and Cardiovascular Disease Were Independently Associated with Metalloproteinase-14 in Patients with Type 1 Diabetes: A Cross Sectional Study. *Diabetol. Metab. Syndr.* **2021**, *13*, 118. [CrossRef]
37. Johnson, J.L.; Jenkins, N.P.; Huang, W.-C.; Di Gregoli, K.; Sala-Newby, G.B.; Scholtes, V.P.W.; Moll, F.L.; Pasterkamp, G.; Newby, A.C. Relationship of MMP-14 and TIMP-3 Expression with Macrophage Activation and Human Atherosclerotic Plaque Vulnerability. *Mediators Inflamm.* **2014**, *2014*, 276457. [CrossRef]
38. Lu, Y.; Thavarajah, T.; Gu, W.; Cai, J.; Xu, Q. Impact of MiRNA in Atherosclerosis. *Arterioscler. Thromb. Vasc. Biol.* **2018**, *38*, e159–e170. [CrossRef]
39. Yuan, M.; Zhang, L.; You, F.; Zhou, J.; Ma, Y.; Yang, F.; Tao, L. MiR-145-5p Regulates Hypoxia-Induced Inflammatory Response and Apoptosis in Cardiomyocytes by Targeting CD40. *Mol. Cell Biochem.* **2017**, *431*, 123–131. [CrossRef]
40. Zhang, X.; Zai, L.; Tao, Z.; Wu, D.; Lin, M.; Wan, J. MiR-145-5p Affects Autophagy by Targeting CaMKIIδ in Atherosclerosis. *Int. J. Cardiol.* **2022**, *360*, 68–75. [CrossRef]
41. Kumar, A.; Priyadarshini, G.; Parameswaran, S.; Ramesh, A.; Rajappa, M. Evaluation of MicroRNA 145 and MicroRNA 155 as Markers of Cardiovascular Risk in Chronic Kidney Disease. *Cureus* **2024**, *16*, e66494. [CrossRef] [PubMed]
42. Gatsiou, A.; Georgiopoulos, G.; Vlachogiannis, N.I.; Pfisterer, L.; Fischer, A.; Sachse, M.; Laina, A.; Bonini, F.; Delialis, D.; Tual-Chalot, S.; et al. Additive Contribution of MicroRNA-34a/b/c to Human Arterial Ageing and Atherosclerosis. *Atherosclerosis* **2021**, *327*, 49–58. [CrossRef]
43. Raitoharju, E.; Lyytikäinen, L.-P.; Levula, M.; Oksala, N.; Mennander, A.; Tarkka, M.; Klopp, N.; Illig, T.; Kähönen, M.; Karhunen, P.J.; et al. MiR-21, MiR-210, MiR-34a, and MiR-146a/b Are up-Regulated in Human Atherosclerotic Plaques in the Tampere Vascular Study. *Atherosclerosis* **2011**, *219*, 211–217. [CrossRef]
44. Han, H.; Qu, G.; Han, C.; Wang, Y.; Sun, T.; Li, F.; Wang, J.; Luo, S. MiR-34a, MiR-21 and MiR-23a as Potential Biomarkers for Coronary Artery Disease: A Pilot Microarray Study and Confirmation in a 32 Patient Cohort. *Exp. Mol. Med.* **2015**, *47*, e138. [CrossRef] [PubMed]
45. Zhu, N.; Zhang, D.; Chen, S.; Liu, X.; Lin, L.; Huang, X.; Guo, Z.; Liu, J.; Wang, Y.; Yuan, W.; et al. Endothelial Enriched MicroRNAs Regulate Angiotensin II-Induced Endothelial Inflammation and Migration. *Atherosclerosis* **2011**, *215*, 286–293. [CrossRef]
46. Xue, Y.; Wei, Z.; Ding, H.; Wang, Q.; Zhou, Z.; Zheng, S.; Zhang, Y.; Hou, D.; Liu, Y.; Zen, K.; et al. MicroRNA-19b/221/222 Induces Endothelial Cell Dysfunction via Suppression of PGC-1α in the Progression of Atherosclerosis. *Atherosclerosis* **2015**, *241*, 671–681. [CrossRef]
47. Laffont, B.; Rayner, K.J. MicroRNAs in the Pathobiology and Therapy of Atherosclerosis. *Can. J. Cardiol.* **2017**, *33*, 313–324. [CrossRef]
48. Karere, G.M.; Glenn, J.P.; Li, G.; Konar, A.; VandeBerg, J.L.; Cox, L.A. Potential MiRNA Biomarkers and Therapeutic Targets for Early Atherosclerotic Lesions. *Sci. Rep.* **2023**, *13*, 3467. [CrossRef]
49. Faccini, J.; Ruidavets, J.-B.; Cordelier, P.; Martins, F.; Maoret, J.-J.; Bongard, V.; Ferrières, J.; Roncalli, J.; Elbaz, M.; Vindis, C. Circulating MiR-155, MiR-145 and Let-7c as Diagnostic Biomarkers of the Coronary Artery Disease. *Sci. Rep.* **2017**, *7*, 42916. [CrossRef]

50. John, F.O.; Neylon, A.; McGorrian, C.; Blake, G.J. MiRNA-93-5p and Other MiRNAs as Predictors of Coronary Artery Disease and STEMI. *Int. J. Cardiol.* **2016**, *224*, 310–316. [CrossRef]
51. Zhang, L.; Zhang, Y.; Xue, S.; Ding, H.; Wang, Y.; Qi, H.; Wang, Y.; Zhu, W.; Li, P. Clinical Significance of Circulating MicroRNAs as Diagnostic Biomarkers for Coronary Artery Disease. *J. Cell Mol. Med.* **2020**, *24*, 1146–1150. [CrossRef] [PubMed]
52. Saavedra, N.; Rojas, G.; Herrera, J.; Rebolledo, C.; Ruedlinger, J.; Bustos, L.; Bobadilla, B.; Pérez, L.; Saavedra, K.; Zambrano, T.; et al. Circulating MiRNA-23b and MiRNA-143 Are Potential Biomarkers for In-Stent Restenosis. *Biomed. Res. Int.* **2020**, *2020*, 2509039. [CrossRef] [PubMed]
53. Gholipour, A.; Zahedmehr, A.; Arabian, M.; Shakerian, F.; Maleki, M.; Oveisee, M.; Malakootian, M. MiR-6721-5p as a Natural Regulator of Meta-VCL Is Upregulated in the Serum of Patients with Coronary Artery Disease. *Noncoding RNA Res.* **2025**, *10*, 25–34. [CrossRef] [PubMed]
54. Busk, P.K. A Tool for Design of Primers for MicroRNA-Specific Quantitative RT-QPCR. *BMC Bioinform.* **2014**, *15*, 29. [CrossRef]

International Journal of
Molecular Sciences

Review

The Role of Cilostazol, a Phosphodiesterase-3 Inhibitor, in the Development of Atherosclerosis and Vascular Biology: A Review with Meta-Analysis

Minji Sohn and Soo Lim *

Department of Internal Medicine, Seoul National University Bundang Hospital, Seoul National University College of Medicine, Seongnam 13620, Republic of Korea; rainbowmjs@naver.com
* Correspondence: limsoo@snu.ac.kr

Abstract: Atherosclerotic cardiovascular disease (ASCVD) stands as the leading global cause of mortality. Addressing this vital and pervasive condition requires a multifaceted approach, in which antiplatelet intervention plays a pivotal role, together with antihypertensive, antidiabetic, and lipid-lowering therapies. Among the antiplatelet agents available currently, cilostazol, a phosphodiesterase-3 inhibitor, offers a spectrum of pharmacological effects. These encompass vasodilation, the impediment of platelet activation and aggregation, thrombosis inhibition, limb blood flow augmentation, lipid profile enhancement through triglyceride reduction and high-density lipoprotein cholesterol elevation, and the suppression of vascular smooth muscle cell proliferation. However, the role of cilostazol has not been clearly documented in many guidelines for ASCVD. We comprehensively reviewed the cardiovascular effects of cilostazol within randomized clinical trials that compared it to control or active agents and involved individuals with previous coronary artery disease or stroke, as well as those with no previous history of such conditions. Our approach demonstrated that the administration of cilostazol effectively reduced adverse cardiovascular events, although there was less evidence regarding its impact on myocardial infarction. Most studies have consistently reported its favorable effects in reducing intermittent claudication and enhancing ambulatory capacity in patients with peripheral arterial disease. Furthermore, cilostazol has shown promise in mitigating restenosis following coronary stent implantation in patients with acute coronary syndrome. While research from more diverse regions is still needed, our findings shed light on the broader implications of cilostazol in the context of atherosclerosis and vascular biology, particularly for individuals at high risk of ASCVD.

Keywords: atherosclerosis; cardiovascular diseases; cilostazol; platelet aggregation inhibitors; aspirin

1. Introduction

Cardiovascular diseases (CVDs) [1], including coronary artery disease (CAD), cerebrovascular disease, and peripheral artery disease (PAD), are a significant global public health problem [1,2]. Ischemic heart disease is the most common cause of death worldwide [3]. Moreover, cerebrovascular diseases are more prevalent among Asian ethnicities, thus becoming a top priority for intervention. Since 2015, stroke has become the leading cause of death and disability in China, posing a significant public health threat [4]. Atherosclerosis in peripheral arteries is characterized by stenosis or the occlusion of the arteries that supply blood to the lower limbs, resulting in symptoms such as intermittent claudication and ulceration [2]. PAD is also related to a high risk of atherosclerotic cardiovascular disease ASCVD, including myocardial infarction, stroke, and renovascular disease [5]. About 1–3% patients with intermittent claudication exhibit progression to severe limb-related complications within 5 years, which may necessitate limb amputation and result in premature death [5].

These vascular diseases are mainly caused by atherosclerosis, which starts with the development of fibrofatty lesions known as atherosclerotic plaques. Several mechanisms are involved in this process: the accumulation of modified low-density lipoprotein (LDL) in the intima, the attraction of pro-inflammatory monocytes and T lymphocytes to the arterial wall, the proliferation and migration of vascular smooth muscle cells (VSMCs), the aggravation of oxidative stress and the increase in adhesion molecules, and the aggregation of platelets [1]. The rupture of the fibrous cap in an atherosclerotic plaque can result in the development of a life-threatening ASCVD, such as myocardial infarction and stroke, both of which can also lead to various complications that significantly impact the patient's quality of life [6,7]. Furthermore, ASCVD is commonly asymptomatic up until the occurrence of acute coronary syndrome or stroke [8]. Therefore, preventive measures and early interventions aimed at reducing the risk of these conditions are crucial.

Type 2 diabetes mellitus (T2DM) is closely linked to an increased risk of CAD and cerebrovascular disease. Patients with T2DM have a 2–4-fold higher CVD risk compared to that of the general population, regardless of the presence/absence of other risk factors [9]. Thus, diabetes mellitus is regarded as being equivalent to the risk of CAD. Furthermore, ASCVD is the principal cause of death and disability among patients with diabetes mellitus [10]. Diabetes mellitus is characterized by insulin resistance, dyslipidemia, inflammation, and hypercoagulability, which exacerbate the underlying causes of atherosclerosis and heart failure [11]. To date, the cardiovascular benefit of multifactorial risk-reduction approaches using antidiabetic agents, antihypertensive drugs, and lipid-lowering therapy has been proven, thus reducing the incidence of cardiovascular complications [12]. However, the current therapeutic strategies are not sufficient for preventing adverse cardiovascular events, and a substantial number of patients with diabetes mellitus still face a risk of CVD, leading to the term "residual risk" [12].

For the management of the residual risk, international guidelines from the USA and Europe recommend the use of antiplatelet agents as a main management strategy in patients with diabetes and a high CVD risk [13,14]. Hence, antiplatelet agents such as aspirin, clopidogrel, and cilostazol could be contemplated in the management of the residual risk, pending additional supportive evidence.

Cilostazol is an antiplatelet agent that inhibits phosphodiesterase-3 (PDE-3) and increases cyclic adenosine monophosphate (cAMP) concentrations, leading to the inhibition of platelet aggregation and thrombus formation [15]. PDE-3 is expressed in cell populations such as platelets, VSMCs, cardiac myocytes, and adipocytes [16]. Therefore, cilostazol is expected to have some effects in these tissues.

Cilostazol has been approved for improving intermittent claudication symptoms in various countries. In further research, cilostazol treatment reduced the progression of atherosclerosis in patients with carotid artery stenosis [17,18] and the recurrence of stroke in patients with cerebrovascular disease [19,20]. In addition, previous studies have shown that cilostazol therapy is beneficial for CAD when administered immediately after percutaneous coronary intervention or in addition to other antiplatelet agents [21,22].

In 2015, a critical review of the literature regarding cilostazol and its role against CVD was reported [23]. Since then, many basic and clinical studies have been published; however, its role has not been reviewed systematically. Moreover, cilostazol has not been well documented in the literature with regard to its role in CVD and diabetes mellitus. In this review, we discuss the mechanism of action of cilostazol and evaluate the efficacy and safety of the drug based on the results of clinical trials. Furthermore, we comprehensively explore the role of cilostazol in the prevention and treatment of atherosclerosis.

2. Limitations of Aspirin Therapy for Atherosclerotic CVD

Aspirin, which inhibits COX-1 and prevents the formation of thromboxane, thereby exerting antiplatelet effects, remains the most commonly used antiplatelet agent [24]. Recently, controversy has arisen regarding the effectiveness of aspirin in the primary prevention of CVD. Both Asian and European studies that investigated the primary preventive effect of aspirin for CVD in patients with T2DM reported an absence of significant differences in the incidence of CVD between the aspirin treatment group and the non-aspirin group [25,26]. A meta-analysis of several clinical studies in which aspirin was administered for the primary prevention of CVD also showed that aspirin did not reduce the incidence of CVD in patients with diabetes [27]. The six-year follow-up of the primary preventive effect of aspirin against CVD in more than 14,000 Japanese elderly patients also failed to demonstrate the beneficial effect of aspirin on the incidence of CVD [28].

Moreover, it was reported that the use of aspirin not only increased the number of adverse events, such as major bleeding and gastrointestinal discomfort, but also did not reduce the risk of cardiovascular events in primary prevention (Table 1) [25,26,28–34].

There is some evidence from basic studies suggesting that aspirin might not be sufficient to reduce abnormal platelet activation. The platelet multidrug resistance protein 4 (MRP4) is upregulated after aspirin administration, which could represent one of the mechanisms underlying the high residual platelet reactivity after aspirin intake [35]. Importantly, patients with persistent high platelet reactivity while on aspirin therapy exhibited an increased risk of recurrent cardiovascular events [36].

Based on these findings, the role of aspirin in this context has changed drastically since 2018. The US Preventive Services Task Force did not recommend the initiation of low-dose aspirin among patients aged 60 years or older [37]. The American Heart Association (AHA) and American College of Cardiology (ACC) Foundation's statement on aspirin for the primary prevention of cardiovascular events in individuals with diabetes suggests that low-dose aspirin should not be administered to those with a low risk for ASCVD (10-year risk < 5%), but can be considered in patients with an increased cardiovascular risk (10-year risk > 10%) [38,39]. Unfortunately, no direct evidence from a clinical trial supports these risk-based treatment recommendations, resulting in controversy in the primary prevention among patients with a high CVD risk. Moreover, the primary preventive effect of aspirin was not clearly demonstrated, even for high-risk patients, such as those with T2DM (Table 1).

In contrast, the guidelines for the secondary prevention of diabetes recommend aspirin therapy (75–162 mg daily) for individuals with diabetes and a history of ASCVD [13]. Nevertheless, concerns regarding the side effects of this therapy remain unaddressed. In the Aspirin in Reducing Events in the Elderly (ASPREE) study, cancer-related death occurred in 3.1% of the participants in the aspirin group and in 2.3% of those in the placebo group (hazard ratio: 1.31; 95% confidence interval (CI): 1.10–1.56), indicating a higher cancer mortality rate in the aspirin therapy compared with that of the placebo group [33]. Although the risk of cancer development was not confirmed in other studies (Table 1), concerns regarding this issue remain.

Table 1. Randomized controlled studies with aspirin for preventing primary cardiovascular events since 2000.

Bibliographic Information	Trial Information *				Patient's Characteristics	Efficacy and Safety Outcomes		
	Population	Duration **	Patients' Number	Men (%)/Age (Years)	Diabetes Comorbidity	Cardiovascular Events ***	Bleeding Risks	Cancer Risks
PPP study [29]	Participants with at least one already known major cardiovascular risk factor	5 years	4495	42.5/64.4	16.5%	RR of 3P-MACE [a] with aspirin vs. no-aspirin: 0.71 (0.48–1.04)	Severe bleedings more frequent in the aspirin group (1.1% vs. 0.3%; $p <$ 0.0008)	No difference in cancer risks with aspirin vs. no-aspirin (3.9% vs. 3.5%)
WHS study [30]	Female health professionals, aged ≥45 and without a history of cardiovascular disease or cancer	mean 10.1 years	39,876	0/54.6	2.6%	RR of 3P-MACE [a] with aspirin vs. placebo: 0.91 (0.80–1.03)	Any gastrointestinal bleeding: RR 1.22 (1.10–1.34) Requiring transfusion: RR 1.40 (1.07–1.83)	Not reported
JPAD study [25]	Patients with type 2 diabetes	mean 4.37 years	2539	54.6/64	100%	HR of atherosclerotic events [b] with aspirin vs. no-aspirin: 0.80 (0.58–1.10)	No difference in significant gastrointestinal bleeding with aspirin vs. no-aspirin (1.0% vs. 0.3%)	Not reported
POPADAD study [26]	Participants aged ≥40 with type 1 or type 2 diabetes and an ankle brachial pressure index of 0.99 or less but no symptomatic cardiovascular disease	median 6.7 years (4.5~8.6 years)	1276	44.1/60.3	100%	No difference in atherosclerotic events [c] with aspirin vs. no-aspirin: 0.98 (0.76–1.26)	No difference in gastrointestinal bleeding with aspirin vs. no-aspirin: 0.90 (0.53–1.52)	No difference in malignancy with aspirin vs. placebo (8.3% vs. 10.7%)
JPPP study [28]	Participants aged 60 to 85 years, presenting with hypertension, dyslipidemia, or diabetes mellitus without cardiovascular disease	6 years (median 5.02 years)	14,658	42.3/70.5	33.9%	HR of 3P-MACE [a] with aspirin vs. no-aspirin: 0.94 (0.77–1.15)	Major gastrointestinal and extracranial bleedings more frequent in the aspirin group (0.1% vs. 0.07%; $p < 0.001$)	Not reported

Table 1. *Cont.*

Bibliographic Information	Trial Information *				Patient's Characteristics	Efficacy and Safety Outcomes		
	Population	Duration **	Patients' Number	Men (%)/Age (Years)	Diabetes Comorbidity	Cardiovascular Events ***	Bleeding Risks	Cancer Risks
ASCEND study [31]	Patients with type 2 diabetes without cardiovascular disease	at least 7 years (mean 7.4 years)	15,480	62.6/63.3	100%	RR of serious vascular events [d] with aspirin vs. placebo: 0.88 (0.79–0.97)	RR of any major bleeding: 1.29 (1.09–1.52)	RR of any cancer: 1.01 (0.92–1.11)
ARRIVE study [32]	Participants aged ≥55 years (men) or ≥60 years (women) and had moderate cardiovascular risk, without at high risk of bleeding or diabetes	6 years (mean 5 years)	12,546	70.4/63.9	0%	HR of 3P-MACE [a] with aspirin vs. no-aspirin: 0.79 (0.61–1.02)	HR of gastrointestinal bleeding: 2.11 (1.39–3.28)	No difference in cancer with aspirin vs. placebo (not sufficient events)
ASPREE study [33]	Elderly participants who did not have cardiovascular disease, dementia, or disability	6 years (median 4.7 years)	19,114	43.6/median 74	10.8	HR of ischemic events-related deaths with aspirin vs. placebo: 0.82 (0.62–1.08)	HR of major hemorrhage-related deaths with aspirin vs. placebo: 1.13 (0.66–1.94)	HR of cancer-related deaths with aspirin vs. placebo: 1.31 (1.10–1.56)
Yusuf S. et al., 2021 [34]	Participants without cardiovascular disease who had an elevated INTERHEART Risk Score	6 years (mean 4.6 years)	5713	47.1/63.9	36.7%	HR of 3P-MACE [a] by aspirin vs. placebo: 0.86 (0.67–1.10)	No difference in major bleeding with aspirin vs. placebo (1.5% vs. 1.3%)	HR of cancer with aspirin vs. placebo: 0.83 (0.54–1.27)

Abbreviations: 3P-MACE, 3-point major adverse cardiovascular events; HR, hazard ratio; and RR, risk ratio. * Aspirin (100 mg) was compared to placebo or control therapy. ** Study drug was administered during the whole study period. *** Definition of cardiovascular events were different between the groups: [a] 3P-MACE: cardiovascular death, non-fatal, myocardial infarction, and stroke. [b] Composite of sudden death; death from coronary, cerebrovascular, and aortic causes; non-fatal acute myocardial infarction; unstable angina; newly developed exertional angina; nonfatal ischemic and hemorrhagic stroke; transient ischemic attack; or nonfatal aortic and peripheral vascular disease (arteriosclerosis obliterans, aortic dissection, mesenteric arterial thrombosis). [c] Death from coronary heart disease or stroke, non-fatal myocardial infarction or stroke, or above ankle amputation for critical limb ischemia. [d] Composite of nonfatal myocardial infarction, nonfatal stroke (excluding confirmed intracranial hemorrhage) or transient ischemic attack, or death from any vascular cause (excluding confirmed intracranial hemorrhage).

3. Beneficial Role of Cilostazol in the Development of Atherosclerosis

3.1. Antiplatelet Activity

Cilostazol inhibits platelet function by inhibiting PDE-3 and increasing cAMP levels [40] (Figure 1). Platelet reactivity is mediated by the intracellular calcium levels, which induce a molecular cascade including cAMP, resulting in platelet degranulation, conformational changes, and aggregation [41]. Elevated cAMP levels upregulate the activity of protein kinase A (PKA), which phosphorylates key intermediary molecules that are essential for platelet aggregation [42]. PKA has also been tied to the downregulation of platelet adhesion through the phosphorylation of the GP-Ib-IX complex, the inhibition of intracellular calcium store release, thromboxane receptor desensitization, and the inhibition of the phosphorylation of myosin light chain kinase [43].

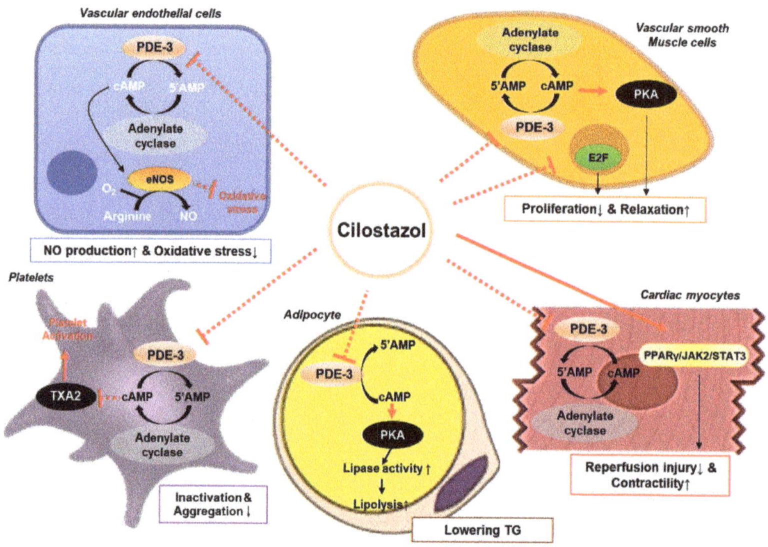

Figure 1. Mechanisms of action of cilostazol. Cilostazol inhibits phosphodiesterase-3 in various cell types including platelets, vascular cells, myocytes, and adipocytes, which affects several pathways resulting in vasodilation and enhanced blood perfusion. Cilostazol induces nitric oxide (NO) release from endothelial cells and activates calcium-dependent potassium channels in vascular smooth muscle cells, leading to vasodilation. This action leads to the upregulation of the protein kinase A (PKA), and eventually causing arterial dilatation and platelet inactivation. Furthermore, cilostazol attenuates the activation of platelets, thus facilitating blood perfusion. Abbreviations: 5′AMP, 5′-adenosine monophosphate; cAMP, cyclic adenosine monophosphate; eNOS, endothelial nitric oxide synthase; JAK2, Janus kinase 2; PDE-3, phosphodiesterase-3; PKA, protein kinase A; PPARγ, peroxisome proliferator-activated receptor gamma; STAT3, signal transducer and activator of transcription 3; TG, triglycerides; and TXA2, thromboxane A2.

Recent evidence has suggested a role for cilostazol in the inhibition of MRP4 [44] and in overcoming a high on-aspirin-treatment residual platelet reactivity in a cAMP-independent manner [45]. MRP4, which is expressed in platelets primarily in the membranes of dense granules [46], promotes platelet aggregation by transporting cyclic nucleotides, including cAMP and cGMP, outside of platelets [47]. MRP4 has also been shown to desensitize platelets to the inhibitory effects of endothelial-derived nitric oxide and sensitize them to ADP-mediated activation [44]. Thus, the inactivation of MRP4 and the inhibition of phosphodiesterase-4 by cilostazol are reported to have synergistic and potent therapeutic antiplatelet effects [46].

The clinical findings of decreased platelet reactivity after cilostazol treatment have been described in various populations, including patients with acute coronary syndrome and ischemic stroke [40,48], and even when administered in addition to aspirin and clopidogrel [49]. Cilostazol is likely to be more effective in inhibiting platelet activation, especially in patients with diabetes mellitus. Platelets themselves have insulin receptors which, when activated, initiate a molecular cascade, leading to increased cAMP levels and platelet inhibition [50]. Insulin resistance is associated with an attenuated P2Y1 response caused by low cAMP levels, which may explain the observation that patients with T2DM are at an increased risk of thrombosis [50]. Another study further established a relatively higher degree of platelet inhibition by cilostazol in patients with diabetes compared with those without this condition [51].

3.2. Increase in Nitric Oxide Secretion

Cilostazol has a potent vasodilatory effect. Cilostazol treatment leads to PKA phosphorylation and the activation of endothelial nitric oxide synthase (eNOS), which increases nitric oxide levels [52]. The vasodilatory effect of cilostazol therapy includes the PKA-mediated phosphorylation of G-protein-coupled receptor kinase 2, the inactivation of G-alpha-q-mediated signaling, and the hyperpolarization of smooth muscle cell membranes through the potentiation of calcium-activated potassium currents [53,54].

Because of its PDE-3-inhibitory function, cilostazol administration resulted in the accumulation of cAMP, thus inducing vasodilation [55]. This process was mediated by the cAMP-dependent secretion of nitrogen oxide (NO) by vascular endothelial cells [56]. The other signaling pathway is endothelium-independent and involves the direct effect of cilostazol on VSMCs. cAMP build-up in these cells induces the PKA-dependent activation of the calcium-dependent potassium channel, leading to vasorelaxation [57]. In addition, cilostazol was shown to inhibit cGMP-specific PDE or PDE-5 [58], which may contribute to its vasorelaxant properties by promoting the accumulation of cGMP in VSMCs [58]. Furthermore, cilostazol treatment attenuated adenosine uptake by several types of cells, thereby leading to adenosine build-up in the interstitial fluid and vascular circulation [59]. The increase in extracellular adenosine potentiates adenosine receptor A2 activity in endothelial cells, causing arterial dilatation [60].

3.3. Antiproliferative Activity, Including Alterations in Adhesion Molecules

Cilostazol exhibited an antiproliferative effect on the vasculature by reducing neointima formation in animal models [61,62]. This antiproliferative effect of cilostazol is likely mediated by its effects on cAMP elevation and PKA inhibition, which are responsible for the decrease in the transcription of genes encoding cellular adhesion molecules and the proliferation of VSMCs [63] (Figure 1). The administration of cilostazol also decreased the levels of the vascular cell adhesion molecule, intercellular adhesion molecule, and E-selectin [64,65]. A decrease in the expression of these cellular adhesion molecules disrupts neointimal proliferation through the reduction in inflammatory cell invasion into the damaged intima [66]. In addition, cilostazol therapy downregulates growth factors, such as the vascular endothelial growth factor and platelet-derived growth factor [62,65]. Furthermore, cilostazol plays a favorable role in the transition to smooth muscle cells from a de-differentiated state [67].

3.4. Improvement in Vascular Endothelial Function

Cilostazol has beneficial effects on endothelial function, which is linked to NO production (Figure 1). Cilostazol treatment increased cAMP levels in endothelial cells, which led to NO production [68]. In aged Wistar rats, endothelial dysfunction was restored by cilostazol treatment [69]. This protective effect of cilostazol could be attributed to its favorable actions on arterial walls, including a reduction in oxidative stress and an increase in NO bioavailability [69]. Another study proved that cilostazol treatment decreased intimal thickening and improved the vasodilation capacity [70]. Cilostazol stimulates the production of hepatocyte growth factor, which is known for its favorable role in attenuating the malformation and apoptosis of endothelial cells [71].

Also, in a clinical setting, a three-month intervention using cilostazol improved endothelial function, as measured by flow-mediated dilation, compared with aspirin in patients with stroke (1.0% vs. 0.8%) [72]. Moreover, a six-month treatment with cilostazol improved vasomotor reactivity, as evidenced by an increase in the coronary luminal diameter following the administration of N-monomethyl-L-arginine [73].

3.5. Anti-Inflammatory Effect

In an animal study, cilostazol deactivated the nucleotide-binding domain-like receptor protein 3 (NLRP3) inflammasome [74], which is associated with atherosclerosis and CVD [75,76]. This anti-inflammatory potential was mediated by the downregulation of p65 NF-κB and the enhancement of sirtuin-1, leading to the downregulation of NLRP3, an apoptosis-associated speck-like protein, active caspase-1, and interleukin-1β [74]. In an animal study of hypercholesterolemic rats, cilostazol treatment protected against hypercholesterolemia-induced cardiac damage via molecular mechanisms targeting the crosstalk between Nrf2 induction and NF-κB inhibition in the heart [77]. Another study using the mouse models of myocardial ischemia–reperfusion showed that cilostazol treatment attenuated multiple inflammatory markers through the activation of the peroxisome proliferator-activated receptor-γ (PPARγ), Janus kinase 2 (JAK2), and the signal transducer and activator of transcription 3 (STAT3) pathways [78].

Similar findings were obtained in human studies. In a randomized controlled trial (RCT), treatment with cilostazol (100 mg twice daily) significantly decreased the hsCRP levels by 23.6%, erythrocyte sedimentation rate by 38.7%, and plasma malondialdehyde concentration by 17.6% [79]. Our group also found that treatment with cilostazol (200 mg once daily) decreased hsCRP levels significantly compared with aspirin in patients with T2DM and coronary artery stenosis [80]. It is suggested that the greater anti-inflammatory potency of cilostazol, when added to the standard dual antiplatelet therapy of aspirin and clopidogrel, may have contributed to the inhibition of the progression of carotid intima–media thickness, without raising the risk of hemorrhage [81]. These data are indicative of the deactivation of inflammation by cilostazol therapy.

3.6. Antioxidative Stress Effect

Cilostazol treatment is related to the activation of endothelial nitric oxide synthase (eNOS), which is implicated in the maintenance of endothelial function and the reduction in superoxide-radical-induced injury [52]. Cilostazol upregulates eNOS activity through multiple pathways. The inhibition of adenosine reuptake increases the activation of an adenosine-mediated signaling mechanisms involving the "survival" kinase Akt, which subsequently activates eNOS via phosphorylation [52]. The cilostazol-mediated inhibition of the phosphatase and tensin homolog also upregulates phosphotadidylinositol-3-phosphate, which in turn activates Akt. The cAMP-mediated activation of PKA has also been shown to activate eNOS through phosphorylation at a site distinct from Akt [52].

Through these basic mechanisms, cilostazol has been shown to attenuate ischemia–reperfusion injury in models of myocardial, hepatic, and spinal cord reperfusion injury [82,83]. The administration of cilostazol prior to coronary occlusion and reperfusion was associated with a significantly smaller infarct size in a rabbit model compared with that of the controls [84].

Oxidative stress was also decreased in a clinical trial involving individuals with T2DM and hypertension [79]. Plasma malondialdehyde and blood glutathione markers were improved after a one-month treatment with cilostazol, indicating its potential antioxidative effects in humans [79].

3.7. Improvement in the Lipid Profile

Cilostazol seems to induce this favorable alteration in lipid metabolism through the upregulation of lipoprotein lipase in adipose tissue [85]. The administration of cilostazol increased lipolysis by inhibiting PDE-3 in adipocytes [86] (Figure 1). In an animal study, the administration of cilostazol enhanced LDL receptor-related protein 1 (LRP1) expression in the liver by activating PPARγ through the peroxisome proliferator-responsive elements present in the LRP1 promoter [87]. This upregulation of hepatic LRP1 may play an important role in improving HDL-cholesterol and triglycerides [88]. In the studies of animals fed with a high-cholesterol diet, the administration of cilostazol decreased the triglyceride and cholesterol content in the vascular system [89,90].

It Is noteworthy that the Increase In cAMP triggered by cilostazol treatment affects norepinephrine, thus increasing fat metabolism and exothermic reactions, and consequently increasing energy consumption. Cilostazol can increase uncoupling protein 1 (UCP1) in adipocytes [91]. Regulating the expression of UCP1 and PGC1α through cAMP-responsive element binding (CREB) and increasing free fatty acid release through lipolysis are used as fuel for thermogenesis in mitochondria [92].

Several clinical trials that examined the effects of cilostazol on lipid profiles have reported similar findings [80,93,94]. In these studies, the triglyceride levels decreased by 15–34% in patients with PAD or T2DM. In contrast, HDL-cholesterol was reported to increase by 7–20% [18]. Cilostazol therapy reduced the remnant lipoprotein level, which is associated with an increased risk of CVD [94]. Furthermore, cilostazol treatment reduced apolipoprotein B levels, which are an indirect indicator of LDL particle number [95]. These improvements in lipid profiles afforded by cilostazol therapy help prevent the development and progression of atherosclerosis.

4. Clinical Results of Cilostazol Treatment for Preventing Cardiovascular Events

4.1. Methods for Meta-Analysis of Major Adverse Cardiovascular Outcomes

For clinical interpretation, we systematically reviewed the effects of cilostazol on cardiovascular outcomes, as registered in PROSPERO CRD42023444959. We searched PubMed, Embase, and the Cochrane databases for English-language studies published up to July 2023. The search terms included keywords such as 'cilostazol' for the study intervention; 'major adverse cardiovascular event', 'cardiovascular disease', 'cardiovascular event', 'myocardial infarction', and 'stroke' for the outcomes; and 'randomized controlled trial' for the study design. The full list of search terms can be found in Supplementary Table S1. Using this process, we selected the studies to be included in the present analysis based on the following inclusion criteria: studies that (1) compared cilostazol with placebo, control, aspirin, or clopidogrel; (2) reported composite major adverse cardiovascular events (MACEs); and (3) were RCTs. We excluded studies with a follow-up duration of less than 3 months.

The primary outcome was MACE. Secondary outcomes Included individual cardiovascular events, such as fatal or non-fatal MI, fatal or non-fatal stroke, cardiovascular death, and all-cause mortality. Other adverse events, including major bleeding, discontinuation, headache, and palpitation, were also analyzed.

Study selection and data collection were confirmed by both authors. Logarithmic hazard ratios (HRs) were used to calculate combined estimates with a random-effects model. Random-effects risk ratios were calculated for studies that provided only the event numbers. The included trials were assessed for the risk of bias using the Cochrane Risk of Bias 2 tool (see Supplementary Figure S3). The I^2 statistic was employed to evaluate the overall heterogeneity of all comparisons. Publication bias was assessed using a funnel plot and Egger's test. Sensitivity analyses were performed focusing on the regions of the trials. The meta-analysis was conducted using the 'metafor' statistical package in R software (version 4.1.0; R Development Core Team, Vienna, Austria).

4.2. Meta-Analysis Results of Major Adverse Cardiovascular Outcomes

Out of 496 articles, 34 were selected [18,20,95–125] (Figure 2), with five trials targeting patients with diabetes (patients with diabetes included, ranging from 8.8% to 56.0% in non-targeted trials) (Table 2). A total of 29 studies were conducted for secondary prevention among patients suffering from CAD, stroke, or PAD. Cilostazol was concurrently used with aspirin in 19 studies, and as part of a triple regimen including aspirin and clopidogrel in 13 studies. The bias of the meta-analyses is reported in Supplementary Figures S2 and S3.

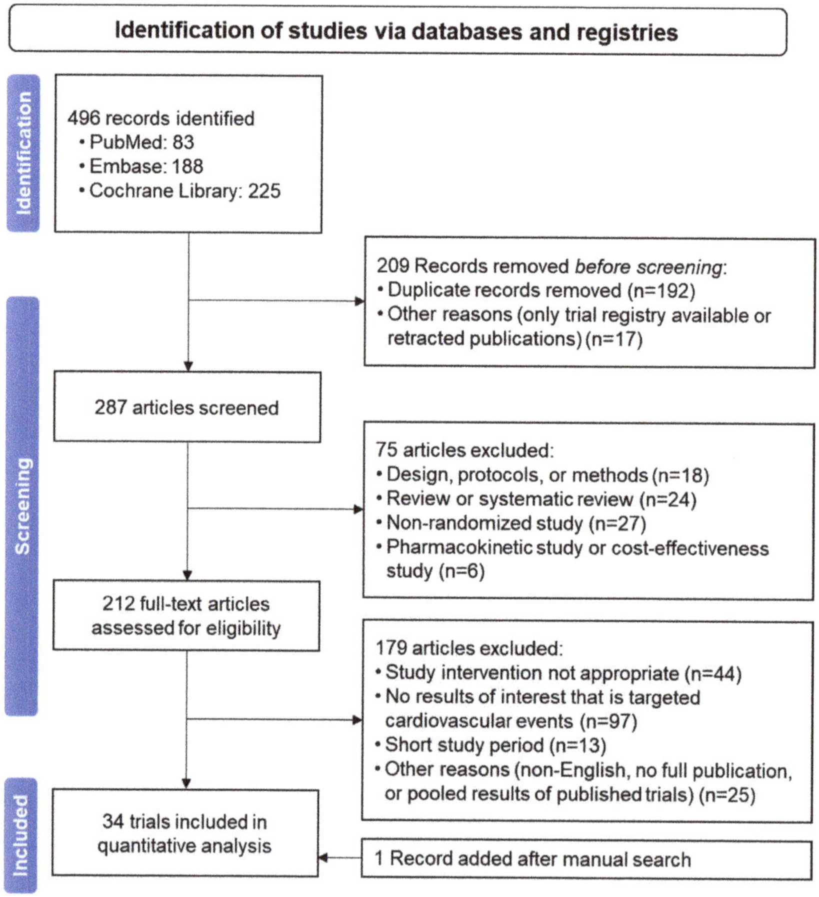

Figure 2. PRISMA flow diagram for studies included in the current meta-analysis.

All 33 studies mentioned above were included in the meta-analysis of cilostazol therapy for the prevention of composite MACE. The definition of MACE varied among the trials, which might be attributed to differences in patient characteristics (Supplementary Table S2). Cilostazol administration effectively reduced the risk of MACE compared with both the control (risk ratio (RR): 0.62; 95% CI: 0.52–0.73) (Figure 3A) and aspirin (RR: 0.74; 95% CI: 0.63–0.87) treatments (Figure 3B). Cilostazol exhibited a superior efficacy over aspirin for secondary prevention, whereas further evidence is needed to draw a solid conclusion regarding its efficacy in primary prevention (Figure 3B). Our results confirmed the favorable effects of cilostazol on stroke, which are even better than those of aspirin [126] (Figure 4B). The beneficial efficacy of cilostazol in reducing the risk of myocardial infarction and cardiovascular death was not demonstrated (Figure 4A,C). The distinction in responses between ischemic stroke and myocardial infarction might lie in their differing associations with underlying etiologies [127]. Ischemic stroke is primarily associated with the clogging of blood vessels. In contrast, in myocardial infarction, multiple blood vessels may be involved, and other risk factors often play a significant role before an attack occurs.

Cilostazol therapy yielded a reduced bleeding risk compared with aspirin (Figure 4E). However, its usage was limited because of adverse events, leading to therapy discontinuation (Figure 4F), such as headache and palpitation (Supplementary Figure S3). This suggests the need for improvements in this medication to address its side effects.

4.3. Coronary Artery Disease (CAD)

To date, the effect of cilostazol on CAD has not been fully elucidated, particularly as a primary prevention. In the ESCAPE study, we investigated the efficacy and safety of cilostazol and aspirin as the primary prevention of CAD in patients with T2DM. This investigation comprehensively evaluated CAD by assessing coronary artery stenosis, plaque composition, and calcium deposition using up-to-date computed tomography angiography [80]. A sustained-release form of cilostazol treatment (200 mg/day) for 12 months reduced the progression of coronary artery stenosis in patients with diabetes compared with aspirin (−3.1% vs. 1.7%). Notably, the noncalcified plaque component was the main portion of atheromatous plaques that was reduced by cilostazol treatment [80].

We extended this observation to investigate the long-term effect of cilostazol and aspirin (ESCAPE-extension study) [123]. In this extension study, we found that cilostazol treatment reduced the incidence of cardiovascular events in the patients with T2DM compared with aspirin over a median follow-up of 5.2 years (hazard ratio: 0.24; 95% CI: 0.07–0.83). This benefit of cilostazol therapy was maintained together with age, sex, blood pressure, LDL-cholesterol, and coronary artery calcium score, without serious adverse events [123].

A previous study that compared cilostazol with aspirin for primary prevention in patients with T2DM failed to observe favorable effects for cilostazol [118]. The overall cardiovascular event rate was very small (<3% in both the aspirin and cilostazol groups), which may have hampered the detection of any significant differences in this population. The overall data suggest the potential beneficial role of cilostazol treatment in the primary prevention of CVD, although additional evidence is still needed.

4.4. Carotid Artery Stenosis and Cerebrovascular Disease

Cilostazol decreased the carotid intima–media thickness (IMT), which is a surrogate indicator of CVD. In the Diabetic Atherosclerosis Prevention by Cilostazol study, which was conducted in patients with T2DM accompanied by arteriosclerosis obliterans, the carotid IMT was increased in the aspirin group (+0.048 mm), whereas the cilostazol group exhibited a decrease in this parameter (–0.024 mm), resulting in a statistically significant difference in carotid IMT within 2 years [18].

The Cilostazol Stroke Prevention Study compared the secondary stroke preventive effects by dividing patients with a history of stroke into a cilostazol group and an aspirin group. As a result, the frequency of stroke recurrence was about 26% lower in the cilostazol group vs. the aspirin group [20]. Moreover, dual antiplatelet therapy using cilostazol together with aspirin or clopidogrel reduced the incidence of ischemic stroke recurrence in patients at high risk of this condition [119]. In that study, the risk of severe or life-threatening bleeding was similar between the cilostazol with aspirin or clopidogrel therapy and the aspirin or clopidogrel alone therapy.

In a network meta-analysis comparing 11 antiplatelet medications, cilostazol monotherapy yielded the most favorable results in stroke recurrence and bleeding risk over other agents in the patients who had experienced a stroke or transient ischemic attack (TIA) [128]. Further studies are needed for directly comparing cilostazol with a therapeutic agent other than aspirin.

Table 2. Randomized controlled studies of cilostazol for preventing cardiovascular outcomes.

Bibliographic Information	Population	Intervention *	Duration (Intervention/Observation)	Patients' Number	Men (%)/Age (Years)	Diabetes
Gotoh F. et al., 2000 [95]	Patients who had cerebral infarction within the previous 1–6 months	cilostazol 200 mg/day vs. placebo	1 year/3 years	1052	65.6/65.1	24.7%
CREST study [96]	Patients with angina or silent myocardial ischemia undergoing coronary stent implantation	cilostazol 200 mg/day + clopidogrel + aspirin vs. placebo + aspirin + clopidogrel	6 months/6 months	526	74.2/60	25.7%
Chen Y.D. et al., 2006 [97]	Patients undergoing bare metal stent implantation	cilostazol 200 mg/day + clopidogrel + aspirin vs. placebo + aspirin + clopidogrel	6 months/9 month	106	61.7/58	29.2%
DECLARE-LONG study [98]	Patients with angina pectoris and/or positive stress test	cilostazol 200 mg/day + clopidogrel + aspirin vs. aspirin + clopidogrel	6 months/9 month	500	64.2/61.1	33.2%
CASTLE study [99]	Patients with clinical diagnosis of PAD and symptoms of claudication	cilostazol 200 mg/day (or 100 mg/day) vs. placebo	3 years/3 years	1435	65.5/66.2	35.7%
CASISP study [100]	Patients who had ischemic stroke within the previous 1–6 months	cilostazol 200 mg/day vs. aspirin 100 mg/day	12–18 months/18 months	719	68.7/60.2	18.2%
DECLARE-DIABETES study [101]	Patients with diabetes and angina pectoris or positive stress test and a native coronary lesion	cilostazol 200 mg/day + clopidogrel + aspirin vs. aspirin + clopidogrel	6 months/9 month	400	58/60.9	100%
Guo J.J. et al., 2009 [102]	Patients who had ischemic stroke during the recent 1–6 months	cilostazol 200 mg/day vs. aspirin 100 mg	1 year/1 year	68	35.3/60.8	8.8%
Han Y. et al., 2009 [103]	Patients with acute coronary syndromes undergoing PCI	cilostazol 200 mg/day + clopidogrel + aspirin vs. aspirin + clopidogrel	6 months/1 year	1212	73.3/59.9	21.7%
Soga Y. et al., 2009 [104]	Patients with intermittent claudication undergoing endovascular therapy	cilostazol 200 mg/day + aspirin 81 or 100 mg/day vs. aspirin 81 mg or 100 mg/day	2 years/2 years	78	83.3/70.7	35.9%
DAPC study [18]	Patients with T2D suspected of PAD	cilostazol 100 mg or 200 mg/day vs. aspirin 81 mg or 100 mg/day	2 years/2 years	297	52.2/63.5	100%
CSPS 2 study [20]	Patients who had cerebral infarction within the previous 26 weeks	cilostazol 200 mg/day vs. aspirin 81 mg/day	1–5 years/5 years	2672	71.7/63.5	29.0%
TOSS-2 study [105]	Patients with acute symptomatic stenosis in the middle cerebral artery or the basilar artery	cilostazol 200 mg/day vs. clopidogrel	7 months/7 months	457	51.2/65.5	42.5%

Table 2. *Cont.*

Bibliographic Information	Population	Intervention *	Duration (Intervention/Observation)	Patients' Number	Men (%)/Age (Years)	Diabetes
DECLARE-LONG II study [106]	Patients with stable angina or acute coronary syndrome and a native long coronary lesion	cilostazol 200 mg/day + clopidogrel + aspirin vs. placebo + aspirin + clopidogrel	8 months/1 year	499	70.6/61.5	35.3%
CAIST study [107]	Patients who had ischemic stroke with neurological deficits	cilostazol 200 mg/day vs. aspirin 300 mg/day	90 days/90 days	458	61.4/63	34.7%
CILON-T study [108]	Patients undergoing drug-eluting stent	cilostazol 200 mg/day + clopidogrel + aspirin vs. aspirin + clopidogrel	6 months/6 months	915	70.7/64.4	33.6%
STOP-IC study [109]	Patients with symptomatic PAD	cilostazol 200 mg/day + aspirin vs. aspirin	12 months/12 months	191	68.6/73	56.0%
Gao W. et al., 2013 [110]	Obese patients undergoing coronary stenting	cilostazol 200 mg/day + clopidogrel + aspirin vs. aspirin + clopidogrel	1 year/1 year	428	80.4/56.5	17.8%
Youn Y.J. et al., 2014 [111]	Patients with CAD implanting drug-eluting stent	cilostazol 200 mg/day + clopidogrel + aspirin vs. aspirin + clopidogrel	3 months/1 year	615	63.6/64.6	31.7%
CATHARSIS study [112]	Patients with intracranial arterial stenosis	cilostazol 200 mg/day + aspirin vs. aspirin	2 years/2 years	163	65.6/68.3	36.8%
CATS-I study [113]	Patients with stable CAD or acute coronary syndrome	cilostazol 200 mg/day + aspirin vs. aspirin	2 year/2 year	514	74.7/69	39.9%
Zheng X.-T. et al., 2016 [114]	Patients with complex lesions undergoing PCI	cilostazol 100 mg/day + clopidogrel + aspirin vs. aspirin + clopidogrel	3 months/1 year	127	70.9/64.6	37.0%
CREATIVE study [115]	Patients undergoing PCI	cilostazol 200 mg/day + aspirin + clopidogrel vs. aspirin + clopidogrel (75 mg or 150 mg)	12 months/18 months	1076	59.9/58.4	33.2%
DECREASE PCI study [116]	Patients undergoing drug-eluting stents for CAD	cilostazol 200 mg/day + aspirin + clopidogrel vs. placebo + aspirin + clopidogrel	1 year/1 year	404	71.3/62.2	30.9%
PICASSO study [117]	Patients with ischemic stroke with intracerebral hemorrhage or multiple microbleeds	cilostazol 200 mg/day vs. aspirin	At least 1 year/median 1.9 years	1512	62/65.7	32.1%
Hong S et al., 2019 [118]	Patients with T2D without macrovascular complications	cilostazol 200 mg/day vs. aspirin	3 years/3 years	415	50.4/59.6	100%

Table 2. *Cont.*

Bibliographic Information	Population	Intervention *	Duration (Intervention/Observation)	Patients' Number	Men (%)/Age (Years)	Diabetes
CSPS.com study [119]	Patients with high-risk non-cardioembolic ischemic stroke	cilostazol 200 mg/day + aspirin or clopidogrel vs. aspirin or clopidogrel	At least 1 year/median 1.4 years	1879	70.3/69.7	37.3%
Chen Y.-C. et al., 2019 [120]	Patients undergoing PCI	cilostazol 200 mg/day + clopidogrel + aspirin vs. aspirin + clopidogrel	6 months/2 years	211	69.7/65.7	25%
Uchiyama S. et al., 2021 [121]	Patients with intracranial arterial stenosis	cilostazol 200 mg/day + aspirin or clopidogrel vs. aspirin or clopidogrel	At least 1 year/median 1.4 years	547	67.1/70	39.5%
Kalantzi K. et al., 2021 [122]	Patients with T2D exhibiting symptomatic lower extremity arterial disease	cilostazol 200 mg/day + clopidogrel vs. clopidogrel	12 months/3 years	794	64/67.8	100%
ESCAPE-Extension: Sohn M. et al., 2022 [123]	Patients with T2D and mild to moderate coronary artery stenosis	cilostazol 200 mg/day vs. aspirin	At least 1 year/median 5.2 years	88	63/61	100%
Lin J.-L. et al., 2022 [124]	Patients with CAD or at a high risk of cardiovascular disease	cilostazol 200 mg/day vs. placebo	mean 2.9 years/mean 2.9 years	266	73.3/65.8	39.5%
LACI-2 study [125]	Patients who had lacunar stroke	cilostazol 200 mg/day ± isosorbide mononitrate vs. isosorbide mononitrate or no study drug	12 months/12 months	363	69.1/64.3	22.0%
Park S. et al., 2023 [129]	Patients who had ST-elevation myocardial infarction	cilostazol 200 mg/day + aspirin or clopidogrel vs. aspirin or clopidogrel	1 or 6 months/12 months	948	81.5/61.6	26.6%

* The standard dosage of other interventions was not specified: aspirin, 100 mg, and clopidogrel, 75 mg. CAD, coronary artery disease; PAD, peripheral arterial disease; PCI, percutaneous coronary intervention; and T2D, type 2 diabetes.

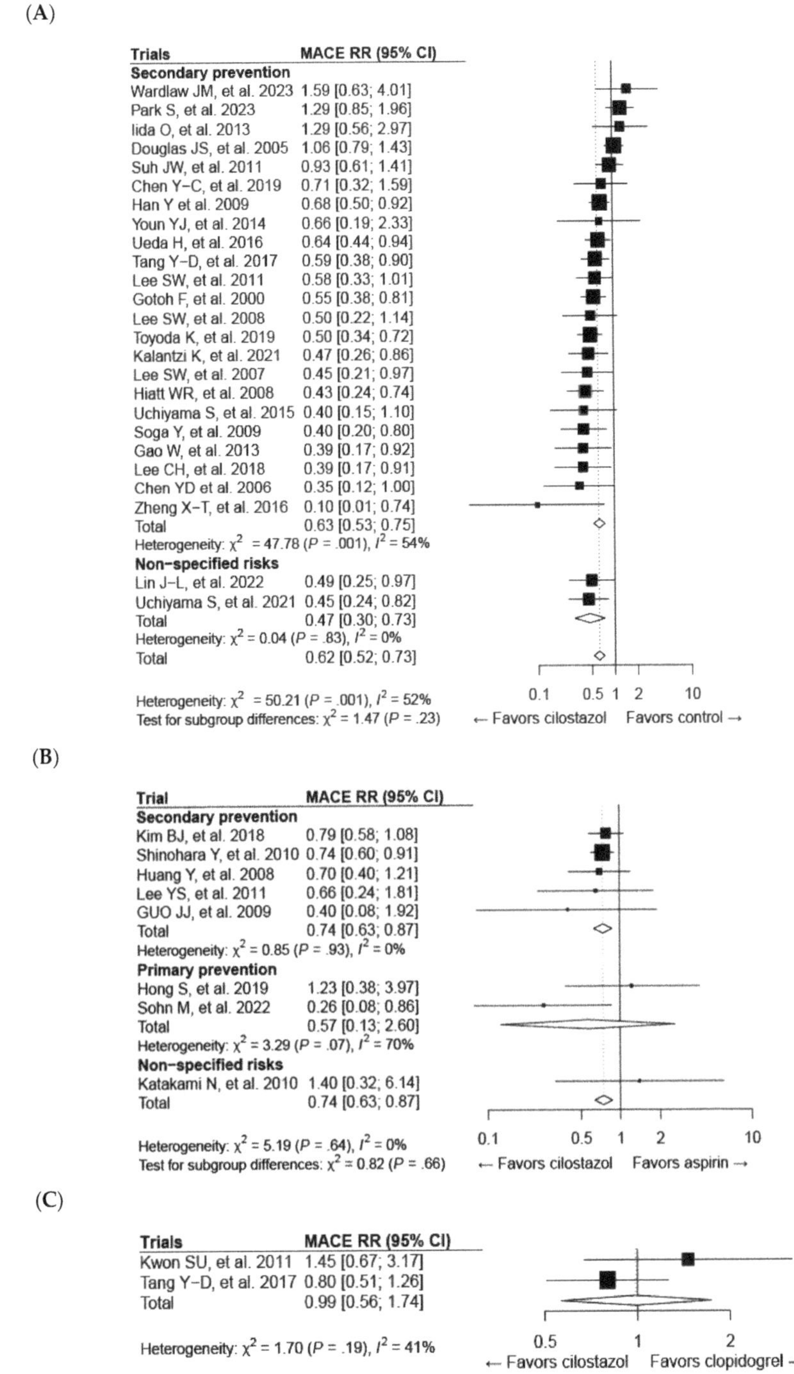

Figure 3. Forest plots of cilostazol in composite major adverse cardiovascular events (MACEs) compared with the following: (**A**) the control, (**B**) aspirin, and (**C**) clopidogrel. CI, confidence interval; RR, risk ratio.

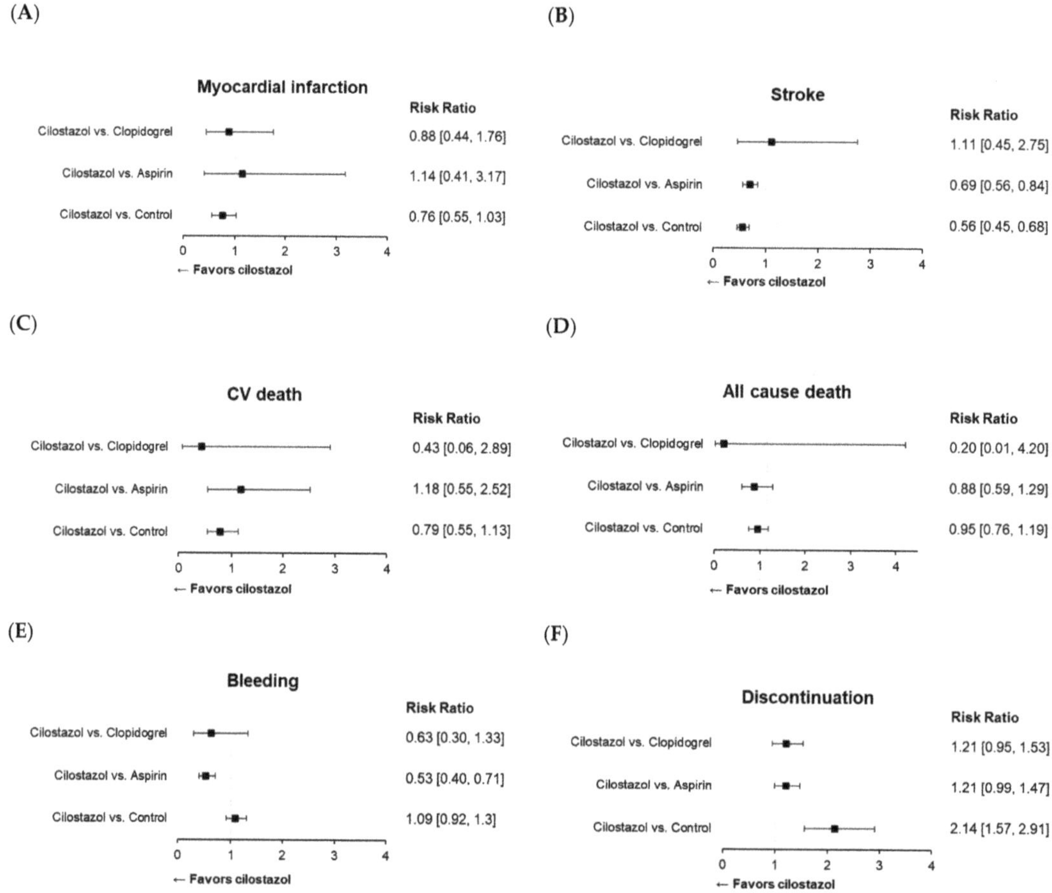

Figure 4. Forest plots of cilostazol in cardiovascular and safety events: (**A**) myocardial infarction, (**B**) stroke, (**C**) cardiovascular death, (**D**) all-cause death, (**E**) bleeding, and (**F**) discontinuation of the study drug.

4.5. Peripheral Artery Disease (PAD)

The clinical excellence of cilostazol is sufficient to recommend it as a first-line drug in PAD, because it increases NO in vascular endothelial cells in a dose-dependent manner, to dilate blood vessels [130]. A meta-analysis of 16 RCTs reported that intermittent claudication was significantly improved by cilostazol therapy (100–300 mg per day) compared with the placebo [131]. An RCT including 698 patients with moderate-to-severe claudication symptoms reported that a 6-month cilostazol therapy improved the maximal walking distance by 54%, compared with pentoxifylline therapy (30% increase) [132]. Another study including 394 patients with intermittent claudication showed that cilostazol treatment for 6 months improved the maximal walking distance compared with the placebo [133]. A 2021 Cochrane Systematic Review and Meta-analysis including 16 double-blind RCTs reported that participants taking cilostazol had a higher initial claudication distance, by 26.5 m (95% CI: 18.9–34.1 m), compared with those taking the placebo [131]. Cilostazol exerted beneficial effects regarding the primary prevention of diabetic foot ulcers via a lowering effect on MMP-9 levels [134].

Recently, a prospective study with 794 participants showed that the adjunctive administration of cilostazol to clopidogrel-treated patients with T2DM with symptomatic

PAD lowered the risk of ischemic events and improved intermittent claudication symptoms, without increasing the bleeding risk [122]. Based on this evidence, the ACC/AHA guidelines provided a class I recommendation for the use of cilostazol in the treatment of intermittent claudication in 2016 and thereafter [135].

5. Potential Benefits of Cilostazol Therapy

Neuroprotective Effect

There is evidence supporting the benefits of cilostazol in neuroprotection. Several studies reported that cilostazol was helpful in preventing symptomatic cerebral vasospasm and in reducing cerebral infarction and intracranial hemorrhage in patients with stroke [136,137]. These effects depended mainly on the anti-inflammatory and antiapoptotic effects of cilostazol, which are mediated by scavenging hydroxyl radicals, decreasing the formation of tumor necrosis factor-α (TNF-α), and inhibiting adenosine diphosphate-ribose polymerase activity [138]. Moreover, cilostazol treatment improved neuronal survival by promoting the Akt and CREB, as well as brain-derived neurotrophic factor content in a rat model [74]. The production of NO triggered by cilostazol therapy via the activation of endothelial NO synthase also contributed to neuroprotection via endothelial protection [139].

It is known that cilostazol reduces blood–brain barrier permeability and the degree of intracerebral cell death via mechanisms involving the inhibition of collagenase [140]. Cilostazol treatment also prevented endothelial cell death and protected collagen type 4, laminin, and vascular endothelial and N-cadherins from collagenase injury, and attenuated blood–brain barrier leakage, resulting in intracranial hemorrhage [141].

In addition, cilostazol had a neuroprotective effect against hypoperfusion and permanent cerebral ischemia [142,143]. Cilostazol treatment in Wistar rats with bilateral carotid artery occlusion decreased apoptosis by downregulating TNF-α, suppressed overly activated astroglia and microglia in the white matter, and increased oligodendrocytes [142]. The protection mechanism was multifactorial in reducing oxidative stress [143].

In a multicenter and double-blind RCT, the administration of cilostazol to participants with moderate or severe white matter changes (WMC), which demonstrates small-vessel disease in the brain, and at least one lacunar infarction significantly reduced the risk of ischemic vascular events compared with aspirin (HR: 0.11; 95% CI: 0.02–0.89) [144]. However, there was no significant difference between the effects of cilostazol and those of aspirin on WMC progression in patients with cerebral small-vessel disease [144]. In a systematic review and meta-analysis of RCTs for stroke and cognitive decline, cilostazol therapy reduced recurrent ischemic stroke; however, the authors failed to prove its efficacy on cognitive dysfunction [126].

6. Considerations in Using Cilostazol Therapy

6.1. Adverse Effects of Cilostazol Therapy

Cilostazol has been reported to cause more headaches, palpitations, and gastrointestinal disorders when compared with a placebo [145]. Headaches were the primary reason for the discontinuation of this medication. Cilostazol significantly increased the cerebral blood flow in patients with chronic cerebral infarction [95]; therefore, the cerebral blood vessels dilated, which may have caused headaches, although the patients would acclimate to it within 1 week. Currently, a sustained-release formulation that reduces the incidence of headache by introducing a technology with controlled dissolution is available in several countries [146].

It is important to understand that cilostazol has the potential to increase the heart rate by about 3–5 beats/min [23,145]. Although this side effect will not necessarily be present in all patients, and the extent of its impact may vary according to the dosage and individual physiological responses, further research is needed to investigate how this outcome may affect the progression of CVDs. Thus, cilostazol is contraindicated in patients with established heart failure [147].

6.2. Effects of Cilostazol Therapy by Regional Background

Although numerous studies have been published on cilostazol's protective effects against atherosclerosis, it is evident that most of these studies have been conducted in Asia (Figure 5). Studies have demonstrated that cilostazol improves major adverse cardiovascular events (MACE) and stroke outcomes, affirming its efficacy. However, limited studies make it hard to interpret its effects in other regions (Figure 5A,C). Moreover, as recent studies have not shown favorable results for myocardial infarction [125,129], further investigation is needed to determine its efficacy in Asian populations as well (Figure 5B).

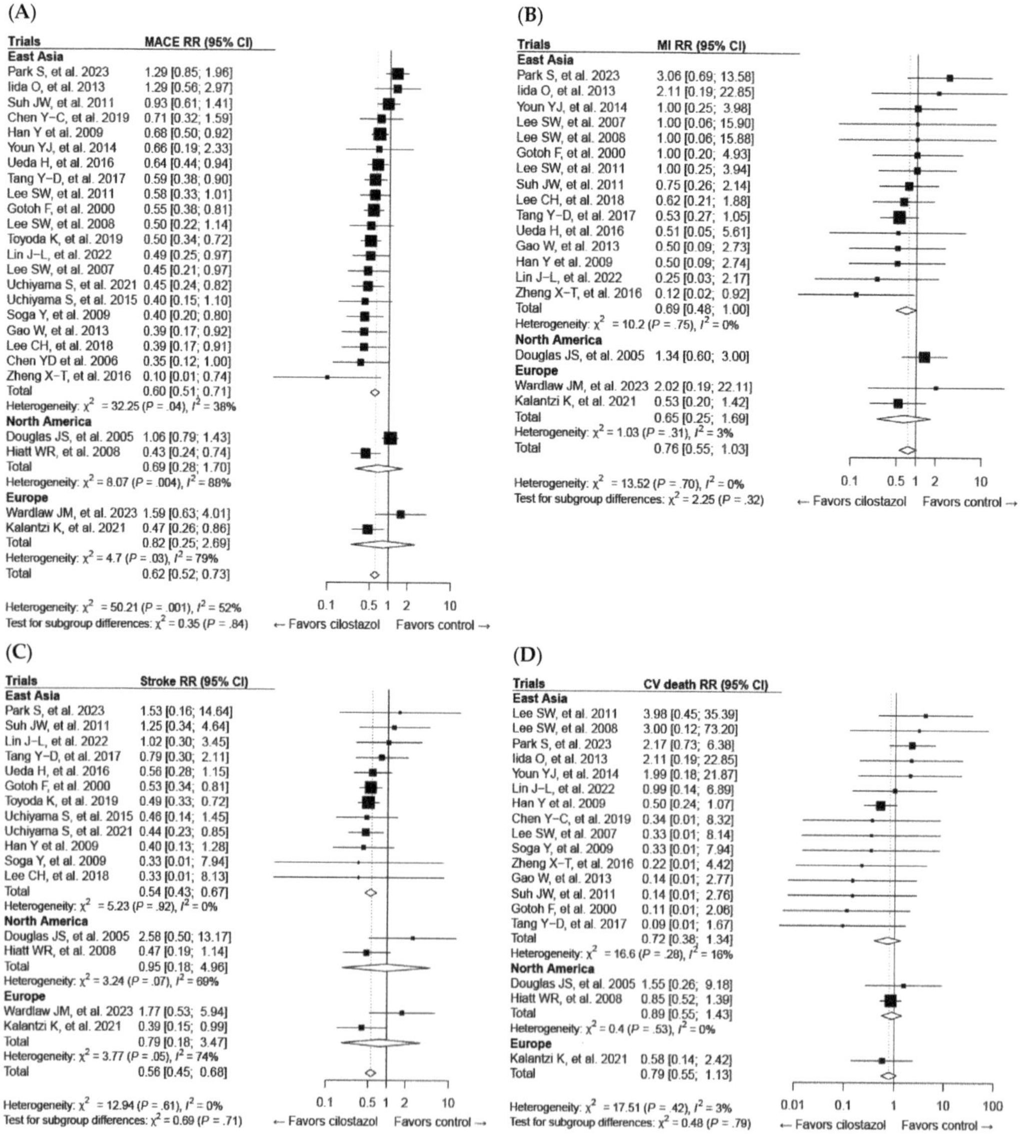

Figure 5. Forest plots of cilostazol's effect on composite major adverse cardiovascular events (MACEs) and individual components categorized by regional background: (**A**) MACE, (**B**) myocardial infarction (MI), (**C**) stroke, and (**D**) cardiovascular death. CI, confidence interval; RR, risk ratio.

7. Conclusions

Cilostazol has multifaceted beneficial effects through various mechanisms, including platelet inhibition, vasodilation via NO production, protective effects on vascular endothelial cells, antiproliferative effects on VSMCs, and favorable changes in lipid profiles (Figure 6). These beneficial effects of cilostazol are attributable to its pleiotropic properties, including its anti-inflammatory and antioxidative actions. A neuroprotective effect was also found in a few clinical studies of cilostazol.

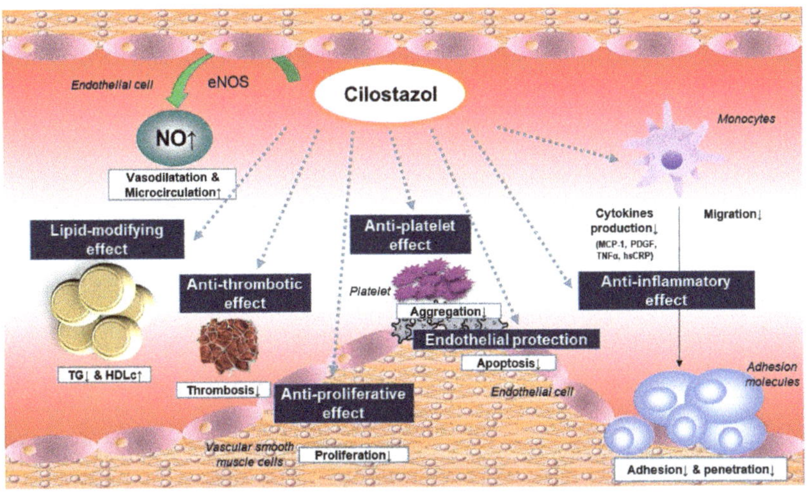

Figure 6. Anti-atherosclerotic effect of cilostazol.

Based on the recent results of large clinical studies suggesting that aspirin should not be recommended in primary prevention settings, cilostazol treatment may be a viable option for preventing the development and progression of vascular diseases. Obviously, cilostazol is effective in PAD, and recent evidence supports its effectiveness in CAD as well as ischemic stroke. Notably, recent studies reported that cilostazol treatment was efficacious in reducing atheromatous plaque progression in coronary arteries and decreasing cardiovascular events compared with aspirin in patients with diabetes and subclinical CAD. Thus, cilostazol might be helpful in the comprehensive vascular management of patients with a high risk of CV. However, it is noteworthy that these results were mainly derived from East-Asian populations. Additional trials including other ethnic groups are needed to generalize the beneficial effects of this drug. Adverse events occurring after cilostazol therapy, such as headache and heart rate increase, have not been completely resolved; therefore, the development of more-advanced PDE-3 inhibitors that do not exhibit these unwanted effects is warranted. Longer-term studies with a robust outcome are needed to confirm the efficacy and safety of cilostazol therapy.

Supplementary Materials: The following supporting information can be downloaded at: https://www.mdpi.com/article/10.3390/ijms25052593/s1.

Author Contributions: Conceptualization, M.S. and S.L.; methodology, M.S. and S.L.; validation, M.S. and S.L.; formal analysis, M.S. and S.L.; investigation, M.S. and S.L.; resources, M.S. and S.L.; data curation, M.S. and S.L.; writing—original draft preparation, M.S. and S.L.; writing—review and editing, M.S. and S.L.; visualization, M.S. and S.L.; supervision, S.L.; project administration, S.L. All authors have read and agreed to the published version of the manuscript.

Funding: This research received no external funding.

Institutional Review Board Statement: This is not applicable as this project did not involve humans or animals.

Informed Consent Statement: Not applicable.

Data Availability Statement: The supporting data for the findings can be obtained from the corresponding author upon a reasonable request.

Conflicts of Interest: The authors declare no conflicts of interest.

References

1. Libby, P.; Buring, J.E.; Badimon, L.; Hansson, G.K.; Deanfield, J.; Bittencourt, M.S.; Tokgozoglu, L.; Lewis, E.F. Atherosclerosis. *Nat. Rev. Dis. Prim.* **2019**, *5*, 56. [CrossRef]
2. Golledge, J. Update on the pathophysiology and medical treatment of peripheral artery disease. *Nat. Rev. Cardiol.* **2022**, *19*, 456–474. [CrossRef] [PubMed]
3. The Top 10 Causes of Death. Available online: https://www.who.int/news-room/fact-sheets/detail/the-top-10-causes-of-death (accessed on 30 September 2023).
4. Wang, Y.; Li, Z.; Zhao, X.; Wang, D.; Li, H.; Xian, Y.; Liu, L.; Wang, Y. Stroke care quality in China: Substantial improvement, and a huge challenge and opportunity. *Int. J. Stroke* **2017**, *12*, 229–235. [CrossRef]
5. Morley, R.L.; Sharma, A.; Horsch, A.D.; Hinchliffe, R.J. Peripheral artery disease. *BMJ* **2018**, *360*, j5842. [CrossRef] [PubMed]
6. Mollon, L.; Bhattacharjee, S. Health related quality of life among myocardial infarction survivors in the United States: A propensity score matched analysis. *Health Qual. Life Outcomes* **2017**, *15*, 235. [CrossRef]
7. Sprigg, N.; Selby, J.; Fox, L.; Berge, E.; Whynes, D.; Bath, P.M.; Efficacy of Nitric Oxide in Stroke Investigators. Very low quality of life after acute stroke: Data from the Efficacy of Nitric Oxide in Stroke trial. *Stroke* **2013**, *44*, 3458–3462. [CrossRef]
8. Jouven, X.; Lemaitre, R.N.; Rea, T.D.; Sotoodehnia, N.; Empana, J.P.; Siscovick, D.S. Diabetes, glucose level, and risk of sudden cardiac death. *Eur. Heart J.* **2005**, *26*, 2142–2147. [CrossRef]
9. Emerging Risk Factors, C.; Sarwar, N.; Gao, P.; Seshasai, S.R.; Gobin, R.; Kaptoge, S.; Di Angelantonio, E.; Ingelsson, E.; Lawlor, D.A.; Selvin, E.; et al. Diabetes mellitus, fasting blood glucose concentration, and risk of vascular disease: A collaborative meta-analysis of 102 prospective studies. *Lancet* **2010**, *375*, 2215–2222. [CrossRef]
10. Beckman, J.A.; Creager, M.A. Vascular Complications of Diabetes. *Circ. Res.* **2016**, *118*, 1771–1785. [CrossRef] [PubMed]
11. Low Wang, C.C.; Hess, C.N.; Hiatt, W.R.; Goldfine, A.B. Clinical Update: Cardiovascular Disease in Diabetes Mellitus: Atherosclerotic Cardiovascular Disease and Heart Failure in Type 2 Diabetes Mellitus—Mechanisms, Management, and Clinical Considerations. *Circulation* **2016**, *133*, 2459–2502. [CrossRef] [PubMed]
12. Patel, K.V.; Pandey, A.; de Lemos, J.A. Conceptual Framework for Addressing Residual Atherosclerotic Cardiovascular Disease Risk in the Era of Precision Medicine. *Circulation* **2018**, *137*, 2551–2553. [CrossRef]
13. ElSayed, N.A.; Aleppo, G.; Aroda, V.R.; Bannuru, R.R.; Brown, F.M.; Bruemmer, D.; Collins, B.S.; Das, S.R.; Hilliard, M.E.; Isaacs, D.; et al. 10. Cardiovascular Disease and Risk Management: Standards of Care in Diabetes—2023. *Diabetes Care* **2023**, *46* (Suppl. S1), S158–S190. [CrossRef]
14. Marx, N.; Federici, M.; Schutt, K.; Muller-Wieland, D.; Ajjan, R.A.; Antunes, M.J.; Christodorescu, R.M.; Crawford, C.; Di Angelantonio, E.; Eliasson, B.; et al. 2023 ESC Guidelines for the management of cardiovascular disease in patients with diabetes. *Eur. Heart J.* **2023**, *44*, 4043–4140. [CrossRef] [PubMed]
15. Kambayashi, J.; Liu, Y.; Sun, B.; Shakur, Y.; Yoshitake, M.; Czerwiec, F. Cilostazol as a unique antithrombotic agent. *Curr. Pharm. Des.* **2003**, *9*, 2289–2302. [CrossRef] [PubMed]
16. Degerman, E.; Belfrage, P.; Manganiello, V.C. Structure, localization, and regulation of cGMP-inhibited phosphodiesterase (PDE3). *J. Biol. Chem.* **1997**, *272*, 6823–6826. [CrossRef] [PubMed]
17. Huh, J.H.; Seok, H.; Lee, B.W.; Kang, E.S.; Lee, H.C.; Cha, B.S. Effect of cilostazol on carotid intima-media thickness in type 2 diabetic patients without cardiovascular event. *Endocrine* **2014**, *47*, 138–145. [CrossRef] [PubMed]
18. Katakami, N.; Kim, Y.S.; Kawamori, R.; Yamasaki, Y. The phosphodiesterase inhibitor cilostazol induces regression of carotid atherosclerosis in subjects with type 2 diabetes mellitus: Principal results of the Diabetic Atherosclerosis Prevention by Cilostazol (DAPC) study: A randomized trial. *Circulation* **2010**, *121*, 2584–2591. [CrossRef] [PubMed]
19. Kwon, S.U.; Cho, Y.J.; Koo, J.S.; Bae, H.J.; Lee, Y.S.; Hong, K.S.; Lee, J.H.; Kim, J.S. Cilostazol prevents the progression of the symptomatic intracranial arterial stenosis: The multicenter double-blind placebo-controlled trial of cilostazol in symptomatic intracranial arterial stenosis. *Stroke* **2005**, *36*, 782–786. [CrossRef] [PubMed]
20. Shinohara, Y.; Katayama, Y.; Uchiyama, S.; Yamaguchi, T.; Handa, S.; Matsuoka, K.; Ohashi, Y.; Tanahashi, N.; Yamamoto, H.; Genka, C.; et al. Cilostazol for prevention of secondary stroke (CSPS 2): An aspirin-controlled, double-blind, randomised non-inferiority trial. *Lancet Neurol.* **2010**, *9*, 959–968. [CrossRef]
21. Biondi-Zoccai, G.G.; Lotrionte, M.; Anselmino, M.; Moretti, C.; Agostoni, P.; Testa, L.; Abbate, A.; Cosgrave, J.; Laudito, A.; Trevi, G.P.; et al. Systematic review and meta-analysis of randomized clinical trials appraising the impact of cilostazol after percutaneous coronary intervention. *Am. Heart J.* **2008**, *155*, 1081–1089. [CrossRef] [PubMed]

22. Angiolillo, D.J.; Capranzano, P.; Goto, S.; Aslam, M.; Desai, B.; Charlton, R.K.; Suzuki, Y.; Box, L.C.; Shoemaker, S.B.; Zenni, M.M.; et al. A randomized study assessing the impact of cilostazol on platelet function profiles in patients with diabetes mellitus and coronary artery disease on dual antiplatelet therapy: Results of the OPTIMUS-2 study. *Eur. Heart J.* **2008**, *29*, 2202–2211. [CrossRef]
23. Rogers, K.C.; Oliphant, C.S.; Finks, S.W. Clinical efficacy and safety of cilostazol: A critical review of the literature. *Drugs* **2015**, *75*, 377–395. [CrossRef]
24. Berger, J.S. Aspirin for Primary Prevention-Time to Rethink Our Approach. *JAMA Netw. Open* **2022**, *5*, e2210144. [CrossRef]
25. Ogawa, H.; Nakayama, M.; Morimoto, T.; Uemura, S.; Kanauchi, M.; Doi, N.; Jinnouchi, H.; Sugiyama, S.; Saito, Y.; Japanese Primary Prevention of Atherosclerosis With Aspirin for Diabetes (JPAD) Trial Investigators. Low-dose aspirin for primary prevention of atherosclerotic events in patients with type 2 diabetes: A randomized controlled trial. *JAMA* **2008**, *300*, 2134–2141. [CrossRef]
26. Belch, J.; MacCuish, A.; Campbell, I.; Cobbe, S.; Taylor, R.; Prescott, R.; Lee, R.; Bancroft, J.; MacEwan, S.; Shepherd, J.; et al. The prevention of progression of arterial disease and diabetes (POPADAD) trial: Factorial randomised placebo controlled trial of aspirin and antioxidants in patients with diabetes and asymptomatic peripheral arterial disease. *BMJ* **2008**, *337*, a1840. [CrossRef] [PubMed]
27. Calvin, A.D.; Aggarwal, N.R.; Murad, M.H.; Shi, Q.; Elamin, M.B.; Geske, J.B.; Fernandez-Balsells, M.M.; Albuquerque, F.N.; Lampropulos, J.F.; Erwin, P.J.; et al. Aspirin for the primary prevention of cardiovascular events: A systematic review and meta-analysis comparing patients with and without diabetes. *Diabetes Care* **2009**, *32*, 2300–2306. [CrossRef] [PubMed]
28. Ikeda, Y.; Shimada, K.; Teramoto, T.; Uchiyama, S.; Yamazaki, T.; Oikawa, S.; Sugawara, M.; Ando, K.; Murata, M.; Yokoyama, K.; et al. Low-dose aspirin for primary prevention of cardiovascular events in Japanese patients 60 years or older with atherosclerotic risk factors: A randomized clinical trial. *JAMA* **2014**, *312*, 2510–2520. [CrossRef] [PubMed]
29. de Gaetano, G.; Collaborative Group of the Primary Prevention Project. Low-dose aspirin and vitamin E in people at cardiovascular risk: A randomised trial in general practice. Collaborative Group of the Primary Prevention Project. *Lancet* **2001**, *357*, 89–95. [PubMed]
30. Ridker, P.M.; Cook, N.R.; Lee, I.M.; Gordon, D.; Gaziano, J.M.; Manson, J.E.; Hennekens, C.H.; Buring, J.E. A randomized trial of low-dose aspirin in the primary prevention of cardiovascular disease in women. *N. Engl. J. Med.* **2005**, *352*, 1293–1304. [CrossRef] [PubMed]
31. Group, A.S.C.; Bowman, L.; Mafham, M.; Wallendszus, K.; Stevens, W.; Buck, G.; Barton, J.; Murphy, K.; Aung, T.; Haynes, R.; et al. Effects of Aspirin for Primary Prevention in Persons with Diabetes Mellitus. *N. Engl. J. Med.* **2018**, *379*, 1529–1539.
32. Gaziano, J.M.; Brotons, C.; Coppolecchia, R.; Cricelli, C.; Darius, H.; Gorelick, P.B.; Howard, G.; Pearson, T.A.; Rothwell, P.M.; Ruilope, L.M.; et al. Use of aspirin to reduce risk of initial vascular events in patients at moderate risk of cardiovascular disease (ARRIVE): A randomised, double-blind, placebo-controlled trial. *Lancet* **2018**, *392*, 1036–1046. [CrossRef]
33. McNeil, J.J.; Nelson, M.R.; Woods, R.L.; Lockery, J.E.; Wolfe, R.; Reid, C.M.; Kirpach, B.; Shah, R.C.; Ives, D.G.; Storey, E.; et al. Effect of Aspirin on All-Cause Mortality in the Healthy Elderly. *N. Engl. J. Med.* **2018**, *379*, 1519–1528. [CrossRef]
34. Yusuf, S.; Joseph, P.; Dans, A.; Gao, P.; Teo, K.; Xavier, D.; Lopez-Jaramillo, P.; Yusoff, K.; Santoso, A.; Gamra, H.; et al. Polypill with or without Aspirin in Persons without Cardiovascular Disease. *N. Engl. J. Med.* **2021**, *384*, 216–228. [CrossRef]
35. Massimi, I.; Lotti, L.V.; Temperilli, F.; Mancone, M.; Sardella, G.; Calcagno, S.; Turriziani, O.; Frati, L.; Pulcinelli, F.M. Enhanced platelet MRP4 expression and correlation with platelet function in patients under chronic aspirin treatment. *Thromb. Haemost.* **2016**, *116*, 1100–1110. [CrossRef] [PubMed]
36. Angiolillo, D.J. Variability in responsiveness to oral antiplatelet therapy. *Am. J. Cardiol.* **2009**, *103* (Suppl. S3), 27A–34A. [CrossRef] [PubMed]
37. Mora, S.; Shufelt, C.L.; Manson, J.E. Whom to Treat for Primary Prevention of Atherosclerotic Cardiovascular Disease: The Aspirin Dilemma. *JAMA Intern. Med.* **2022**, *182*, 587–589. [CrossRef]
38. American Diabetes, A. 8. Cardiovascular Disease and Risk Management. *Diabetes Care* **2016**, *39* (Suppl. S1), S60–S71. [CrossRef]
39. Pignone, M.; Alberts, M.J.; Colwell, J.A.; Cushman, M.; Inzucchi, S.E.; Mukherjee, D.; Rosenson, R.S.; Williams, C.D.; Wilson, P.W.; Kirkman, M.S.; et al. Aspirin for primary prevention of cardiovascular events in people with diabetes: A position statement of the American Diabetes Association, a scientific statement of the American Heart Association, and an expert consensus document of the American College of Cardiology Foundation. *Diabetes Care* **2010**, *33*, 1395–1402. [PubMed]
40. Xue, Y.; Wang, Z.; Wu, H.; Li, X.; Chen, J.; Lv, Q. Cilostazol increases adenosine plasma concentration in patients with acute coronary syndrome. *J. Clin. Pharm. Ther.* **2021**, *46*, 328–332. [CrossRef]
41. Yun, S.H.; Sim, E.H.; Goh, R.Y.; Park, J.I.; Han, J.Y. Platelet Activation: The Mechanisms and Potential Biomarkers. *Biomed. Res. Int.* **2016**, *2016*, 9060143. [CrossRef]
42. Paul, S.; Feoktistov, I.; Hollister, A.S.; Robertson, D.; Biaggioni, I. Adenosine inhibits the rise in intracellular calcium and platelet aggregation produced by thrombin: Evidence that both effects are coupled to adenylate cyclase. *Mol. Pharmacol.* **1990**, *37*, 870–875.
43. Yan, R.; Li, S.; Dai, K. The critical roles of cyclic AMP/cyclic AMP-dependent protein kinase in platelet physiology. *Front. Biol. China* **2009**, *4*, 7–14. [CrossRef]
44. Guarino, M.L.; Massimi, I.; Alemanno, L.; Conti, L.; Angiolillo, D.J.; Pulcinelli, F.M. MRP4 over-expression has a role on both reducing nitric oxide-dependent antiplatelet effect and enhancing ADP induced platelet activation. *J. Thromb. Thrombolysis* **2021**, *51*, 625–632. [CrossRef]

45. Alemanno, L.; Massimi, I.; Klaus, V.; Guarino, M.L.; Maltese, T.; Frati, L.; Angiolillo, D.J.; Pulcinelli, F.M. Impact of Multidrug Resistance Protein-4 Inhibitors on Modulating Platelet Function and High on-Aspirin Treatment Platelet Reactivity. *Thromb. Haemost.* **2018**, *118*, 490–501. [CrossRef]
46. Cheepala, S.B.; Pitre, A.; Fukuda, Y.; Takenaka, K.; Zhang, Y.; Wang, Y.; Frase, S.; Pestina, T.; Gartner, T.K.; Jackson, C.; et al. The ABCC4 membrane transporter modulates platelet aggregation. *Blood* **2015**, *126*, 2307–2319. [CrossRef] [PubMed]
47. Borgognone, A.; Pulcinelli, F.M. Reduction of cAMP and cGMP inhibitory effects in human platelets by MRP4-mediated transport. *Thromb. Haemost.* **2012**, *108*, 955–962. [CrossRef] [PubMed]
48. Ohnuki, Y.; Ohnuki, Y.; Kohara, S.; Shimizu, M.; Takizawa, S. Dual Therapy with Aspirin and Cilostazol May Improve Platelet Aggregation in Noncardioembolic Stroke Patients: A Pilot Study. *Intern. Med.* **2017**, *56*, 1307–1313. [CrossRef]
49. Jeong, Y.H.; Hwang, J.Y.; Kim, I.S.; Park, Y.; Hwang, S.J.; Lee, S.W.; Kwak, C.H.; Park, S.W. Adding cilostazol to dual antiplatelet therapy achieves greater platelet inhibition than high maintenance dose clopidogrel in patients with acute myocardial infarction: Results of the adjunctive cilostazol versus high maintenance dose clopidogrel in patients with AMI (ACCEL-AMI) study. *Circ. Cardiovasc. Interv.* **2010**, *3*, 17–26.
50. Angiolillo, D.J. Antiplatelet therapy in type 2 diabetes mellitus. *Curr. Opin. Endocrinol. Diabetes Obes.* **2007**, *14*, 124–131. [CrossRef] [PubMed]
51. Capranzano, P.; Ferreiro, J.L.; Ueno, M.; Capodanno, D.; Dharmashankar, K.; Darlington, A.; Desai, B.; Tello-Montoliu, A.; Rollini, F.; Angiolillo, D.J. Pharmacodynamic effects of adjunctive cilostazol therapy in patients with coronary artery disease on dual antiplatelet therapy: Impact of high on-treatment platelet reactivity and diabetes mellitus status. *Catheter. Cardiovasc. Interv.* **2013**, *81*, 42–49. [CrossRef]
52. Manickavasagam, S.; Ye, Y.; Lin, Y.; Perez-Polo, R.J.; Huang, M.H.; Lui, C.Y.; Hughes, M.G.; McAdoo, D.J.; Uretsky, B.F.; Birnbaum, Y. The cardioprotective effect of a statin and cilostazol combination: Relationship to Akt and endothelial nitric oxide synthase activation. *Cardiovasc. Drugs Ther.* **2007**, *21*, 321–330. [CrossRef] [PubMed]
53. Tanaka, T.; Ishikawa, T.; Hagiwara, M.; Onoda, K.; Itoh, H.; Hidaka, H. Effects of cilostazol, a selective cAMP phosphodiesterase inhibitor on the contraction of vascular smooth muscle. *Pharmacology* **1988**, *36*, 313–320. [CrossRef] [PubMed]
54. Wu, S.N.; Liu, S.I.; Huang, M.H. Cilostazol, an inhibitor of type 3 phosphodiesterase, stimulates large-conductance, calcium-activated potassium channels in pituitary GH3 cells and pheochromocytoma PC12 cells. *Endocrinology* **2004**, *145*, 1175–1184. [CrossRef] [PubMed]
55. Dindyal, S.; Kyriakides, C. A review of cilostazol, a phosphodiesterase inhibitor, and its role in preventing both coronary and peripheral arterial restenosis following endovascular therapy. *Recent. Pat. Cardiovasc. Drug Discov.* **2009**, *4*, 6–14. [CrossRef] [PubMed]
56. Nakamura, T.; Houchi, H.; Minami, A.; Sakamoto, S.; Tsuchiya, K.; Niwa, Y.; Minakuchi, K.; Nakaya, Y. Endothelium-dependent relaxation by cilostazol, a phosphodiesteras III inhibitor, on rat thoracic aorta. *Life Sci.* **2001**, *69*, 1709–1715. [CrossRef]
57. Li, H.; Hong, D.H.; Son, Y.K.; Na, S.H.; Jung, W.K.; Bae, Y.M.; Seo, E.Y.; Kim, S.J.; Choi, I.W.; Park, W.S. Cilostazol induces vasodilation through the activation of $Ca^{(2+)}$-activated $K^{(+)}$ channels in aortic smooth muscle. *Vasc. Pharmacol.* **2015**, *70*, 15–22. [CrossRef]
58. Liu, Y.; Shakur, Y.; Yoshitake, M.; Kambayashi Ji, J. Cilostazol (pletal): A dual inhibitor of cyclic nucleotide phosphodiesterase type 3 and adenosine uptake. *Cardiovasc. Drug Rev.* **2001**, *19*, 369–386. [CrossRef]
59. Liu, Y.; Fong, M.; Cone, J.; Wang, S.; Yoshitake, M.; Kambayashi, J. Inhibition of adenosine uptake and augmentation of ischemia-induced increase of interstitial adenosine by cilostazol, an agent to treat intermittent claudication. *J. Cardiovasc. Pharmacol.* **2000**, *36*, 351–360. [CrossRef]
60. Shryock, J.C.; Belardinelli, L. Adenosine and adenosine receptors in the cardiovascular system: Biochemistry, physiology, and pharmacology. *Am. J. Cardiol.* **1997**, *79*, 2–10. [CrossRef]
61. Chancharoenthana, W.; Leelahavanichkul, A.; Taratummarat, S.; Wongphom, J.; Tiranathanagul, K.; Eiam-Ong, S. Cilostazol attenuates intimal hyperplasia in a mouse model of chronic kidney disease. *PLoS ONE* **2017**, *12*, e0187872. [CrossRef]
62. Takahashi, S.; Oida, K.; Fujiwara, R.; Maeda, H.; Hayashi, S.; Takai, H.; Tamai, T.; Nakai, T.; Miyabo, S. Effect of cilostazol, a cyclic AMP phosphodiesterase inhibitor, on the proliferation of rat aortic smooth muscle cells in culture. *J. Cardiovasc. Pharmacol.* **1992**, *20*, 900–906. [CrossRef]
63. Kim, M.J.; Park, K.G.; Lee, K.M.; Kim, H.S.; Kim, S.Y.; Kim, C.S.; Lee, S.L.; Chang, Y.C.; Park, J.Y.; Lee, K.U.; et al. Cilostazol inhibits vascular smooth muscle cell growth by downregulation of the transcription factor E2F. *Hypertension* **2005**, *45*, 552–556. [CrossRef]
64. Takigawa, T.; Tsurushima, H.; Suzuki, K.; Tsuruta, W.; Nakamura, K.; Matsumura, A. Cilostazol suppression of arterial intimal hyperplasia is associated with decreased expression of sialyl Lewis X homing receptors on mononuclear cells and E-selectin in endothelial cells. *J. Vasc. Surg.* **2012**, *55*, 506–516. [CrossRef] [PubMed]
65. Omi, H.; Okayama, N.; Shimizu, M.; Fukutomi, T.; Nakamura, A.; Imaeda, K.; Okouchi, M.; Itoh, M. Cilostazol inhibits high glucose-mediated endothelial-neutrophil adhesion by decreasing adhesion molecule expression via NO production. *Microvasc. Res.* **2004**, *68*, 119–125. [CrossRef]
66. Deglise, S.; Bechelli, C.; Allagnat, F. Vascular smooth muscle cells in intimal hyperplasia, an update. *Front. Physiol.* **2022**, *13*, 1081881. [CrossRef] [PubMed]

67. Chen, W.J.; Chen, Y.H.; Lin, K.H.; Ting, C.H.; Yeh, Y.H. Cilostazol promotes vascular smooth muscles cell differentiation through the cAMP response element-binding protein-dependent pathway. *Arter. Thromb. Vasc. Biol.* **2011**, *31*, 2106–2113. [CrossRef] [PubMed]
68. Hashimoto, A.; Miyakoda, G.; Hirose, Y.; Mori, T. Activation of endothelial nitric oxide synthase by cilostazol via a cAMP/protein kinase A- and phosphatidylinositol 3-kinase/Akt-dependent mechanism. *Atherosclerosis* **2006**, *189*, 350–357. [CrossRef]
69. Moreira, H.S.; Lima-Leal, G.A.; Santos-Rocha, J.; Gomes-Pereira, L.; Duarte, G.P.; Xavier, F.E. Phosphodiesterase-3 inhibitor cilostazol reverses endothelial dysfunction with ageing in rat mesenteric resistance arteries. *Eur. J. Pharmacol.* **2018**, *822*, 59–68. [CrossRef] [PubMed]
70. Suzuki, K.; Uchida, K.; Nakanishi, N.; Hattori, Y. Cilostazol activates AMP-activated protein kinase and restores endothelial function in diabetes. *Am. J. Hypertens.* **2008**, *21*, 451–457. [CrossRef] [PubMed]
71. Morishita, R.; Higaki, J.; Hayashi, S.I.; Yo, Y.; Aoki, M.; Nakamura, S.; Moriguchi, A.; Matsushita, H.; Matsumoto, K.; Nakamura, T.; et al. Role of hepatocyte growth factor in endothelial regulation: Prevention of high D-glucose-induced endothelial cell death by prostaglandins and phosphodiesterase type 3 inhibitor. *Diabetologia* **1997**, *40*, 1053–1061. [CrossRef]
72. Lee, S.J.; Lee, J.S.; Choi, M.H.; Lee, S.E.; Shin, D.H.; Hong, J.M. Cilostazol improves endothelial function in acute cerebral ischemia patients: A double-blind placebo controlled trial with flow-mediated dilation technique. *BMC Neurol.* **2017**, *17*, 169. [CrossRef]
73. Watanabe, K.; Ikeda, S.; Komatsu, J.; Inaba, S.; Suzuki, J.; Sueda, S.; Funada, J.; Kitakaze, M.; Sekiya, M. Effect of cilostazol on vasomotor reactivity in patients with vasospastic angina pectoris. *Am. J. Cardiol.* **2003**, *92*, 21–25. [CrossRef]
74. Zaki, O.S.; Nassar, N.N.; Abdallah, D.M.; Safar, M.M.; Mohammed, R.A. Cilostazol Alleviates NLRP3 Inflammasome-Induced Allodynia/Hyperalgesia in Murine Cerebral Cortex Following Transient Ischemia: Focus on TRPA1/Glutamate and Akt/Dopamine/BDNF/Nrf2 Trajectories. *Mol. Neurobiol.* **2022**, *59*, 7194–7211. [CrossRef]
75. Hoseini, Z.; Sepahvand, F.; Rashidi, B.; Sahebkar, A.; Masoudifar, A.; Mirzaei, H. NLRP3 inflammasome: Its regulation and involvement in atherosclerosis. *J. Cell Physiol.* **2018**, *233*, 2116–2132. [CrossRef] [PubMed]
76. Grebe, A.; Hoss, F.; Latz, E. NLRP3 Inflammasome and the IL-1 Pathway in Atherosclerosis. *Circ. Res.* **2018**, *122*, 1722–1740. [CrossRef] [PubMed]
77. de Oliveira Lopes, R.; Lima, G.F.; Mendes, A.B.A.; Autran, L.J.; de Assis Pereira, N.C.; Brazao, S.C.; Alexandre-Santos, B.; Frantz, E.D.C.; Scaramello, C.B.V.; Brito, F.C.F.; et al. Cilostazol attenuates cardiac oxidative stress and inflammation in hypercholesterolemic rats. *Naunyn Schmiedebergs Arch. Pharmacol.* **2022**, *395*, 789–801. [CrossRef] [PubMed]
78. Li, J.; Xiang, X.; Gong, X.; Shi, Y.; Yang, J.; Xu, Z. Cilostazol protects mice against myocardium ischemic/reperfusion injury by activating a PPARgamma/JAK2/STAT3 pathway. *Biomed. Pharmacother.* **2017**, *94*, 995–1001. [CrossRef] [PubMed]
79. Agrawal, N.K.; Maiti, R.; Dash, D.; Pandey, B.L. Cilostazol reduces inflammatory burden and oxidative stress in hypertensive type 2 diabetes mellitus patients. *Pharmacol. Res.* **2007**, *56*, 118–123. [CrossRef] [PubMed]
80. Lee, D.H.; Chun, E.J.; Oh, T.J.; Kim, K.M.; Moon, J.H.; Choi, S.H.; Park, K.S.; Jang, H.C.; Lim, S. Effect of cilostazol, a phosphodiesterase-3 inhibitor, on coronary artery stenosis and plaque characteristics in patients with type 2 diabetes: ESCAPE study. *Diabetes Obes. Metab.* **2019**, *21*, 1409–1418. [CrossRef] [PubMed]
81. Ahn, C.M.; Hong, S.J.; Park, J.H.; Kim, J.S.; Lim, D.S. Cilostazol reduces the progression of carotid intima-media thickness without increasing the risk of bleeding in patients with acute coronary syndrome during a 2-year follow-up. *Heart Vessel.* **2011**, *26*, 502–510. [CrossRef]
82. Gendy, A.M.; Amin, M.M.; Al-Mokaddem, A.K.; Abd Ellah, M.F. Cilostazol mitigates mesenteric ischemia/reperfusion-induced lung lesion: Contribution of PPAR-gamma, NF-kappaB, and STAT3 crosstalk. *Life Sci.* **2021**, *266*, 118882. [CrossRef]
83. Fujii, T.; Obara, H.; Matsubara, K.; Fujimura, N.; Yagi, H.; Hibi, T.; Abe, Y.; Kitago, M.; Shinoda, M.; Itano, O.; et al. Oral administration of cilostazol improves survival rate after rat liver ischemia/reperfusion injury. *J. Surg. Res.* **2017**, *213*, 207–214. [CrossRef]
84. Bai, Y.; Muqier; Murakami, H.; Iwasa, M.; Sumi, S.; Yamada, Y.; Ushikoshi, H.; Aoyama, T.; Nishigaki, K.; Takemura, G.; et al. Cilostazol protects the heart against ischaemia reperfusion injury in a rabbit model of myocardial infarction: Focus on adenosine, nitric oxide and mitochondrial ATP-sensitive potassium channels. *Clin. Exp. Pharmacol. Physiol.* **2011**, *38*, 658–665. [CrossRef]
85. Tani, T.; Uehara, K.; Sudo, T.; Marukawa, K.; Yasuda, Y.; Kimura, Y. Cilostazol, a selective type III phosphodiesterase inhibitor, decreases triglyceride and increases HDL cholesterol levels by increasing lipoprotein lipase activity in rats. *Atherosclerosis* **2000**, *152*, 299–305. [CrossRef] [PubMed]
86. Hirose, T.; Kurebayashi, S.; Kasayama, S. Antiplatelet agent cilostazol potentiates adipocyte differentiation of 3T3-L1 cells. *Atherosclerosis* **2001**, *158*, 19–22. [CrossRef] [PubMed]
87. Kim, H.J.; Moon, J.H.; Kim, H.M.; Yun, M.R.; Jeon, B.H.; Lee, B.; Kang, E.S.; Lee, H.C.; Cha, B.S. The hypolipidemic effect of cilostazol can be mediated by regulation of hepatic low-density lipoprotein receptor-related protein 1 (LRP1) expression. *Metabolism* **2014**, *63*, 112–119. [CrossRef] [PubMed]
88. Oldoni, F.; van Capelleveen, J.C.; Dalila, N.; Wolters, J.C.; Heeren, J.; Sinke, R.J.; Hui, D.Y.; Dallinga-Thie, G.M.; Frikke-Schmidt, R.; Hovingh, K.G.; et al. Naturally Occurring Variants in LRP1 (Low-Density Lipoprotein Receptor-Related Protein 1) Affect HDL (High-Density Lipoprotein) Metabolism Through ABCA1 (ATP-Binding Cassette A1) and SR-B1 (Scavenger Receptor Class B Type 1) in Humans. *Arter. Thromb. Vasc. Biol.* **2018**, *38*, 1440–1453. [CrossRef] [PubMed]

89. Ito, H.; Uehara, K.; Matsumoto, Y.; Hashimoto, A.; Nagano, C.; Niimi, M.; Miyakoda, G.; Nagano, K. Cilostazol inhibits accumulation of triglyceride in aorta and platelet aggregation in cholesterol-fed rabbits. *PLoS ONE* **2012**, *7*, e39374. [CrossRef] [PubMed]
90. da Motta, N.A.; de Brito, F.C. Cilostazol exerts antiplatelet and anti-inflammatory effects through AMPK activation and NF-kB inhibition on hypercholesterolemic rats. *Fundam. Clin. Pharmacol.* **2016**, *30*, 327–337. [CrossRef] [PubMed]
91. Seo, D.H.; Shin, E.; Lee, Y.H.; Park, S.E.; Nam, K.T.; Kim, J.W.; Cha, B.S. Effects of a Phosphodiesterase inhibitor on the Browning of Adipose Tissue in Mice. *Biomedicines* **2022**, *10*, 1852. [CrossRef] [PubMed]
92. Nedergaard, J.; Golozoubova, V.; Matthias, A.; Asadi, A.; Jacobsson, A.; Cannon, B. UCP1: The only protein able to mediate adaptive non-shivering thermogenesis and metabolic inefficiency. *Biochim. Biophys. Acta* **2001**, *1504*, 82–106. [CrossRef]
93. Thompson, P.D.; Zimet, R.; Forbes, W.P.; Zhang, P. Meta-analysis of results from eight randomized, placebo-controlled trials on the effect of cilostazol on patients with intermittent claudication. *Am. J. Cardiol.* **2002**, *90*, 1314–1319. [CrossRef]
94. Rizzo, M.; Corrado, E.; Patti, A.M.; Rini, G.B.; Mikhailidis, D.P. Cilostazol and atherogenic dyslipidemia: A clinically relevant effect? *Expert. Opin. Pharmacother.* **2011**, *12*, 647–655. [CrossRef]
95. Gotoh, F.; Tohgi, H.; Hirai, S.; Terashi, A.; Fukuuchi, Y.; Otomo, E.; Shinohara, Y.; Itoh, E.; Matsuda, T.; Sawada, T.; et al. Cilostazol stroke prevention study: A placebo-controlled double-blind trial for secondary prevention of cerebral infarction. *J. Stroke Cerebrovasc. Dis.* **2000**, *9*, 147–157. [CrossRef]
96. Douglas, J.S., Jr.; Holmes, D.R., Jr.; Kereiakes, D.J.; Grines, C.L.; Block, E.; Ghazzal, Z.M.; Morris, D.C.; Liberman, H.; Parker, K.; Jurkovitz, C.; et al. Coronary stent restenosis in patients treated with cilostazol. *Circulation* **2005**, *112*, 2826–2832. [CrossRef] [PubMed]
97. Chen, Y.D.; Lu, Y.L.; Jin, Z.N.; Yuan, F.; Lu, S.Z. A prospective randomized antiplatelet trial of cilostazol versus clopidogrel in patients with bare metal stent. *Chin. Med. J.* **2006**, *119*, 360–366. [CrossRef] [PubMed]
98. Lee, S.W.; Park, S.W.; Kim, Y.H.; Yun, S.C.; Park, D.W.; Lee, C.W.; Hong, M.K.; Kim, H.S.; Ko, J.K.; Park, J.H.; et al. Comparison of triple versus dual antiplatelet therapy after drug-eluting stent implantation (from the DECLARE-Long trial). *Am. J. Cardiol.* **2007**, *100*, 1103–1108. [CrossRef] [PubMed]
99. Hiatt, W.R.; Money, S.R.; Brass, E.P. Long-term safety of cilostazol in patients with peripheral artery disease: The CASTLE study (Cilostazol: A Study in Long-term Effects). *J. Vasc. Surg.* **2008**, *47*, 330–336. [CrossRef] [PubMed]
100. Huang, Y.; Cheng, Y.; Wu, J.; Li, Y.; Xu, E.; Hong, Z.; Li, Z.; Zhang, W.; Ding, M.; Gao, X.; et al. Cilostazol as an alternative to aspirin after ischaemic stroke: A randomised, double-blind, pilot study. *Lancet Neurol.* **2008**, *7*, 494–499. [CrossRef] [PubMed]
101. Lee, S.W.; Park, S.W.; Kim, Y.H.; Yun, S.C.; Park, D.W.; Lee, C.W.; Hong, M.K.; Kim, H.S.; Ko, J.K.; Park, J.H.; et al. Drug-eluting stenting followed by cilostazol treatment reduces late restenosis in patients with diabetes mellitus the DECLARE-DIABETES Trial (A Randomized Comparison of Triple Antiplatelet Therapy with Dual Antiplatelet Therapy after Drug-Eluting Stent Implantation in Diabetic Patients). *J. Am. Coll. Cardiol.* **2008**, *51*, 1181–1187. [PubMed]
102. Guo, J.J.; Xu, E.; Lin, Q.Y.; Zeng, G.L.; Xie, H.F. Effect of cilostazol on cerebral arteries in secondary prevention of ischemic stroke. *Neurosci. Bull.* **2009**, *25*, 383–390. [CrossRef] [PubMed]
103. Han, Y.; Li, Y.; Wang, S.; Jing, Q.; Wang, Z.; Wang, D.; Shu, Q.; Tang, X. Cilostazol in addition to aspirin and clopidogrel improves long-term outcomes after percutaneous coronary intervention in patients with acute coronary syndromes: A randomized, controlled study. *Am. Heart J.* **2009**, *157*, 733–739. [CrossRef]
104. Soga, Y.; Yokoi, H.; Kawasaki, T.; Nakashima, H.; Tsurugida, M.; Hikichi, Y.; Nobuyoshi, M. Efficacy of cilostazol after endovascular therapy for femoropopliteal artery disease in patients with intermittent claudication. *J. Am. Coll. Cardiol.* **2009**, *53*, 48–53. [CrossRef] [PubMed]
105. Kwon, S.U.; Hong, K.S.; Kang, D.W.; Park, J.M.; Lee, J.H.; Cho, Y.J.; Yu, K.H.; Koo, J.S.; Wong, K.S.; Lee, S.H.; et al. Efficacy and safety of combination antiplatelet therapies in patients with symptomatic intracranial atherosclerotic stenosis. *Stroke* **2011**, *42*, 2883–2890. [CrossRef]
106. Lee, S.W.; Park, S.W.; Kim, Y.H.; Yun, S.C.; Park, D.W.; Lee, C.W.; Kang, S.J.; Park, S.J.; Lee, J.H.; Choi, S.W.; et al. A randomized, double-blind, multicenter comparison study of triple antiplatelet therapy with dual antiplatelet therapy to reduce restenosis after drug-eluting stent implantation in long coronary lesions: Results from the DECLARE-LONG II (Drug-Eluting Stenting Followed by Cilostazol Treatment Reduces Late Restenosis in Patients with Long Coronary Lesions) trial. *J. Am. Coll. Cardiol.* **2011**, *57*, 1264–1270.
107. Lee, Y.S.; Bae, H.J.; Kang, D.W.; Lee, S.H.; Yu, K.; Park, J.M.; Cho, Y.J.; Hong, K.S.; Kim, D.E.; Kwon, S.U.; et al. Cilostazol in Acute Ischemic Stroke Treatment (CAIST Trial): A randomized double-blind non-inferiority trial. *Cerebrovasc. Dis.* **2011**, *32*, 65–71. [CrossRef] [PubMed]
108. Suh, J.W.; Lee, S.P.; Park, K.W.; Lee, H.Y.; Kang, H.J.; Koo, B.K.; Cho, Y.S.; Youn, T.J.; Chae, I.H.; Choi, D.J.; et al. Multicenter randomized trial evaluating the efficacy of cilostazol on ischemic vascular complications after drug-eluting stent implantation for coronary heart disease: Results of the CILON-T (influence of CILostazol-based triple antiplatelet therapy ON ischemic complication after drug-eluting stenT implantation) trial. *J. Am. Coll. Cardiol.* **2011**, *57*, 280–289. [PubMed]
109. Iida, O.; Yokoi, H.; Soga, Y.; Inoue, N.; Suzuki, K.; Yokoi, Y.; Kawasaki, D.; Zen, K.; Urasawa, K.; Shintani, Y.; et al. Cilostazol reduces angiographic restenosis after endovascular therapy for femoropopliteal lesions in the Sufficient Treatment of Peripheral Intervention by Cilostazol study. *Circulation* **2013**, *127*, 2307–2315. [CrossRef]

110. Gao, W.; Zhang, Q.; Ge, H.; Guo, Y.; Zhou, Z. Efficacy and safety of triple antiplatelet therapy in obese patients undergoing stent implantation. *Angiology* **2013**, *64*, 554–558. [CrossRef]
111. Youn, Y.J.; Lee, J.W.; Ahn, S.G.; Lee, S.H.; Choi, H.; Yu, C.W.; Hong, Y.J.; Kwon, H.M.; Hong, M.K.; Jang, Y.; et al. Multicenter randomized trial of 3-month cilostazol use in addition to dual antiplatelet therapy after biolimus-eluting stent implantation for long or multivessel coronary artery disease. *Am. Heart J.* **2014**, *167*, 241–248.e1. [CrossRef]
112. Uchiyama, S.; Sakai, N.; Toi, S.; Ezura, M.; Okada, Y.; Takagi, M.; Nagai, Y.; Matsubara, Y.; Minematsu, K.; Suzuki, N.; et al. Final Results of Cilostazol-Aspirin Therapy against Recurrent Stroke with Intracranial Artery Stenosis (CATHARSIS). *Cerebrovasc. Dis. Extra* **2015**, *5*, 1–13. [CrossRef] [PubMed]
113. Ueda, H.; Kido, A.; Matsuhisa, S.; Asawa, K.; Yoshida, N.; Tsujimoto, M.; Sasaki, Y.; Kuga, Y.; Yamasaki, M.; Ueda, K.; et al. Addition of cilostazol to aspirin therapy for secondary prevention of cardiovascular and cerebrovascular disease in patients undergoing percutaneous coronary intervention: A randomized, open-label trial. *Am. Heart J.* **2016**, *173*, 134–142. [CrossRef]
114. Zheng, X.T.; Chen, K.Y.; Liu, T.; Xu, L.X.; Che, J.J.; Rha, S.W.; Li, G.P. Low-dose adjunctive cilostazol in patients with complex lesions undergoing percutaneous coronary intervention. *Clin. Exp. Pharmacol. Physiol.* **2016**, *43*, 29–33. [CrossRef]
115. Tang, Y.D.; Wang, W.; Yang, M.; Zhang, K.; Chen, J.; Qiao, S.; Yan, H.; Wu, Y.; Huang, X.; Xu, B.; et al. Randomized Comparisons of Double-Dose Clopidogrel or Adjunctive Cilostazol Versus Standard Dual Antiplatelet in Patients with High Posttreatment Platelet Reactivity: Results of the CREATIVE Trial. *Circulation* **2018**, *137*, 2231–2245. [CrossRef]
116. Lee, C.H.; Lee, J.Y.; Park, G.M.; Lee, S.W.; Kim, H.S.; Choi, Y.J.; Nam, C.W.; Cho, J.H.; Shin, W.Y.; Seo, J.B.; et al. Comparison of 1-Year Outcomes of Triple (Aspirin + Clopidogrel + Cilostazol) Versus Dual Antiplatelet Therapy (Aspirin + Clopidogrel + Placebo) after Implantation of Second-Generation Drug-Eluting Stents into One or More Coronary Arteries: From the DECREASE-PCI Trial. *Am. J. Cardiol.* **2018**, *121*, 423–429.
117. Kim, B.J.; Lee, E.J.; Kwon, S.U.; Park, J.H.; Kim, Y.J.; Hong, K.S.; Wong, L.K.S.; Yu, S.; Hwang, Y.H.; Lee, J.S.; et al. Prevention of cardiovascular events in Asian patients with ischaemic stroke at high risk of cerebral haemorrhage (PICASSO): A multicentre, randomised controlled trial. *Lancet Neurol.* **2018**, *17*, 509–518. [CrossRef] [PubMed]
118. Hong, S.; Nam, M.; Little, B.B.; Paik, S.; Lee, K.; Woo, J.; Kim, D.; Kang, J.; Chun, M.; Park, Y. Randomized control trial comparing the effect of cilostazol and aspirin on changes in carotid intima-medial thickness. *Heart Vessel.* **2019**, *34*, 1758–1768. [CrossRef] [PubMed]
119. Toyoda, K.; Uchiyama, S.; Yamaguchi, T.; Easton, J.D.; Kimura, K.; Hoshino, H.; Sakai, N.; Okada, Y.; Tanaka, K.; Origasa, H.; et al. Dual antiplatelet therapy using cilostazol for secondary prevention in patients with high-risk ischaemic stroke in Japan: A multicentre, open-label, randomised controlled trial. *Lancet Neurol.* **2019**, *18*, 539–548. [CrossRef]
120. Chen, Y.C.; Lin, F.Y.; Lin, Y.W.; Cheng, S.M.; Lin, R.H.; Chuang, C.L.; Sheu, J.S.; Chen, S.M.; Chang, C.C.; Tsai, C.S. DAPT Plus Cilostazol is Better Than Traditional DAPT or Aspirin Plus Ticagrelor as Elective PCI for Intermediate-to-Highly Complex Cases: Prospective, Randomized, PRU-Based Study in Taiwan. *Am. J. Cardiovasc. Drugs* **2019**, *19*, 75–86. [CrossRef]
121. Uchiyama, S.; Toyoda, K.; Omae, K.; Saita, R.; Kimura, K.; Hoshino, H.; Sakai, N.; Okada, Y.; Tanaka, K.; Origasa, H.; et al. Dual Antiplatelet Therapy Using Cilostazol in Patients with Stroke and Intracranial Arterial Stenosis. *J. Am. Heart Assoc.* **2021**, *10*, e022575. [CrossRef]
122. Kalantzi, K.; Tentolouris, N.; Melidonis, A.J.; Papadaki, S.; Peroulis, M.; Amantos, K.A.; Andreopoulos, G.; Bellos, G.I.; Boutel, D.; Bristianou, M.; et al. Efficacy and Safety of Adjunctive Cilostazol to Clopidogrel-Treated Diabetic Patients with Symptomatic Lower Extremity Artery Disease in the Prevention of Ischemic Vascular Events. *J. Am. Heart Assoc.* **2021**, *10*, e018184. [CrossRef]
123. Sohn, M.; Chun, E.J.; Lim, S. Cilostazol treatment for preventing adverse cardiovascular events in patients with type 2 diabetes and coronary atherosclerosis: Long-term follow-up of the ESCAPE study. *J. Diabetes* **2022**, *14*, 524–531. [CrossRef] [PubMed]
124. Lin, J.L.; Tseng, W.K.; Lee, P.T.; Lee, C.H.; Tseng, S.Y.; Chen, P.W.; Chang, H.Y.; Chao, T.H. A Randomized Controlled Trial Evaluating Outcome Impact of Cilostazol in Patients with Coronary Artery Disease or at a High Risk of Cardiovascular Disease. *J. Pers. Med.* **2022**, *12*, 938. [CrossRef] [PubMed]
125. Wardlaw, J.M.; Woodhouse, L.J.; Mhlanga, I.I.; Oatey, K.; Heye, A.K.; Bamford, J.; Cvoro, V.; Doubal, F.N.; England, T.; Hassan, A.; et al. Isosorbide Mononitrate and Cilostazol Treatment in Patients with Symptomatic Cerebral Small Vessel Disease: The Lacunar Intervention Trial-2 (LACI-2) Randomized Clinical Trial. *JAMA Neurol.* **2023**, *80*, 682–692. [CrossRef]
126. McHutchison, C.; Blair, G.W.; Appleton, J.P.; Chappell, F.M.; Doubal, F.; Bath, P.M.; Wardlaw, J.M. Cilostazol for Secondary Prevention of Stroke and Cognitive Decline: Systematic Review and Meta-Analysis. *Stroke* **2020**, *51*, 2374–2385. [CrossRef] [PubMed]
127. Muhammad, I.F.; Borne, Y.; Zaigham, S.; Soderholm, M.; Johnson, L.; Persson, M.; Melander, O.; Engstrom, G. Comparison of risk factors for ischemic stroke and coronary events in a population-based cohort. *BMC Cardiovasc. Disord.* **2021**, *21*, 536. [CrossRef]
128. Xie, W.; Zheng, F.; Zhong, B.; Song, X. Long-Term Antiplatelet Mono- and Dual Therapies after Ischemic Stroke or Transient Ischemic Attack: Network Meta-Analysis. *J. Am. Heart Assoc.* **2015**, *4*, e002259. [CrossRef] [PubMed]
129. Park, S.; Rha, S.W.; Choi, B.G.; Kim, W.; Choi, W.G.; Lee, S.J.; Lee, J.B.; Park, J.Y.; Park, S.M.; Jeong, M.H.; et al. Efficacy and safety of cilostazol-based triple antiplatelet therapy compared with clopidogrel-based dual antiplatelet therapy in patients with acute ST-elevation myocardial infarction undergoing percutaneous coronary intervention: A multicenter, randomized, open-label, phase 4 trial. *Am. Heart J.* **2023**, *265*, 11–21.
130. Kherallah, R.Y.; Khawaja, M.; Olson, M.; Angiolillo, D.; Birnbaum, Y. Cilostazol: A Review of Basic Mechanisms and Clinical Uses. *Cardiovasc. Drugs Ther.* **2022**, *36*, 777–792. [CrossRef]

131. Brown, T.; Forster, R.B.; Cleanthis, M.; Mikhailidis, D.P.; Stansby, G.; Stewart, M. Cilostazol for intermittent claudication. *Cochrane Database Syst. Rev.* **2021**, *6*, CD003748. [CrossRef]
132. Dawson, D.L.; Cutler, B.S.; Hiatt, W.R.; Hobson, R.W., 2nd; Martin, J.D.; Bortey, E.B.; Forbes, W.P.; Strandness, D.E., Jr. A comparison of cilostazol and pentoxifylline for treating intermittent claudication. *Am. J. Med.* **2000**, *109*, 523–530. [CrossRef]
133. Strandness, D.E., Jr.; Dalman, R.L.; Panian, S.; Rendell, M.S.; Comp, P.C.; Zhang, P.; Forbes, W.P. Effect of cilostazol in patients with intermittent claudication: A randomized, double-blind, placebo-controlled study. *Vasc. Endovasc. Surg.* **2002**, *36*, 83–91. [CrossRef] [PubMed]
134. de Franciscis, S.; Gallelli, L.; Battaglia, L.; Molinari, V.; Montemurro, R.; Stillitano, D.M.; Buffone, G.; Serra, R. Cilostazol prevents foot ulcers in diabetic patients with peripheral vascular disease. *Int. Wound J.* **2015**, *12*, 250–253. [CrossRef] [PubMed]
135. Gerhard-Herman, M.D.; Gornik, H.L.; Barrett, C.; Barshes, N.R.; Corriere, M.A.; Drachman, D.E.; Fleisher, L.A.; Fowkes, F.G.R.; Hamburg, N.M.; Kinlay, S.; et al. 2016 AHA/ACC Guideline on the Management of Patients with Lower Extremity Peripheral Artery Disease: Executive Summary: A Report of the American College of Cardiology/American Heart Association Task Force on Clinical Practice Guidelines. *J. Am. Coll. Cardiol.* **2017**, *69*, 1465–1508. [CrossRef]
136. Senbokuya, N.; Kinouchi, H.; Kanemaru, K.; Ohashi, Y.; Fukamachi, A.; Yagi, S.; Shimizu, T.; Furuya, K.; Uchida, M.; Takeuchi, N.; et al. Effects of cilostazol on cerebral vasospasm after aneurysmal subarachnoid hemorrhage: A multicenter prospective, randomized, open-label blinded end point trial. *J. Neurosurg.* **2013**, *118*, 121–130. [CrossRef]
137. Takagi, T.; Hara, H. Protective effects of cilostazol against hemorrhagic stroke: Current and future perspectives. *J. Pharmacol. Sci.* **2016**, *131*, 155–161. [CrossRef]
138. Lee, J.H.; Park, S.Y.; Shin, H.K.; Kim, C.D.; Lee, W.S.; Hong, K.W. Protective effects of cilostazol against transient focal cerebral ischemia and chronic cerebral hypoperfusion injury. *CNS Neurosci. Ther.* **2008**, *14*, 143–152. [CrossRef] [PubMed]
139. Lim, J.H.; Woo, J.S.; Shin, Y.W. Cilostazol protects endothelial cells against lipopolysaccharide-induced apoptosis through ERK1/2- and P38 MAPK-dependent pathways. *Korean J. Intern. Med.* **2009**, *24*, 113–122. [CrossRef] [PubMed]
140. Watanabe, T.; Zhang, N.; Liu, M.; Tanaka, R.; Mizuno, Y.; Urabe, T. Cilostazol protects against brain white matter damage and cognitive impairment in a rat model of chronic cerebral hypoperfusion. *Stroke* **2006**, *37*, 1539–1545. [CrossRef]
141. Takagi, T.; Imai, T.; Mishiro, K.; Ishisaka, M.; Tsujimoto, M.; Ito, H.; Nagashima, K.; Matsukawa, H.; Tsuruma, K.; Shimazawa, M.; et al. Cilostazol ameliorates collagenase-induced cerebral hemorrhage by protecting the blood-brain barrier. *J. Cereb. Blood Flow. Metab.* **2017**, *37*, 123–139. [CrossRef]
142. Lee, J.H.; Park, S.Y.; Shin, Y.W.; Hong, K.W.; Kim, C.D.; Sung, S.M.; Kim, K.Y.; Lee, W.S. Neuroprotection by cilostazol, a phosphodiesterase type 3 inhibitor, against apoptotic white matter changes in rat after chronic cerebral hypoperfusion. *Brain Res.* **2006**, *1082*, 182–191. [CrossRef] [PubMed]
143. Shichinohe, H.; Tan, C.; Abumiya, T.; Nakayama, N.; Kazumata, K.; Hokari, M.; Houkin, K.; Kuroda, S. Neuroprotective effects of cilostazol are mediated by multiple mechanisms in a mouse model of permanent focal ischemia. *Brain Res.* **2015**, *1602*, 53–61. [CrossRef] [PubMed]
144. Kim, B.C.; Youn, Y.C.; Jeong, J.H.; Han, H.J.; Kim, J.H.; Lee, J.H.; Park, K.H.; Park, K.W.; Kim, E.J.; Oh, M.S.; et al. Cilostazol Versus Aspirin on White Matter Changes in Cerebral Small Vessel Disease: A Randomized Controlled Trial. *Stroke* **2022**, *53*, 698–709. [CrossRef] [PubMed]
145. Pratt, C.M. Analysis of the cilostazol safety database. *Am. J. Cardiol.* **2001**, *87*, 28D–33D. [CrossRef]
146. Lee, D.H.; Chun, E.J.; Moon, J.H.; Yun, H.M.; Lim, S. Effect of cilostazol on carotid plaque volume measured by three-dimensional ultrasonography in patients with type 2 diabetes: The FANCY study. *Diabetes Obes. Metab.* **2020**, *22*, 2257–2266. [CrossRef]
147. Otsuka. *Pletal—Highlights of Prescribing Information*; Otsuka: Tokyo, Japan, 1999.

International Journal of
Molecular Sciences

Review

Coronary Plaque Erosion: Epidemiology, Diagnosis, and Treatment

Panagiotis Theofilis [1], Panayotis K. Vlachakis [1], Aggelos Papanikolaou [1], Paschalis Karakasis [2], Evangelos Oikonomou [3], Konstantinos Tsioufis [1] and Dimitris Tousoulis [1,*]

1 1st Department of Cardiology, "Hippokration" General Hospital, National and Kapodistrian University of Athens, 11527 Athens, Greece; panos.theofilis@hotmail.com (P.T.); vlachakispanag@gmail.com (P.K.V.); agepap25@otenet.gr (A.P.); kptsioufis@gmail.com (K.T.)
2 2nd Department of Cardiology, "Hippokration" General Hospital, Aristotle University of Thessaloniki, 54642 Thessaloniki, Greece; pakar15@hotmail.com
3 3rd Department of Cardiology, Thoracic Diseases General Hospital "Sotiria", National and Kapodistrian University of Athens, 11527 Athens, Greece; boikono@gmail.com
* Correspondence: drtousoulis@hotmail.com

Abstract: Plaque erosion (PE), a distinct etiology of acute coronary syndromes (ACSs), is often overshadowed by plaque ruptures (PRs). Concerning its epidemiology, PE has garnered increasing recognition, with recent studies revealing its prevalence to be approximately 40% among ACS patients, challenging earlier assumptions based on autopsy data. Notably, PE exhibits distinct epidemiological features, preferentially affecting younger demographics, particularly women, and often manifesting as a non-ST-segment elevation myocardial infarction. There are seasonal variations, with PE events being less common in winter, potentially linked to physiological changes and cholesterol solidification, while peaking in summer, warranting further investigation. Moving to molecular mechanisms, PE presents a unique profile characterized by a lesser degree of inflammation compared to PR, with endothelial shear stress emerging as a plausible molecular mechanism. Neutrophil activation, toll-like receptor-2 pathways, and hyaluronidase 2 expression are among the factors implicated in PE pathophysiology, underscoring its multifactorial nature. Advancements in intravascular imaging diagnostics, particularly optical coherence tomography and near-infrared spectroscopy coupled with intravascular ultrasound, offer unprecedented insights into plaque composition and morphology. Artificial intelligence algorithms show promise in enhancing diagnostic accuracy and streamlining image interpretation, augmenting clinician decision-making. Therapeutically, the management of PE evolves, with studies exploring less invasive approaches such as antithrombotic therapy without stenting, particularly in cases identified early through intravascular imaging. Additionally, the potential role of drug-coated balloons in reducing thrombus burden and minimizing future major adverse cardiovascular events warrants further investigation. Looking ahead, the integration of advanced imaging modalities, biomarkers, and artificial intelligence promises to revolutionize the diagnosis and treatment of coronary PE, ushering in a new era of personalized and precise cardiovascular care.

Keywords: atherosclerosis; coronary artery disease; acute coronary syndrome; plaque erosion; molecular mechanisms; optical coherence tomography

1. Introduction

Acute coronary syndromes (ACSs) constitute a significant burden on global healthcare systems and remain a leading cause of morbidity and mortality worldwide. Within the spectrum of ACS, plaque rupture (PR) has traditionally garnered considerable attention as the predominant etiology, shaping therapeutic strategies and research agendas. The management of ACS has evolved with the introduction of newer antiplatelet agents, more potent statins, and novel therapies targeting inflammation and plaque stabilization. Additionally, early invasive strategies like coronary angiography and percutaneous coronary intervention (PCI) have become the standard of care.

Although the existing therapeutic advances in this field have been based on the concept of ruptured plaques, recent insights have illuminated the role of another distinct culprit: plaque erosion (PE). While often overshadowed by PR, PE represents a substantial portion of ACS cases, with its epidemiology, diagnosis, and management offering a rich terrain for exploration and innovation. Advances in intravascular imaging techniques have improved our ability to detect and characterize PE. Interestingly, such precise plaque characterization might have therapeutic implications, with personalized approaches to PE management. Therefore, in this review article, we delve into the multifaceted landscape of coronary PE, aiming to provide a comprehensive overview of its epidemiology, diagnostic modalities, and therapeutic considerations.

2. Plaque Phenotypes

2.1. Plaque Rupture

Coronary thrombosis driven by PR constitutes a significant portion, approximately 75%, of all ACSs. Various conventional cardiovascular risk factors like hypertension, smoking, diabetes, hyperlipidemia, and obesity, alongside non-traditional factors like inflammation, infection, and genetic predisposition, collectively contribute to the development of vulnerable plaques. For instance, hypertension imposes mechanical strain on the arterial wall, accelerating plaque formation and elevating the likelihood of rupture. Diabetes and smoking exacerbate plaque inflammation, compromise endothelial function, and foster plaque instability.

The inception of PR occurs within a vulnerable plaque, characterized by a thin fibrous cap overlaying a lipid-laden core [1]. Beneath this cap lies a cluster of inflammatory cells, including macrophages and T lymphocytes, actively involved in ongoing plaque inflammation and restructuring [1]. The breach of the fibrous cap exposes the lipid core to the bloodstream, initiating a cascade of events [1]. Mechanical stress, inflammation, and degradation of the extracellular matrix are among the factors precipitating PR. Hemodynamic factors like shear stress and cyclic strain exert mechanical strain on the plaque, leading to cap thinning and eventual rupture. Moreover, prolonged inflammation within the plaque prompts the release of proteolytic enzymes, particularly matrix metalloproteinases (MMPs), which degrade components of the extracellular matrix [2]. An imbalance between MMPs and their inhibitors weakens the fibrous cap, rendering it more susceptible to rupture [2]. Inflammation plays a pivotal role in both the initiation and progression of PR. Circulating monocytes adhere to activated endothelial cells, infiltrating into the intima where they differentiate into macrophages [3]. These macrophages, upon internalizing oxidized low-density lipoproteins, transform into foam cells, contributing to the formation of the lipid core [3]. Inflammatory cytokines such as interleukin-6 (IL-6) and tumor necrosis factor-alpha (TNF-α) heighten plaque vulnerability by perpetuating inflammation [4]. Additionally, local inflammatory mediators such as C-reactive protein (CRP) significantly contribute to plaque destabilization, elevating the risk of rupture [4].

2.2. Calcified Nodule

The role of calcified nodules in ACS has gained increasing attention. Calcified nodules refer to discrete calcified structures within the coronary arteries that can contribute to luminal narrowing and subsequent ischemic events. The formation of calcified nodules in coronary arteries involves a complex interplay of biological processes, including inflammation, osteogenic transformation, and matrix remodeling [5]. Chronic inflammation within atherosclerotic plaques triggers the release of pro-inflammatory cytokines and growth factors, stimulating the migration and differentiation of vascular smooth muscle cells (VSMCs) into osteoblast-like cells. These VSMCs promote the deposition of calcium phosphate crystals, leading to the development of calcified nodules. Matrix remodeling, characterized by altered expression of matrix metalloproteinases and their inhibitors, further contributes to the process. Calcified nodules are responsible for 5.3% of ACS [6]. Several traditional risk factors for atherosclerosis, including advanced age, male gender, hypertension, dyslipidemia, and diabetes mellitus, are associated with an increased likelihood of calcified nodules [7]. In addition, emerging risk factors such as chronic kidney disease and genetic predisposition have been implicated [7]. These risk factors promote vascular calcification by disrupting the balance between calcification inhibitors and promoters, favoring the deposition of calcium within the arterial wall.

2.3. Plaque Erosion

While calcified nodules are characterized by the presence of focal calcifications within the atherosclerotic plaque and PR involves the rupture of an atherosclerotic plaque's fibrous cap, PE predominantly involves superficial erosion of the denuded endothelium without extensive calcification (Figure 1). The presence of PE in culprit coronary arteries of patients with ACS has been increasingly more common over the years. Two main factors could be responsible for this observation. First and foremost, although early studies have noted a PE prevalence in approximately 20% of ACS patients, they were based on autopsy studies of fatal acute cardiovascular events that may be more commonly associated with PR [8]. Invasive vascular imaging was not widely used; thus, these rates could have been falsely low. Moreover, the increased awareness regarding the management of major cardiovascular risk factors may have accounted for the attenuation of atherosclerosis progression and the stabilization of atherosclerotic plaques [8]. Specifically, aggressive lipid-lowering therapies (statins, ezetimibe, bempedoic acid, and proprotein convertase subtilisin/kexin type 9 (PCSK9) inhibitors including inclisiran) [9–13], novel antidiabetic agents with pleiotropic effects (sodium-glucose cotransporter-2 inhibitors, glucagon-like peptide-1 receptor agonists) [14,15], and contemporary antihypertensive medications (renin-angiotensin-aldosterone system blockers) are common approaches with significant anti-atherosclerotic effects. Smoking cessation and adaptation of a healthier lifestyle in terms of diet and exercise could be essential determinants of atherosclerosis stabilization [16–18]. The importance of inflammation should be also stressed, as the residual inflammatory risk is a crucial aspect of the atherosclerotic process that could be medically managed with agents such as colchicine [19], sodium-glucose cotransporter-2 inhibitors [20], and others. As a result, the regression of atherosclerosis could prevent vulnerable, rupture-prone plaque formations and lead to more cases of non-ST-segment elevation myocardial infarction (NSTEMI) with PE. We should also mention that the use of invasive vascular imaging methods and the establishment of possible PE criteria could have contributed to a greater degree of PE detection. It is, therefore, unsurprising that contemporary studies in the field have produced PE rates of approximately 40% [8]. However, even such rates may not reflect the true prevalence of PE, since only a limited proportion of patients with ACS undergo invasive coronary imaging with optical coherence tomography (OCT) or intravascular ultrasound (IVUS).

The epidemiology of PE has distinct characteristics. To begin with, it appears that men and women are equally affected overall, presenting with PE in 40% of ACS based on the study of Seegers et al. (Figure 2) [21]. When looking at the trends of PE prevalence according to age, a stepwise decrease is noted, with higher rates being recorded in those <70 years of age (<50: 55%, 51–60: 43%, 61–70: 41%, Figure 2). The evidence is lacking regarding racial differences in PE prevalence, with one study showing similar rates in Asian and White patients after adjustment for confounders [22].

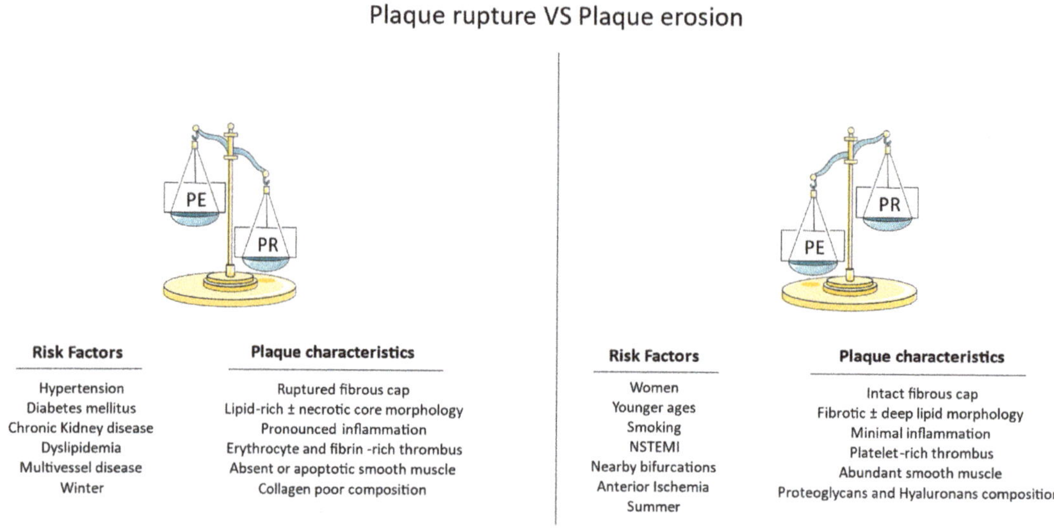

Figure 1. Risk factors and plaque characteristics in plaque erosion (PE) vs. plaque rupture (PR). NSTEMI—non-ST-segment elevation myocardial infarction.

Concerning additional age-related characteristics of patients with ACS caused by PE, younger patients present more commonly with thrombus (and a STEMI), while the elderly more frequently have greater percentage diameter stenoses and lipid-rich and calcified plaques [23]. In an attempt to better characterize PE prevalence and risk factors solely in women with ACS, Seegers et al. performed OCT prior to PCI in 382 women and found that PE was more common in younger women (<60 years old) and in NSTE-ACS [24]. Among the examined factors, a family history of CAD was predictive of PE presence [24]. Additionally, ACS events triggered by PE occur at lower rates during the winter season compared to the summer season (odds ratio (OR): 0.62, 95% confidence interval (CI): 0.43–0.91, $p = 0.013$). This interesting observation could potentially be explained by the increases in blood pressure at lower temperatures due to the stimulation of cold skin receptors and the rise in circulating catecholamines [25], together with cholesterol solidification [26], rendering a coronary plaque more prone to rupture. On the contrary, a greater incidence of PE during the summer season is a finding that mandates further research regarding its pathophysiologic basis.

Eroded plaques are less likely to cause STEMIs but are frequently implicated in cases of NSTEMI [27]. Several studies have found that PE is preferentially localized in the left anterior descending artery (LAD), notably in the proximal and mid segments, which are grouped around a bifurcation [28–30]. This usual distribution may represent distinct local hemodynamic pressures working within the coronary circulation, such as altered endothelial shear stress, which may be more prominent in a conduit that has side branches, such as the LAD [31]. In terms of angiographic properties, PE is associated with a less complicated and widespread atherosclerotic pattern than PR [28–30]. PE was associated with a lower prevalence of multivessel CAD (28.5% vs. 49.6%, $p < 0.001$), a lower Gensini score (21.3 vs. 25.6, $p = 0.014$), and a lower Syntax score (8.9 vs. 11.5, $p < 0.001$) compared to PR in a cohort of NSTE-ACS patients [28]. These characteristics are consistent with OCT evidence revealing decreased pancoronary vulnerability in patients with PE, and may help to explain why these individuals have a better prognosis than those with PR [32,33]. PE lesions are less commonly related with a baseline thrombolysis in myocardial infarction (TIMI) flow grade 1. Furthermore, PE is frequently linked with a simpler angiographic lesion phenotype. PE generally exhibits a more "simple" A/B1 lesion phenotype when using the ACC/AHA lesion categorization, as opposed to PR, which typically exhibits a "complex" B2/C lesion phenotype [34]. PE is more commonly linked with a concentric type I lesion, whereas PR is associated with an eccentric type II lesion, according to the Ambrose lesion classification [34]. PE, unlike PR, is less usually associated with angiographic signs of calcification and thrombus [34]. However, PE could be on a background of a lipid-rich plaque (maximal lipid arc >180°), which may share similarities with PR, such as the presentation (STEMI), peak creatine kinase level, and small dense low-density lipoprotein cholesterol levels of affected patients, as opposed to PE of a fibrous plaque [35].

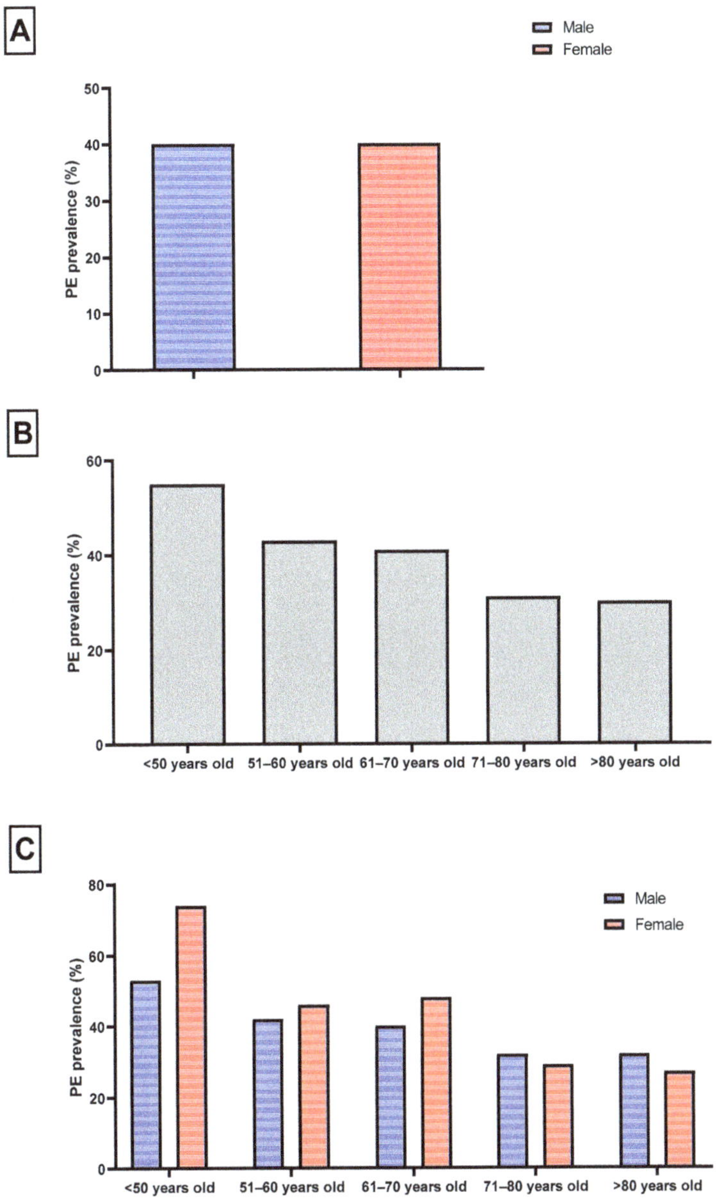

Figure 2. Trends in plaque erosion (PE) prevalence according to (**A**) sexes, (**B**) age categories, and (**C**) age-sex categories.

Prognosis also differs between PR and PE. In an analysis of 398 consecutive ACS patients (62% PR, 25% PE), major adverse cardiovascular events (cardiac mortality, recurrent ACS, hospitalization for unstable angina, and target vessel revascularization) occurred less frequently in patients with PE (14.3% vs. 26.7%, $p = 0.02$) [36]. In another analysis of 702 ACS patients treated with OCT-guided PCI, the subgroup of patients with PE as the underlying pathophysiology faced the lowest proportion of major adverse cardiac events at 1 year when compared to PR and calcified nodules (6.2% vs. 12.4% vs. 32.1%, $p < 0.0001$) [37]. Specifically, patients with PR and calcified nodules have a 2.18-fold and 4.49-fold higher risk of 1-year major adverse cardiac events, respectively, with PE as the reference [37].

Last but not least, patients with PE frequently exhibit less extensive non-coronary atherosclerosis compared to PR as evidenced by peripheral plaque prevalence (79.1% vs. 93.4%, $p < 0.001$), as well as a lower number of peripheral atherosclerotic plaques [38]. Characteristics of peripheral lesion vulnerability (surface irregularity, plaque heterogeneity, and calcification) are also less commonly seen in patients with ACS caused by PE [38].

3. Molecular Mechanisms of PE

Histologically, eroded plaques exhibit distinct features that differentiate them from ruptured plaques. Eroded plaques often have a thick fibrous cap without evidence of cap disruption. Instead of a lipid core, they commonly demonstrate superficial platelet-rich (white) thrombi adherent to an intact endothelial surface. Eroded plaques were rich in extracellular matrix components, such as proteoglycans and glycosaminoglycans, rather than lipids. Eroded lesions had fewer inflammatory cells and more vascular smooth muscle cells than ruptured plaques. The absence of a fibrous cap rupture and the presence of adherent thrombi are key histopathological characteristics distinguishing PE from PR.

Regarding the molecular mechanisms implicated in PE pathophysiology, an inflammatory process of a lesser magnitude is described in PE compared to PR, as shown by a lower inflammatory expression of NLRP3 inflammasome downstream products such as IL-1β-associated proteins and IL-6 [36].

The role of endothelial sheer stress has been increasingly speculated as a molecular mechanism of PE development. Based on the study of Hakim et al. in patients who underwent coronary angiography and OCT examination, maximal endothelial sheer stress (OR: 1.32, 95% CI: 1.06–1.65, $p = 0.014$) and maximal endothelial sheer stress gradient in any direction (OR: 1.22, 95% CI: 1.03–1.45, $p = 0.009$) were independent predictors of PE development [39]. Those parameters appear largely unchanged during a 12-month follow-up in 23 patients treated with a no-stent strategy and dual antiplatelet therapy for 1 year after the index ACS [40], suggesting the persistence of the prothrombotic state due to augmented endothelial sheer stress and potentially a need for prolonged intense antithrombotic treatment. While the presence of PE near bifurcations could serve as a simple explanation of the enhanced endothelial sheer stress, a significant proportion of PE leading to ACS arise from vessel areas away from bifurcations (~30%) based on the OPTICO-ACS study [41]. This could be partially explained by the presence of coronary microevaginations, which could serve as a medium of coronary flow disruption and adverse vascular remodeling [42]. Moreover, in such instances, there is a more pronounced activation of the innate immune system, especially $CD14^{+}CD16^{-}$ classical monocytes [42].

A recently proposed prevailing theory regarding PE suggests that it involves multiple hits, including distinct activation of neutrophils dependent on toll-like receptor-2 (TLR2) [43]. This activation is believed to be sustained by an increased local expression of hyaluronidase 2, leading to heightened cleavage of hyaluronic acid at the coronary culprit eroded lesion [43]. Consequently, this results in the intensified release of active MMP9 by neutrophils, exacerbating the detachment of luminal endothelial cells under disturbed flow conditions [43]. Besides the significance of the TLR2 pathway in patients with PE, there is a general exacerbation of neutrophil cytotoxicity towards endothelial cells independent of TLR2, which may contribute to the progression of PE [43]. MMP9 may also play a role in bridging innate and adaptive immunity, potentially triggering a complementary T-cell-mediated response in individuals with PE [43].

4. Diagnostic Approach toward Plaque Erosion

Understanding the diagnostic approach towards coronary PE necessitates a comprehensive integration of evolving methodologies, such as circulating biomarkers and intravascular imaging techniques, in particular (Figure 3). In this section, we discuss the current advances in the field of PE diagnosis.

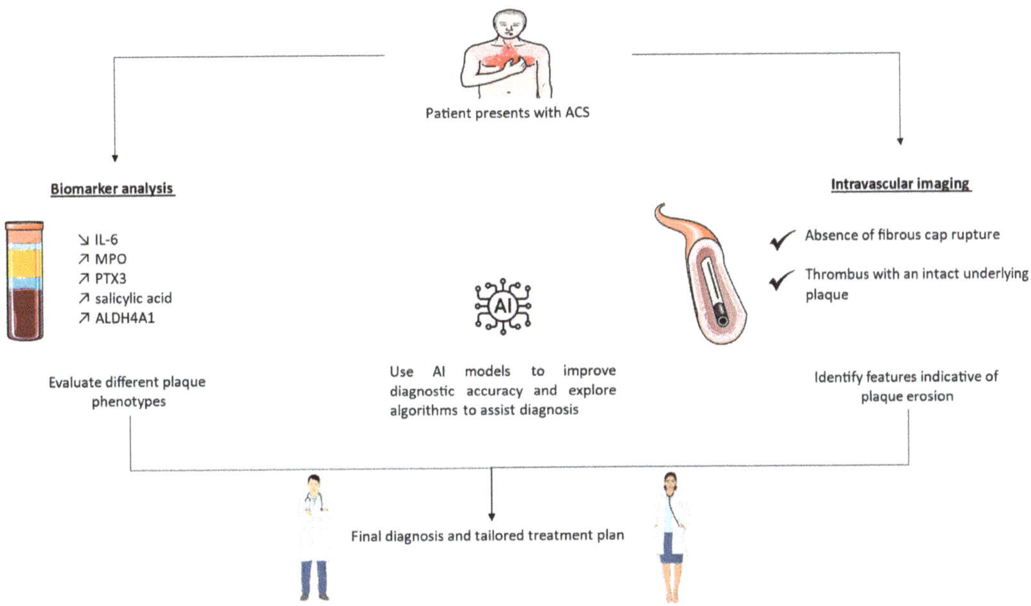

Figure 3. Diagnostic pathway to identify coronary plaque erosion. ACS—acute coronary syndrome, AI—artificial intelligence, IL-6—interleukin-6, MPO—myeloperoxidase, PTX3—pentraxin 3, ALDH4A1—Aldehyde dehydrogenase 4A1.

4.1. Biomarkers

In the field of biomarkers, several research efforts have been made in trying to differentiate between plaque phenotypes. Beginning with inflammatory biomarkers, and according to the OPTICO-ACS study, peripheral blood concentration of IL-6 was significantly lower in patients with PE compared to PR (3.6 ± 3.9 pg/mL vs. 1.4 ± 1.9 pg/mL, $p = 0.006$), but no difference in other common inflammatory biomarkers (CRP, IL-1β) were noted [36]. Importantly, this study found no alterations in inflammatory biomarkers for patients with PE at follow-up examinations [36]. These findings are in line with previous reports showcasing a lower systemic inflammatory burden in PE compared to PR [44]. With regards to CRP, the most widely used circulating inflammatory biomarker, multiple studies have failed to identify differences in its concentration according to plaque phenotype [36,45,46].

Myeloperoxidase (MPO) has been suggested as a systemic biomarker of PE. MPO, serving as an indicator of neutrophil activation, has the potential to promote thrombosis by producing reactive oxygen species, leading to endothelial cell apoptosis and a decrease in nitric oxide levels [47]. Consequently, this exacerbates the deterioration of the endothelial layer in eroded plaques [47]. In a study of 25 consecutive ACS patients (PE: 28%), MPO levels were significantly elevated in PE compared to PR (2500 ng/mL vs. 707 ng/mL, $p = 0.001$) [45]. Similar findings were replicated in a cohort of patients with NSTE-ACS or stable angina, where MPO levels were considerably higher in subjects with PE compared to the other entities (PE: 685.9 ng/mL vs. PR: 340.0 ng/mL vs. stable angina: 272.5 ng/mL, $p < 0.001$) [48]. According to this study, MPO was an independent predictor of PE presence (OR: 1.04, 95% CI: 1.01–1.05, $p = 0.04$) [48]. In the largest prospective study to date in 172 STEMI patients (PE: 46.5%), plasma MPO was higher in PE compared to PR (96.3 ng/mL vs. 41.7 ng/mL, $p < 0.001$), representing an independent predictor (OR: 3.25, 95% CI: 1.37–7.76, $p = 0.008$) but with moderate discriminative ability (area under ROC curve: 0.75, optimal cutoff: 74.2 ng/mL with sensitivity: 64% and specificity: 82%) [49].

Pentraxin 3 (PTX3) is another marker with potentially prognostic significance in the setting of ACS [50]. When considering patients with PE, a high PTX3 concentration (≥6.6 ng/mL) was associated with a higher incidence of the composite endpoint (all-cause death, recurrence of myocardial infarction, stroke, and unplanned revascularization of any coronary artery) during a 1.9-year follow-up (hazard ratio (HR): 5.44, 95% CI: 1.46–20.29, $p = 0.012$) [51]. Based on the study of Zhao et al., PTX3 was associated with fibrous and healing plaques in patients with PE [52]. Prognostically, PTX3 was associated with an over 8-fold increase in the incidence of adverse endpoints in patients with PE, independently of confounders [52].

Apart from inflammation, dyslipidemia is a major mediator of atherosclerosis. While lipid biomarkers, such as Apolipoprotein A-I (ApoA-I) and Apolipoprotein B (ApoB), are strongly associated with the development and progression of atherosclerosis, there is no evidence suggesting their ability to differentiate between PR and PE. A study has previously suggested the presence of plaque instability in cases of high ApoB/A-I ratio [53]. Moreover, given that ApoB/A-I was negatively correlated with fibrous cap thickness [54], we may assume that a lower ratio in the setting of ACS could identify patients with PE. However, this remains to be proven in future studies.

Moving to other less studied markers, in the study of Luo et al. in 123 patients with STEMI, increased salicylic acid was associated with PE presence [55]. However, we should note the mediocre area under the receiver operating characteristic (<0.8) [55]. Given that thrombi in eroded plaques are white, consisting of highly activated platelets, this finding may indicate the existence of disordered salicylic acid metabolism and consequent platelet hyperactivity. Moreover, increased concentrations of salicylic could identify patients with PE who could benefit from intensified antiplatelet therapy regimens, a concept which needs to be further tested.

MicroRNAs are another category of molecules with diagnostic and therapeutic potential in cardiovascular diseases [56–58]. Concerning plaque phenotyping, however, evidence remains scarce. Dong et al. studied 76 culprit lesions (32.6% PE) in STEMI patients and in a subanalysis of 16 patients with PE or RP, they found dysregulated expression of 34 microRNAs [59]. Among them, only a higher expression of circulating microRNA-3667-3p remained predictive of PE even after multivariable adjustment (OR: 2.28, 95% CI 1.19–4.35, $p = 0.01$) [59]. Li et al. examined a pool of 24 differentially expressed microRNAs, which was subsequently narrowed to 5 based on the results of the validation cohort [60]. In a replication cohort, the investigators noted lower expression of microRNAs-744-3p, -324-3p, -330-3p, -641, and -4435 in PE compared to PR [60].

Finally, a potential role of Aldehyde dehydrogenase 4A1 (ALDH4A1) was suggested by the study of Li et al. in 312 patients with STEMI (151 with PE) [61]. The circulating plasma ALDH4A1 was significantly increased in subjects with PE compared to PR (4.6 ng/mL vs. 3.5 ng/mL $p = 0.005$), while its abundance in PE was confirmed after immunofluorescence in aspirated coronary thrombus samples [61].

4.2. Intravascular Imaging

4.2.1. Optical Coherence Tomography

Intravascular imaging is perhaps the method of choice in identifying PE, namely with OCT, as it has a 10-fold higher spatial resolution than IVUS. OCT is unable to view the endothelium monolayer directly. Because endothelial cell loss is a pathological characteristic of PE, this constraint prevents the use of endothelial cell absence as an OCT criterion for identifying PE. OCT has developed a plaque classification algorithm as a result of this. In patients with ACS, the absence of a fibrous cap rupture at the culprit lesion on OCT implies PE, according to this strategy (Figure 4). Identification of a thrombus with an intact underlying plaque is required for a definitive diagnosis of PE. If the luminal surface of the plaque appears sloppy in the absence of a thrombus or if there is a thrombus that hinders the visibility of an underlying plaque without a subjacent lipid accumulation or calcium proximal or distal to the lesion, PE is suspected. This exclusionary approach leads to significant discrepancies in the reported prevalence of PE across various OCT studies. To this end, artificial intelligence may have the potential to improve diagnostic accuracy. Park et al. tested two different deep learning algorithms, convolutional neural networks and transformers, regarding their diagnostic accuracy for PE [62]. They found that the transformer model had slightly superior accuracy at the lesion level (sensitivity: 91.9%, specificity: 81.6%) [62]. When compared to human diagnosticians, the model was superior to less experienced operators but inferior to more experienced operators [62]. Importantly, when it was supplied to less experienced operators, it could assist in improving their diagnostic capabilities toward PE and ultimately outperform the model [62]. Therefore, artificial intelligence could be of critical assistance to flatten out the learning curve in this field.

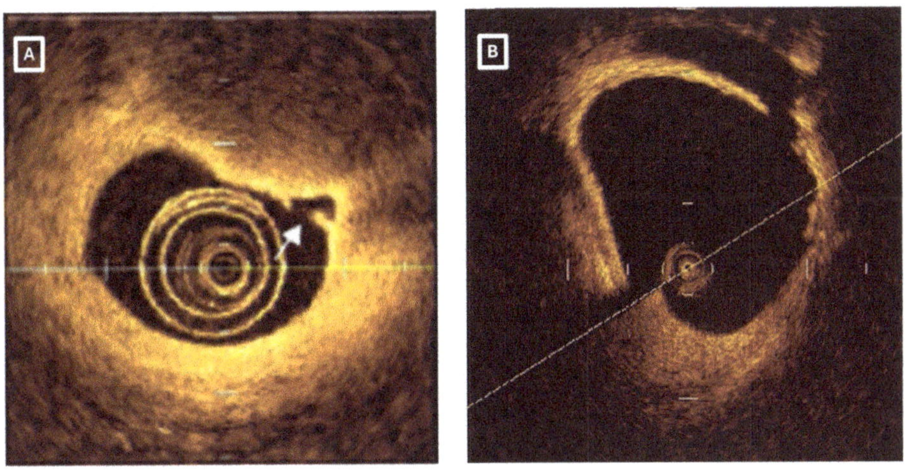

Figure 4. Optical coherence tomography of (**A**) plaque rupture (white arrow) and (**B**) and plaque erosion.

Concerning prognostic features, an increased abundance of lipids proximally to the erosion site was independently related to a higher incidence of major adverse cardiovascular (HR: 3.74, 95% CI: 1.22–11.5, $p = 0.02$) after a median follow-up of 2.97 years in a cohort of 152 STEMI patients with PE [63]. Proximal lipid content above the median value was associated with a higher fibrous cap thickness, thin cap fibroatheroma prevalence, and the presence of macrophages [63].

4.2.2. Intravascular Ultrasound-Near-Infrared Spectroscopy

High-definition intravascular ultrasound (IVUS) enables detailed examination of the luminal surface and holds potential for detecting PE. Several case series highlight the usefulness of high-definition IVUS in assessing PE [64]. The absence of significant vessel wall abnormalities alongside minor intimal irregularities, with or without thrombus, may indicate PE. Additionally, the presence of fibrotic or lipid plaques exhibiting surface irregularities or layered images, without evidence of cap rupture, could suggest PE. IVUS can also demonstrate the negative vascular remodeling process in the cases of PE compared to the positive remodeling in PR, a finding which is also indicative of the diagnosis [65]. Nonetheless, it is important to acknowledge the inherent difficulty in diagnosing PE using IVUS, since it lacks the resolution necessary for directly visualizing fibrous cap thickness. However, IVUS can be particularly beneficial in cases where PE is suspected and OCT cannot be performed, such as patients with significant renal dysfunction at risk of contrast-associated acute kidney injury. The addition of virtual histology may further aid in characterizing the tissue underneath the plaque by identifying white thrombus and fibrosis [65].

Near-infrared spectroscopy (NIRS), when added to IVUS (IVUS-NIRS), has the ability to quantify lipid core burdens through the lipid core burden index (LCBI). IVUS-NIRS has recently been assessed in 244 patients with ACS regarding its ability to discriminate between PR, PE, and calcified nodule, with an OCT diagnosis as the reference standard [66]. Based on their analysis with a development cohort and a validation cohort, the investigators proposed a three-step approach regarding plaque phenotyping with IVUS-NIRS [66]. Initially, the presence of convex calcium signifies the presence of a calcified nodule (sensitivity 100%, specificity: 99%) [66]. Next, the occurrence of plaque cavitation is a distinct characteristic of definite PR (sensitivity: 97%, specificity: 96%) [66]. In its absence, the maximal LCBI at 4 mm should be assessed, with values below 426 indicating PE (sensitivity: 93%, specificity: 99%, positive predictive value: 93%, negative predictive value 99%) [66].

4.3. Non-Invasive Imaging

Coronary computed tomography angiography (CCTA) has recently gained attention as a method for characterizing the plaque phenotype of patients with ACS. While the features of vulnerable coronary atherosclerotic plaques that are prone to rupture have been well-established in previous studies [1], its role in identifying PE has not been thoroughly investigated. PE may exhibit lower coronary artery inflammation as assessed by the CCTA-derived pericoronary adipose tissue (PCAT) attenuation, which is considerably higher in cases of PR [67]. Moreover, a recently published study suggested that the absence of vulnerable plaque features (low attenuation, napkin-ring sign, PCAT attenuation in culprit vessel >-70.3) and a zero coronary artery calcium score are independent predictors of PE presence, with an increasing frequency when multiple criteria were fulfilled [68]. In another study, total plaque volume was another variable that related to the presence of PE (OR: 0.995, 95% CI: 0.99–1, $p = 0.038$), with values ≤ 116 mm^3 determined as the optimal cutoff.

5. Treatment of Plaque Erosion: Contemporary Practice and Future Considerations

As previously stated, patients with PE often have a better prognosis and a lower risk of adverse cardiovascular events compared to those with PR. Since clinical studies showed favorable outcomes in ACS patients with PE versus rupture and thrombi associated with eroded plaques are platelet-rich, it is plausible that a less invasive management strategy (antithrombotic therapy without stenting) may be safe and effective in these patients. In the EROSION trial, 60 ACS patients with PE diagnosed by OCT (96.7% with STEMI), residual diameter stenosis <70%, and thrombolysis in myocardial infarction flow grade 3 on angiography were treated with antithrombotic therapy alone without stent implantation [69]. The use of a glycoprotein IIb/IIIa inhibitor (tirofiban) and manual aspiration thrombectomy was significant (63% and 85%, respectively). After one month, all patients had a repeat coronary angiography and OCT. At 1 month, 78% of these patients attained the main goal of a >50% decrease in thrombus volume. A one-year follow-up study revealed a substantial decrease in median thrombus volume from one month to one year, with 92.5% of patients free of serious adverse cardiovascular events [70]. These findings implied that antithrombotic treatment without stenting may be an option for selected individuals with ACS caused by PE. However, according to the EROSION study's 4-year follow-up analysis, the incidence of MACE increased to 23%, primarily due to nonurgent target lesion revascularization that was not associated with death, heart failure, stroke, recurrent myocardial infarction, unstable angina-induced rehospitalization, or coronary artery bypass grafting [71]. In an observational analysis of 232 patients, including a fraction from the initial EROSION trial, Yin and colleagues expanded our understanding of this field [72]. During a median follow-up of 2.9 years, 50 of 232 patients (21.6%) developed MACE (6 patients died, 3 patients had nonfatal reinfarction, 29 patients had target lesion revascularization, 36 patients required rehospitalization for angina pectoris, 2 patients had severe bleeding, and 5 patients had a stroke). MACE was predicted by age, percentage of area stenosis, and thrombus load, according to multivariate Cox regression analysis. The threshold values for predictors were age ≥60 years, percentage of area stenosis ≥63.5%, and thrombus load ≥18.5%, respectively, and when all three were present, the risk of MACE spiked to a very high level of 58%. Despite the progress made with the investigation of a no-stent approach in this subset of patients with ACS, large-scale randomized clinical trials are required before recommendations can be made for a routine conservative management with intensive antiplatelet therapy of patients with ACS and PE as the underlying mechanism.

Finally, another open question is whether drug-coated balloon (DCB) angioplasty, might be effective for PE; such an approach might still avoid a stent-based strategy for the majority of patients, but provide a lower area of stenosis, a driver of future MACE. In a retrospective study of consecutive ACS patients with OCT-guided DCB management, target lesion failure was the lowest in the subset of patients with confirmed PE at 3 years [73]. Critically, plaque phenotype (PE) was an independent predictor of target lesion failure [73]. Another observation of this study concerned the post-PCI thrombus burden, with PE and PR having similar target lesion failure rates in cases of residual thrombus burden below 8.4% [73].

Despite their significance in cardiovascular events, ongoing studies on tailored, personalized management of coronary plaque erosions remain sparse. This gap impedes the optimization of treatment strategies, potentially limiting advancements in preventive care and therapeutic interventions for individuals at risk of plaque-related complications. Consequently, universal stenting persists as the standard of care, owing to the absence of additional robust data supporting alternative approaches. However, it should be noted that such approaches may not be adequate in PE, since the findings of a previous study revealed that stents placed on erosion sites exhibit inferior healing, with increased uncovered struts observed at the 6-month mark [74]. These results imply that underlying plaque morphology influences post-stenting vascular response, impacting neointimal coverage and potentially necessitating personalized antiplatelet therapy durations.

6. Conclusions and Future Directions

In conclusion, PE has emerged as a significant etiology of ACS, challenging previous assumptions about its prevalence and demographics. With distinct epidemiological features and seasonal variations, PE often affects younger individuals, particularly women, and presents as NSTEMI. Molecular mechanisms highlight reduced inflammation and endothelial shear stress as key factors, while advancements in intravascular imaging offer unprecedented insights into plaque morphology. Artificial intelligence shows promise in enhancing diagnostic accuracy. Therapeutically, less invasive approaches such as antithrombotic therapy without stenting are being explored, alongside the potential of drug-coated balloons to reduce thrombus burden.

The future directions in the diagnosis and treatment of coronary PE are likely to be shaped by advancements in technology, a deeper understanding of molecular mechanisms, and innovative therapeutic strategies. Concerning their diagnosis, continued refinement of intravascular imaging modalities (OCT, NIRS) is expected to enhance the detection and characterization of PE with higher resolution and specificity. Moreover, the determination of specific biomarkers associated with PE for non-invasive diagnosis through blood tests may offer a more accessible and less invasive approach for risk stratification and monitoring. Integration of multiple imaging modalities, including molecular imaging and functional imaging, along with blood-based biomarkers could provide a comprehensive assessment of plaque composition, inflammation, and vulnerability.

The importance of artificial intelligence should not be overlooked. Machine learning (ML) and artificial intelligence-based methods offer promising avenues for biomarker discovery and validations in coronary PE by leveraging diverse data sources, including genomic, proteomic, imaging, and clinical data. ML algorithms excel in integrating multi-omics data, including genomics, transcriptomics, proteomics, and metabolomics, to capture the complex molecular signatures associated with coronary PE. By analyzing these integrated datasets, ML models can identify patterns and interactions among various molecular features, facilitating the discovery of novel biomarkers. Rigorous validation is essential to ensure the reliability and generalizability of ML-based biomarkers for coronary PE. Cross-validation within training datasets and external validation using independent cohorts are critical steps to assess the robustness and reproducibility of identified biomarkers.

ML algorithms can analyze intravascular imaging data to identify subtle features indicative of PE, such as superficial irregularities or thrombus formation, aiding in the identification of imaging-based biomarkers. Deep learning techniques, particularly convolutional neural networks, have demonstrated remarkable capabilities in analyzing medical images for diagnostic purposes. By training on large datasets of coronary imaging scans, convolutional neural networks can learn complex patterns associated with PE, enabling automated detection and characterization of erosive plaques from imaging data. ML techniques can also analyze electronic health records and clinical databases to extract relevant features associated with coronary PE, such as patient demographics, medical history, laboratory results, and medication usage. By identifying patterns and associations within these clinical datasets, ML models can uncover potential biomarkers and risk factors for PE.

Author Contributions: Conceptualization, D.T.; literature review, P.T.; visualization, P.K.V.; writing—original draft preparation, P.T.; writing—review and editing, P.K.V., A.P., P.K., E.O., K.T. and D.T. All authors have read and agreed to the published version of the manuscript.

Funding: This research received no external funding.

Conflicts of Interest: The authors declare no conflicts of interest.

Abbreviations

ACS	acute coronary syndrome
PR	plaque rupture
PCI	percutaneous coronary intervention
PE	plaque erosion
MMP	matrix metalloproteinase
IL-6	interleukin-6
TNF-α	tumor necrosis factor-alpha
CRP	C reactive protein
VSMC	vascular smooth muscle cell
PCSK9	proprotein convertase subtilisin/kexin type 9
OCT	optical coherence tomography
IVUS	intravascular ultrasound
OR	odds ratio
LAD	left anterior descending
TLR2	toll-like receptor-2
MPO	myeloperoxidase
PTX3	pentraxin-3
HR	hazard ratio
ALDH4A1	aldehyde dehydrogenase 4A1
NIRS	near-infrared spectroscopy
LCBI	lipid core burden index
CCTA	coronary computed tomography angiography
PCAT	pericoronary adipose tissue
DCB	drug-coated balloon
ML	machine learning

References

1. Theofilis, P.; Sagris, M.; Antonopoulos, A.S.; Oikonomou, E.; Tsioufis, K.; Tousoulis, D. Non-Invasive Modalities in the Assessment of Vulnerable Coronary Atherosclerotic Plaques. *Tomography* **2022**, *8*, 1742–1758. [CrossRef] [PubMed]
2. Theofilis, P.; Sagris, M.; Oikonomou, E.; Antonopoulos, A.S.; Lazaros, G.; Theofilis, A.; Papastamos, C.; Papaioannou, S.; Siasos, G.; Tsioufis, K.; et al. Extracellular Matrix Remodeling Biomarkers in Coronary Artery Disease. *Curr. Top. Med. Chem.* **2022**, *22*, 2355–2367. [CrossRef] [PubMed]
3. Theofilis, P.; Oikonomou, E.; Tsioufis, K.; Tousoulis, D. The Role of Macrophages in Atherosclerosis: Pathophysiologic Mechanisms and Treatment Considerations. *Int. J. Mol. Sci.* **2023**, *24*, 9568. [CrossRef] [PubMed]
4. Tsioufis, P.; Theofilis, P.; Tsioufis, K.; Tousoulis, D. The Impact of Cytokines in Coronary Atherosclerotic Plaque: Current Therapeutic Approaches. *Int. J. Mol. Sci.* **2022**, *23*, 15937. [CrossRef] [PubMed]
5. Theofilis, P.; Oikonomou, E.; Chasikidis, C.; Tsioufis, K.; Tousoulis, D. Pathophysiology of Acute Coronary Syndromes-Diagnostic and Treatment Considerations. *Life* **2023**, *13*, 1543. [CrossRef] [PubMed]
6. Sugane, H.; Kataoka, Y.; Otsuka, F.; Nakaoku, Y.; Nishimura, K.; Nakano, H.; Murai, K.; Honda, S.; Hosoda, H.; Matama, H.; et al. Cardiac outcomes in patients with acute coronary syndrome attributable to calcified nodule. *Atherosclerosis* **2021**, *318*, 70–75. [CrossRef] [PubMed]
7. Torii, S.; Sato, Y.; Otsuka, F.; Kolodgie, F.D.; Jinnouchi, H.; Sakamoto, A.; Park, J.; Yahagi, K.; Sakakura, K.; Cornelissen, A.; et al. Eruptive Calcified Nodules as a Potential Mechanism of Acute Coronary Thrombosis and Sudden Death. *J. Am. Coll. Cardiol.* **2021**, *77*, 1599–1611. [CrossRef] [PubMed]
8. Fahed, A.C.; Jang, I.K. Plaque erosion and acute coronary syndromes: Phenotype, molecular characteristics and future directions. *Nat. Rev. Cardiol.* **2021**, *18*, 724–734. [CrossRef] [PubMed]
9. Ueda, Y.; Hiro, T.; Hirayama, A.; Komatsu, S.; Matsuoka, H.; Takayama, T.; Ishihara, M.; Hayashi, T.; Saito, S.; Kodama, K.; et al. Effect of Ezetimibe on Stabilization and Regression of Intracoronary Plaque—The ZIPANGU Study. *Circ. J.* **2017**, *81*, 1611–1619. [CrossRef]
10. Ota, H.; Omori, H.; Kawasaki, M.; Hirakawa, A.; Matsuo, H. Clinical impact of PCSK9 inhibitor on stabilization and regression of lipid-rich coronary plaques: A near-infrared spectroscopy study. *Eur. Heart J. Cardiovasc. Imaging* **2022**, *23*, 217–228. [CrossRef]
11. van Rosendael, A.R.; van den Hoogen, I.J.; Gianni, U.; Ma, X.; Tantawy, S.W.; Bax, A.M.; Lu, Y.; Andreini, D.; Al-Mallah, M.H.; Budoff, M.J.; et al. Association of Statin Treatment with Progression of Coronary Atherosclerotic Plaque Composition. *JAMA Cardiol.* **2021**, *6*, 1257–1266. [CrossRef] [PubMed]
12. Tummala, R.; Gupta, M.; Devanabanda, A.R.; Bandyopadhyay, D.; Aronow, W.S.; Ray, K.K.; Mamas, M.; Ghosh, R.K. Bempedoic acid and its role in contemporary management of hyperlipidemia in atherosclerosis. *Ann. Med.* **2022**, *54*, 1287–1296. [CrossRef] [PubMed]
13. Kong, N.; Xu, Q.; Cui, W.; Feng, X.; Gao, H. PCSK9 inhibitor inclisiran for treating atherosclerosis via regulation of endothelial cell pyroptosis. *Ann. Transl. Med.* **2022**, *10*, 1205. [CrossRef] [PubMed]
14. Chen, Y.C.; Jandeleit-Dahm, K.; Peter, K. Sodium-Glucose Co-Transporter 2 (SGLT2) Inhibitor Dapagliflozin Stabilizes Diabetes-Induced Atherosclerotic Plaque Instability. *J. Am. Heart Assoc.* **2022**, *11*, e022761. [CrossRef] [PubMed]
15. Gaspari, T.; Welungoda, I.; Widdop, R.E.; Simpson, R.W.; Dear, A.E. The GLP-1 receptor agonist liraglutide inhibits progression of vascular disease via effects on atherogenesis, plaque stability and endothelial function in an $ApoE^{-/-}$ mouse model. *Diabetes Vasc. Dis. Res.* **2013**, *10*, 353–360. [CrossRef] [PubMed]
16. Pellegrin, M.; Miguet-Alfonsi, C.; Bouzourene, K.; Aubert, J.F.; Deckert, V.; Berthelot, A.; Mazzolai, L.; Laurant, P. Long-term exercise stabilizes atherosclerotic plaque in ApoE knockout mice. *Med. Sci. Sports Exerc.* **2009**, *41*, 2128–2135. [CrossRef]
17. Goncalves, I.; Andersson Georgiadou, E.; Mattsson, S.; Skog, G.; Pedro, L.; Fernandes, E.F.J.; Dias, N.; Engstrom, G.; Nilsson, J.; Stenstrom, K. Direct association between diet and the stability of human atherosclerotic plaque. *Sci. Rep.* **2015**, *5*, 15524. [CrossRef] [PubMed]
18. Gambardella, J.; Sardu, C.; Sacra, C.; Del Giudice, C.; Santulli, G. Quit smoking to outsmart atherogenesis: Molecular mechanisms underlying clinical evidence. *Atherosclerosis* **2017**, *257*, 242–245. [CrossRef] [PubMed]
19. Cecconi, A.; Vilchez-Tschischke, J.P.; Mateo, J.; Sanchez-Gonzalez, J.; Espana, S.; Fernandez-Jimenez, R.; Lopez-Melgar, B.; Fernandez Friera, L.; Lopez-Martin, G.J.; Fuster, V.; et al. Effects of Colchicine on Atherosclerotic Plaque Stabilization: A Multimodality Imaging Study in an Animal Model. *J. Cardiovasc. Transl. Res.* **2021**, *14*, 150–160. [CrossRef]
20. Theofilis, P.; Sagris, M.; Oikonomou, E.; Antonopoulos, A.S.; Siasos, G.; Tsioufis, K.; Tousoulis, D. The impact of SGLT2 inhibitors on inflammation: A systematic review and meta-analysis of studies in rodents. *Int. Immunopharmacol.* **2022**, *111*, 109080. [CrossRef]
21. Seegers, L.M.; Araki, M.; Nakajima, A.; Yonetsu, T.; Minami, Y.; Ako, J.; Soeda, T.; Kurihara, O.; Higuma, T.; Kimura, S.; et al. Sex Differences in Culprit Plaque Characteristics Among Different Age Groups in Patients With Acute Coronary Syndromes. *Circ. Cardiovasc. Interv.* **2022**, *15*, e011612. [CrossRef] [PubMed]
22. Russo, M.; Kim, H.O.; Thondapu, V.; Kurihara, O.; Araki, M.; Shinohara, H.; Yamamoto, E.; Lee, H.; Yonetsu, T.; Minami, Y.; et al. Ethnic Differences in the Pathobiology of Acute Coronary Syndromes Between Asians and Whites. *Am. J. Cardiol.* **2020**, *125*, 1757–1764. [CrossRef] [PubMed]
23. Araki, M.; Yonetsu, T.; Kurihara, O.; Nakajima, A.; Lee, H.; Soeda, T.; Minami, Y.; Higuma, T.; Kimura, S.; Takano, M.; et al. Age and Phenotype of Patients with Plaque Erosion. *J. Am. Heart Assoc.* **2021**, *10*, e020691. [CrossRef] [PubMed]

24. Seegers, L.M.; Yeh, D.D.; Wood, M.J.; Yonetsu, T.; Minami, Y.; Araki, M.; Nakajima, A.; Yuki, H.; Ako, J.; Soeda, T.; et al. Cardiovascular Risk Factors and Culprit Plaque Characteristics in Women with Acute Coronary Syndromes. *Am. J. Cardiol.* **2023**, *207*, 13–20. [CrossRef] [PubMed]
25. Claeys, M.J.; Rajagopalan, S.; Nawrot, T.S.; Brook, R.D. Climate and environmental triggers of acute myocardial infarction. *Eur. Heart J.* **2017**, *38*, 955–960. [CrossRef] [PubMed]
26. Abela, G.S.; Aziz, K. Cholesterol crystals rupture biological membranes and human plaques during acute cardiovascular events--a novel insight into plaque rupture by scanning electron microscopy. *Scanning* **2006**, *28*, 1–10. [CrossRef] [PubMed]
27. Yamamoto, E.; Yonetsu, T.; Kakuta, T.; Soeda, T.; Saito, Y.; Yan, B.P.; Kurihara, O.; Takano, M.; Niccoli, G.; Higuma, T.; et al. Clinical and Laboratory Predictors for Plaque Erosion in Patients With Acute Coronary Syndromes. *J. Am. Heart Assoc.* **2019**, *8*, e012322. [CrossRef] [PubMed]
28. Kim, H.O.; Kim, C.J.; Kurihara, O.; Thondapu, V.; Russo, M.; Yamamoto, E.; Sugiyama, T.; Fracassi, F.; Lee, H.; Yonetsu, T.; et al. Angiographic features of patients with coronary plaque erosion. *Int. J. Cardiol.* **2019**, *288*, 12–16. [CrossRef] [PubMed]
29. Tian, J.; Vergallo, R.; Jia, H.; Soeda, T.; Lee, H.; Yu, B.; Jang, I.K. Morphologic characteristics of eroded coronary plaques: A combined angiographic, optical coherence tomography, and intravascular ultrasound study. *Int. J. Cardiol.* **2014**, *176*, e137–e139. [CrossRef]
30. Dai, J.; Xing, L.; Jia, H.; Zhu, Y.; Zhang, S.; Hu, S.; Lin, L.; Ma, L.; Liu, H.; Xu, M.; et al. In vivo predictors of plaque erosion in patients with ST-segment elevation myocardial infarction: A clinical, angiographical, and intravascular optical coherence tomography study. *Eur. Heart J.* **2018**, *39*, 2077–2085. [CrossRef]
31. Yamamoto, E.; Thondapu, V.; Poon, E.; Sugiyama, T.; Fracassi, F.; Dijkstra, J.; Lee, H.; Ooi, A.; Barlis, P.; Jang, I.K. Endothelial Shear Stress and Plaque Erosion: A Computational Fluid Dynamics and Optical Coherence Tomography Study. *JACC Cardiovasc. Imaging* **2019**, *12*, 374–375. [CrossRef] [PubMed]
32. Niccoli, G.; Montone, R.A.; Di Vito, L.; Gramegna, M.; Refaat, H.; Scalone, G.; Leone, A.M.; Trani, C.; Burzotta, F.; Porto, I.; et al. Plaque rupture and intact fibrous cap assessed by optical coherence tomography portend different outcomes in patients with acute coronary syndrome. *Eur. Heart J.* **2015**, *36*, 1377–1384. [CrossRef] [PubMed]
33. Sugiyama, T.; Yamamoto, E.; Bryniarski, K.; Xing, L.; Lee, H.; Isobe, M.; Libby, P.; Jang, I.K. Nonculprit Plaque Characteristics in Patients with Acute Coronary Syndrome Caused by Plaque Erosion vs Plaque Rupture: A 3-Vessel Optical Coherence Tomography Study. *JAMA Cardiol.* **2018**, *3*, 207–214. [CrossRef] [PubMed]
34. Vergallo, R.; Porto, I.; De Maria, G.L.; D'Amario, D.; Annibali, G.; Galli, M.; Migliaro, S.; Buccimazza, G.; Aurigemma, C.; Leone, A.M.; et al. Dual quantitative coronary angiography accurately quantifies intracoronary thrombotic burden in patients with acute coronary syndrome: Comparison with optical coherence tomography imaging. *Int. J. Cardiol.* **2019**, *292*, 25–31. [CrossRef] [PubMed]
35. Sekimoto, T.; Mori, H.; Koba, S.; Arai, T.; Matsukawa, N.; Sakai, R.; Yokota, Y.; Sato, S.; Tanaka, H.; Masaki, R.; et al. Clinical features and lipid profiles of plaque erosion over lipid-rich plaque versus fibrous plaque in patients with acute coronary syndrome. *Atherosclerosis* **2022**, *360*, 47–52. [CrossRef] [PubMed]
36. Gerhardt, T.; Seppelt, C.; Abdelwahed, Y.S.; Meteva, D.; Wolfram, C.; Stapmanns, P.; Erbay, A.; Zanders, L.; Nelles, G.; Musfeld, J.; et al. Culprit plaque morphology determines inflammatory risk and clinical outcomes in acute coronary syndrome. *Eur. Heart J.* **2023**, *44*, 3911–3925. [CrossRef] [PubMed]
37. Kondo, S.; Mizukami, T.; Kobayashi, N.; Wakabayashi, K.; Mori, H.; Yamamoto, M.H.; Sambe, T.; Yasuhara, S.; Hibi, K.; Nanasato, M.; et al. Diagnosis and Prognostic Value of the Underlying Cause of Acute Coronary Syndrome in Optical Coherence Tomography-Guided Emergency Percutaneous Coronary Intervention. *J. Am. Heart Assoc.* **2023**, *12*, e030412. [CrossRef]
38. Weng, Z.; Zhao, C.; Qin, Y.; Liu, C.; Pan, W.; Hu, S.; He, L.; Xu, Y.; Zeng, M.; Feng, X.; et al. Peripheral atherosclerosis in acute coronary syndrome patients with plaque rupture vs plaque erosion: A prospective coronary optical coherence tomography and peripheral ultrasound study. *Am. Heart J.* **2023**, *263*, 159–168. [CrossRef] [PubMed]
39. Hakim, D.; Pinilla-Echeverri, N.; Coskun, A.U.; Pu, Z.; Kajander, O.A.; Rupert, D.; Maynard, C.; Cefalo, N.; Siasos, G.; Papafaklis, M.I.; et al. The role of endothelial shear stress, shear stress gradient, and plaque topography in plaque erosion. *Atherosclerosis* **2023**, *376*, 11–18. [CrossRef]
40. Kim, H.O.; Jiang, B.; Poon, E.K.W.; Thondapu, V.; Kim, C.J.; Kurihara, O.; Araki, M.; Nakajima, A.; Mamon, C.; Dijkstra, J.; et al. High endothelial shear stress and stress gradient at plaque erosion persist up to 12 months. *Int. J. Cardiol.* **2022**, *357*, 1–7. [CrossRef]
41. Leistner, D.M.; Krankel, N.; Meteva, D.; Abdelwahed, Y.S.; Seppelt, C.; Stahli, B.E.; Rai, H.; Skurk, C.; Lauten, A.; Mochmann, H.C.; et al. Differential immunological signature at the culprit site distinguishes acute coronary syndrome with intact from acute coronary syndrome with ruptured fibrous cap: Results from the prospective translational OPTICO-ACS study. *Eur. Heart J.* **2020**, *41*, 3549–3560. [CrossRef] [PubMed]
42. Seppelt, C.; Abdelwahed, Y.S.; Meteva, D.; Nelles, G.; Stahli, B.E.; Erbay, A.; Krankel, N.; Sieronski, L.; Skurk, C.; Haghikia, A.; et al. Coronary microevaginations characterize culprit plaques and their inflammatory microenvironment in a subtype of acute coronary syndrome with intact fibrous cap: Results from the prospective translational OPTICO-ACS study. *Eur. Heart J. Cardiovasc. Imaging* **2024**, *25*, 175–184. [CrossRef] [PubMed]

43. Meteva, D.; Vinci, R.; Seppelt, C.; Abdelwahed, Y.S.; Pedicino, D.; Nelles, G.; Skurk, C.; Haghikia, A.; Rauch-Krohnert, U.; Gerhardt, T.; et al. Toll-like receptor 2, hyaluronan, and neutrophils play a key role in plaque erosion: The OPTICO-ACS study. *Eur. Heart J.* **2023**, *44*, 3892–3907. [CrossRef] [PubMed]
44. Koganti, S.; Karanasos, A.; Regar, E.; Rakhit, R.D. Association of systemic inflammatory biomarkers with morphological characteristics of coronary atherosclerotic plaque by intravascular optical coherence tomography. *Hell. J. Cardiol.* **2021**, *62*, 101–106. [CrossRef] [PubMed]
45. Ferrante, G.; Nakano, M.; Prati, F.; Niccoli, G.; Mallus, M.T.; Ramazzotti, V.; Montone, R.A.; Kolodgie, F.D.; Virmani, R.; Crea, F. High levels of systemic myeloperoxidase are associated with coronary plaque erosion in patients with acute coronary syndromes: A clinicopathological study. *Circulation* **2010**, *122*, 2505–2513. [CrossRef] [PubMed]
46. Burke, A.P.; Tracy, R.P.; Kolodgie, F.; Malcom, G.T.; Zieske, A.; Kutys, R.; Pestaner, J.; Smialek, J.; Virmani, R. Elevated C-reactive protein values and atherosclerosis in sudden coronary death: Association with different pathologies. *Circulation* **2002**, *105*, 2019–2023. [CrossRef] [PubMed]
47. Sugiyama, S.; Kugiyama, K.; Aikawa, M.; Nakamura, S.; Ogawa, H.; Libby, P. Hypochlorous acid, a macrophage product, induces endothelial apoptosis and tissue factor expression: Involvement of myeloperoxidase-mediated oxidant in plaque erosion and thrombogenesis. *Arterioscler. Thromb. Vasc. Biol.* **2004**, *24*, 1309–1314. [CrossRef] [PubMed]
48. Niccoli, G.; Montone, R.A.; Cataneo, L.; Cosentino, N.; Gramegna, M.; Refaat, H.; Porto, I.; Burzotta, F.; Trani, C.; Leone, A.M.; et al. Morphological-biohumoral correlations in acute coronary syndromes: Pathogenetic implications. *Int. J. Cardiol.* **2014**, *171*, 463–466. [CrossRef] [PubMed]
49. Tan, Y.; Yang, S.; Chen, R.; Sheng, Z.; Zhou, P.; Liu, C.; Zhao, H.; Song, L.; Li, J.; Zhou, J.; et al. High Plasma Myeloperoxidase Is Associated with Plaque Erosion in Patients with ST-Segment Elevation Myocardial Infarction. *J. Cardiovasc. Transl. Res.* **2020**, *13*, 908–915. [CrossRef]
50. Latini, R.; Maggioni, A.P.; Peri, G.; Gonzini, L.; Lucci, D.; Mocarelli, P.; Vago, L.; Pasqualini, F.; Signorini, S.; Soldateschi, D.; et al. Prognostic significance of the long pentraxin PTX3 in acute myocardial infarction. *Circulation* **2004**, *110*, 2349–2354. [CrossRef]
51. Wang, Y.; Zhao, X.; Zhou, P.; Liu, C.; Sheng, Z.; Li, J.; Zhou, J.; Chen, R.; Chen, Y.; Song, L.; et al. Plasma Pentraxin-3 Combined with Plaque Characteristics Predict Cardiovascular Risk in ST-Segment Elevated Myocardial Infarction: An Optical Coherence Tomography Study. *J. Inflamm. Res.* **2021**, *14*, 4409–4419. [CrossRef] [PubMed]
52. Zhao, X.; Song, L.; Wang, Y.; Li, J.; Zhou, J.; Chen, R.; Liu, C.; Zhou, P.; Sheng, Z.; Chen, Y.; et al. Proprotein Convertase Subtilisin/Kexin Type 9 and Systemic Inflammatory Biomarker Pentraxin 3 for Risk Stratification Among STEMI Patients Undergoing Primary PCI. *J. Inflamm. Res.* **2021**, *14*, 5319–5335. [CrossRef] [PubMed]
53. Du, Y.; Zhu, B.; Liu, Y.; Du, Z.; Zhang, J.; Yang, W.; Li, H.; Gao, C. Association between apolipoprotein B/A1 ratio and quantities of tissue prolapse on optical coherence tomography examination in patients with atherosclerotic cardiovascular disease. *Int. J. Cardiovasc. Imaging* **2024**, *40*, 545–555. [CrossRef] [PubMed]
54. Deng, F.; Li, D.; Lei, L.; Yang, Q.; Li, Q.; Wang, H.; Deng, J.; Zheng, Q.; Jiang, W. Association between apolipoprotein B/A1 ratio and coronary plaque vulnerability in patients with atherosclerotic cardiovascular disease: An intravascular optical coherence tomography study. *Cardiovasc. Diabetol.* **2021**, *20*, 188. [CrossRef]
55. Luo, X.; Liu, M.; Wang, S.; Chen, Y.; Bao, X.; Lv, Y.; Zhang, S.; Xu, B.; Weng, X.; Bai, X.; et al. Combining metabolomics and OCT to reveal plasma metabolic profiling and biomarkers of plaque erosion and plaque rupture in STEMI patients. *Int. J. Cardiol.* **2023**, *390*, 131223. [CrossRef] [PubMed]
56. Theofilis, P.; Vogiatzi, G.; Oikonomou, E.; Gazouli, M.; Siasos, G.; Katifelis, H.; Perrea, D.; Vavuranakis, M.; Iliopoulos, D.C.; Tsioufis, C.; et al. The Effect of MicroRNA-126 Mimic Administration on Vascular Perfusion Recovery in an Animal Model of Hind Limb Ischemia. *Front. Mol. Biosci.* **2021**, *8*, 724465. [CrossRef] [PubMed]
57. Theofilis, P.; Oikonomou, E.; Vogiatzi, G.; Sagris, M.; Antonopoulos, A.S.; Siasos, G.; Iliopoulos, D.C.; Perrea, D.; Vavouranakis, M.; Tsioufis, K.; et al. The Role of MicroRNA-126 in Atherosclerotic Cardiovascular Diseases. *Curr. Med. Chem.* **2023**, *30*, 1902–1921. [CrossRef] [PubMed]
58. Theofilis, P.; Oikonomou, E.; Vogiatzi, G.; Antonopoulos, A.S.; Siasos, G.; Iliopoulos, D.C.; Perrea, D.; Tsioufis, C.; Tousoulis, D. The impact of proangiogenic microRNA modulation on blood flow recovery following hind limb ischemia. A systematic review and meta-analysis of animal studies. *Vasc. Pharmacol.* **2021**, *141*, 106906. [CrossRef]
59. Dong, H.; Hu, S.; Sun, R.; Wang, C.; Dai, J.; Pan, W.; Xing, L.; Liu, X.; Wu, J.; Liu, J.; et al. High Levels of Circulating MicroRNA-3667-3p Are Associated with Coronary Plaque Erosion in Patients with ST-Segment Elevation Myocardial Infarction. *Int. Heart J.* **2019**, *60*, 1061–1069. [CrossRef]
60. Li, J.; Tan, Y.; Sheng, Z.; Zhou, P.; Liu, C.; Zhao, H.; Song, L.; Zhou, J.; Chen, R.; Chen, Y.; et al. RNA-seq identifies circulating miRNAs as potential biomarkers for plaque rupture in patients with ST-segment elevation myocardial infarction. *Genomics* **2021**, *113*, 1–10. [CrossRef]
61. Li, J.; Chen, R.; Zhou, J.; Wang, Y.; Zhao, X.; Liu, C.; Zhou, P.; Chen, Y.; Song, L.; Li, N.; et al. Atherosclerotic Autoantigen ALDH4A1 as a Novel Immunological Indicator for Plaque Erosion in Patients with ST Segment Elevated Myocardial Infarction. *Thromb. Haemost.* **2023**, *124*, 584–594. [CrossRef] [PubMed]
62. Park, S.; Araki, M.; Nakajima, A.; Lee, H.; Fuster, V.; Ye, J.C.; Jang, I.K. Enhanced Diagnosis of Plaque Erosion by Deep Learning in Patients with Acute Coronary Syndromes. *JACC Cardiovasc. Interv.* **2022**, *15*, 2020–2031. [CrossRef] [PubMed]

63. Li, J.; Chen, R.; Zhou, J.; Wang, Y.; Zhao, X.; Liu, C.; Zhou, P.; Chen, Y.; Song, L.; Yan, S.; et al. Lipid Content Distribution and its Clinical Implication in Patients with Acute Myocardial Infarction-Plaque Erosion: Results from the Prospective OCTAMI Study. *J. Atheroscler. Thromb.* **2024**, *31*, 23–35. [CrossRef] [PubMed]
64. Cuesta, J.; Antuna, P.; Jimenez, C.; Rivero, F.; Bastante, T.; Garcia-Guimaraes, M.; Alfonso, F. Can Plaque Erosion Be Visualized by High-Definition Intravascular Ultrasound? *JACC Cardiovasc. Interv.* **2020**, *13*, e57–e61. [CrossRef] [PubMed]
65. Higuma, T.; Soeda, T.; Abe, N.; Yamada, M.; Yokoyama, H.; Shibutani, S.; Vergallo, R.; Minami, Y.; Ong, D.S.; Lee, H.; et al. A Combined Optical Coherence Tomography and Intravascular Ultrasound Study on Plaque Rupture, Plaque Erosion, and Calcified Nodule in Patients With ST-Segment Elevation Myocardial Infarction: Incidence, Morphologic Characteristics, and Outcomes After Percutaneous Coronary Intervention. *JACC Cardiovasc. Interv.* **2015**, *8*, 1166–1176. [CrossRef] [PubMed]
66. Terada, K.; Kubo, T.; Kameyama, T.; Matsuo, Y.; Ino, Y.; Emori, H.; Higashioka, D.; Katayama, Y.; Khalifa, A.K.M.; Takahata, M.; et al. NIRS-IVUS for Differentiating Coronary Plaque Rupture, Erosion, and Calcified Nodule in Acute Myocardial Infarction. *JACC Cardiovasc. Imaging* **2021**, *14*, 1440–1450. [CrossRef] [PubMed]
67. Nakajima, A.; Sugiyama, T.; Araki, M.; Seegers, L.M.; Dey, D.; McNulty, I.; Lee, H.; Yonetsu, T.; Yasui, Y.; Teng, Y.; et al. Plaque Rupture, Compared with Plaque Erosion, Is Associated with a Higher Level of Pancoronary Inflammation. *JACC Cardiovasc. Imaging* **2022**, *15*, 828–839. [CrossRef] [PubMed]
68. Nagamine, T.; Hoshino, M.; Yonetsu, T.; Sugiyama, T.; Kanaji, Y.; Matsuda, K.; Sayama, K.; Ueno, H.; Nogami, K.; Hanyu, Y.; et al. Identification of Optical Coherence Tomography-Defined Coronary Plaque Erosion by Preprocedural Computed Tomography Angiography. *J. Am. Heart Assoc.* **2023**, *12*, e029239. [CrossRef] [PubMed]
69. Jia, H.; Dai, J.; Hou, J.; Xing, L.; Ma, L.; Liu, H.; Xu, M.; Yao, Y.; Hu, S.; Yamamoto, E.; et al. Effective anti-thrombotic therapy without stenting: Intravascular optical coherence tomography-based management in plaque erosion (the EROSION study). *Eur. Heart J.* **2017**, *38*, 792–800. [CrossRef]
70. Xing, L.; Yamamoto, E.; Sugiyama, T.; Jia, H.; Ma, L.; Hu, S.; Wang, C.; Zhu, Y.; Li, L.; Xu, M.; et al. EROSION Study (Effective Anti-Thrombotic Therapy without Stenting: Intravascular Optical Coherence Tomography-Based Management in Plaque Erosion): A 1-Year Follow-Up Report. *Circ. Cardiovasc. Interv.* **2017**, *10*, e005860. [CrossRef]
71. He, L.; Qin, Y.; Xu, Y.; Hu, S.; Wang, Y.; Zeng, M.; Feng, X.; Liu, Q.; Syed, I.; Demuyakor, A.; et al. Predictors of non-stenting strategy for acute coronary syndrome caused by plaque erosion: Four-year outcomes of the EROSION study. *EuroIntervention* **2021**, *17*, 497–505. [CrossRef] [PubMed]
72. Yin, Y.; Lei, F.; Fang, C.; Jiang, S.; Xu, X.; Sun, S.; Pei, X.; Jia, R.; Tang, C.; Peng, C.; et al. Predictors of Adverse Prognosis in Patients with Acute Coronary Syndrome Caused by Plaque Erosion with a Nonstent Strategy. *J. Am. Heart Assoc.* **2022**, *11*, e026414. [CrossRef] [PubMed]
73. Yamamoto, T.; Kawamori, H.; Toba, T.; Kakizaki, S.; Nakamura, K.; Fujimoto, D.; Sasaki, S.; Fujii, H.; Hamana, T.; Osumi, Y.; et al. Clinical impact of optical coherence tomography findings after drug-coated balloon treatment for patients with acute coronary syndromes. *Int. J. Cardiol.* **2023**, *387*, 131149. [CrossRef]
74. Hu, S.; Wang, C.; Zhe, C.; Zhu, Y.; Yonetsu, T.; Jia, H.; Hou, J.; Zhang, S.; Jang, I.K.; Yu, B. Plaque erosion delays vascular healing after drug eluting stent implantation in patients with acute coronary syndrome: An In Vivo Optical Coherence Tomography Study. *Catheter. Cardiovasc. Interv.* **2017**, *89*, 592–600. [CrossRef] [PubMed]

International Journal of
Molecular Sciences

MDPI

Article

Glycoprotein Acetyls Is a Novel Biomarker Predicting Cardiovascular Complications in Rheumatoid Arthritis

Melody Kasher [1], Maxim B. Freidin [2,†], Frances M. K. Williams [3,†], Stacey S. Cherny [4,5], Shai Ashkenazi [1] and Gregory Livshits [1,3,4,*]

[1] Department of Morphological Sciences, Adelson School of Medicine, Ariel University, Ariel 4070000, Israel; melodykasher@mail.tau.ac.il (M.K.); shaias@ariel.ac.il (S.A.)
[2] Department of Biology, School of Biological and Behavioural Sciences, Queen Mary University of London, London E1 4NS, UK; m.freydin@qmul.ac.uk
[3] Department of Twin Research and Genetic Epidemiology, School of Life Course Sciences, King's College London, London WC2R 2LS, UK; frances.williams@kcl.ac.uk
[4] Human Population Biology Research Unit, Department of Anatomy and Anthropology, School of Medicine, Tel Aviv University, Tel Aviv 69978, Israel; cherny@tauex.tau.ac.il
[5] Department of Epidemiology and Preventive Medicine, Sackler Faculty of Medicine, Tel Aviv University, Tel Aviv 69978, Israel
* Correspondence: zviliv@ariel.ac.il
† These authors contributed equally to this work.

Abstract: The relationship between rheumatoid arthritis (RA) and early onset atherosclerosis is well depicted, each with an important inflammatory component. Glycoprotein acetyls (GlycA), a novel biomarker of inflammation, may play a role in the manifestation of these two inflammatory conditions. The present study examined a potential mediating role of GlycA within the RA–atherosclerosis relationship to determine whether it accounts for the excess risk of cardiovascular disease over that posed by lipid risk factors. The UK Biobank dataset was acquired to establish associations among RA, atherosclerosis, GlycA, and major lipid factors: total cholesterol (TC), high- and low-density lipoprotein (HDL, LDL) cholesterol, and triglycerides (TGs). Genome-wide association study summary statistics were collected from various resources to perform genetic analyses. Causality among variables was tested using Mendelian Randomization (MR) analysis. Genes of interest were identified using colocalization analysis and gene enrichment analysis. MR results appeared to indicate that the genetic relationship between GlycA and RA and also between RA and atherosclerosis was explained by horizontal pleiotropy (p-value = 0.001 and <0.001, respectively), while GlycA may causally predict atherosclerosis (p-value = 0.017). Colocalization analysis revealed several functionally relevant genes shared between GlycA and all the variables assessed. Two loci were apparent in all relationships tested and included the HLA region as well as *SLC22A1*. GlycA appears to mediate the RA–atherosclerosis relationship through several possible pathways. GlycA, although pleiotropically related to RA, appears to causally predict atherosclerosis. Thus, GlycA is suggested as a significant factor in the etiology of atherosclerosis development in RA.

Keywords: rheumatoid arthritis; atherosclerosis; lipid factors; GlycA; inflammation; pleiotropy

1. Introduction

Rheumatoid arthritis (RA) is an inflammatory, autoimmune joint disease whose manifestation and progression are caused by a variety of genetic, metabolic, and environmental factors [1,2]. RA patients experience increased risk of cardiovascular disease (CVD) as well as other comorbidities [3], leading to higher mortality, disability, and disease burden [4,5].

CVD is a major comorbidity of RA [6], affecting over 50% of patients with cardiovascular complications [7,8]. Atherosclerosis, a key CVD phenotype, is an inflammatory condition promoting arterial plaque formation, prevalent in both clinical and sub-clinical

RA cases [9]. Atherosclerosis involves significant lipid profile changes, heart failure, myocardial infarction (MI), and other cardiovascular complications [10,11]. Examining lipid profile abnormalities and inflammatory markers can shed light on the distinctive RA–atherosclerosis relationship [10,11].

Both RA and atherosclerosis involve genetic factors, with RA's heritability estimated at approximately 0.60 in twin studies [12]. Atherosclerosis, in a study of 20,966 twins, showed heritability estimates of 0.38 in females and 0.57 in males [13]. Shared genetic components between RA and atherosclerosis include TNFA, CCR5, MTHFR, and the HLA region, though the extent of their shared effects is yet to be determined [14,15].

A novel inflammation biomarker, glycoprotein acetyls (GlycA), has been proposed for assessing inflammation in RA and other autoimmune conditions, along with the evaluation of the CVD risk [16]. GlycA appears to reflect the clinical profile of RA patients, indicating both the inflammatory status and CVD risk [17]. It captures acute and chronic inflammation and correlates with disease severity under inflammatory conditions [16]. The inflammatory mechanism of GlycA may differ from that of C-reactive protein (CRP), though it significantly correlates with CRP and other inflammatory markers like the erythrocyte sedimentation rate [17].

The correlation between atherosclerosis-related phenotypes and RA has been explored previously, emphasizing their shared inflammatory nature [18,19]. However, the potential pathway underlying these relationships remains incompletely understood and is a major focus of this study. Using large datasets, we investigated the underlying shared genetic architecture between RA and atherosclerosis, assessing pleiotropy and possible causal relationships. Furthermore, we examined the role of inflammation by assessing the involvement of GlycA in these diseases as well as in lipid profile components. The present study was carried out in two stages: (1) assessing GlycA's relationship with RA, atherosclerotic phenotypes, and lipid factors and (2) analyzing the relationship between RA and atherosclerotic phenotypes, excluding lipid factors. The underlying genetic architecture between RA and lipid factors was previously examined by us and reported elsewhere [20].

2. Results

2.1. Phenotypic Association

The UKBB dataset, comprising 273,294 females and 229,062 males with a mean age of 56.53 ± 0.01 years, was analyzed. First, potential predictors of GlycA variation were examined in a multiple linear regression model (Table 1). GlycA was highly and significantly correlated with all the variables examined ($p < 10^{-16}$), and the regression model explained about 40% of the variation in the circulating GlycA levels ($R^2 = 0.4374$, $p < 2.0 \times 10^{-16}$). Importantly, the presence of disease (RA and atherosclerosis) as well as lipid factors (except total cholesterol) also exhibited an independent association. The association of TGs was particularly strong (β = 0.5772 ± 0.0019). Lastly, males had elevated GlycA compared to females (β = 0.3197 ± 0.0152). Although the multiple regression results of the lipid factors appear promising, it should be noted that TCH may cause collinearity with the other lipid factors as TCH is a culmination of TGs, LDL, and HDL.

Table 1. Risk factors for GlycA assessed through multiple linear regression analysis *.

Independent Variables	Estimate	SE	t-Value	*p*-Value
Intercept	−0.2497	0.0184	−13.6	$<2.00 \times 10^{-16}$
RA	0.2740	0.0088	31.1	$<2.00 \times 10^{-16}$
Atherosclerosis	0.3197	0.0152	21.0	$<2.00 \times 10^{-16}$
Total Cholesterol	−0.5652	0.0101	−56.2	$<2.00 \times 10^{-16}$
Triglycerides	0.5772	0.0019	298.7	$<2.00 \times 10^{-16}$
HDL	0.2066	0.0037	55.3	$<2.00 \times 10^{-16}$

Table 1. *Cont.*

Independent Variables	Estimate	SE	t-Value	*p*-Value
LDL	0.5970	0.0087	68.8	$<2.00 \times 10^{-16}$
BMI	0.1956	0.0016	125.7	$<2.00 \times 10^{-16}$
Age	0.0642	0.0015	44.3	$<2.00 \times 10^{-16}$
Sex	−0.2442	0.0033	−74.4	$<2.00 \times 10^{-16}$

* These variables were tested as dummy variables. For both RA and atherosclerosis, the presence of the condition was defined as 1 vs. no disease—0. Sex included 0 for males and 1 for females. All quantitative variables were standardized prior to analysis. General goodness-of-fit measure for the model, $R^2 = 0.4374$, $p < 2.00 \times 10^{-16}$.

Subsequently, multiple logistic regression analysis assessed whether and to what extent RA is associated with GlycA and atherosclerosis, while adjusting for age, sex, and BMI. RA appeared significantly and independently associated with GlycA ($\beta = 0.0079 \pm 0.0003$, $p < 2.0 \times 10^{-16}$) and atherosclerosis ($\beta = 0.0202 \pm 0.0033$, $p = 8.30 \times 10^{-10}$). (Table S1, Supplementary Materials).

2.2. Genetic Association Study

Genetic correlations were used to investigate whether a potential underlying genetic framework depicts the relationship between GlycA and RA, as well as those between GlycA and the atherosclerotic phenotypes. The results summarized in Table 2 show that GlycA was significantly genetically correlated with RA, atherosclerosis, CAD, heart failure, heart attack/MI, and all tested lipids except LDL. The genetic correlation between GlycA and RA, although statistically significant, was modest (Rg = 0.0724 ± 0.0344). The most impressive genetic correlations were detected between GlycA and TGs (Rg = 0.6046 ± 0.0751), while others ranged between 0.2311 and 0.3479. Subsequently, the genetic correlation was examined between RA and atherosclerotic phenotypes, with no genetic correlation with any of the atherosclerotic phenotypes detected by LDSC (Table 2).

Table 2. Pairwise genetic correlation using LDSC.

Phenotype Pairs	Rg	SE	*p*-Value
GlycA, RA	0.0724	0.0344	3.56×10^{-2}
GlycA, Atherosclerosis	0.2311	0.0468	8.09×10^{-7}
GlycA, CAD	0.2934	0.0393	7.82×10^{-14}
GlycA, Heart Failure	0.3232	0.0383	3.34×10^{-17}
GlycA, Heart Attack/MI	0.3108	0.0494	3.11×10^{-10}
GlycA, HDL	−0.2910	0.0611	1.94×10^{-6}
GlycA, LDL	0.3244	0.2425	1.81×10^{-1}
GlycA, TC	0.3479	0.1402	1.31×10^{-2}
GlycA, TGs	0.6046	0.0751	8.27×10^{-16}
RA, Atherosclerosis	0.0152	0.0476	7.49×10^{-1}
RA, CAD	0.0285	0.0342	4.06×10^{-1}
RA, Heart Failure	0.0981	0.0560	7.98×10^{-2}
RA, Heart Attack/MI	0.0291	0.0562	6.04×10^{-1}

In addition, the genetic correlations between the atherosclerosis-related phenotypes and lipid factors were estimated to potentially decipher the nature of the relationships from all directions. Interestingly, the four atherosclerotic variables showed consistent significant correlations with HDL and TGs (Table S2): atherosclerosis with HDL (Rg = −0.18 ± 0.08) and TGs (Rg = 0.27 ± 0.10); CAD with HDL (Rg = −0.22 ± 0.07) and TGs (Rg = 0.31 ± 0.08); and heart failure with HDL (Rg = −0.26 ± 0.06) and TGs (Rg = 0.26 ± 0.06); lastly, heart attack/MI genetically correlated with HDL (Rg = −0.20 ± 0.08) and TGs (Rg = 0.35 ± 0.09).

2.3. *Mendelian Randomization Analysis*

Mendelian randomization was implemented to assess potential causality between GlycA and all other phenotypes. GlycA served as the exposure variable while RA, atherosclerotic phenotypes, and lipid factors were the outcome variables. The reverse scenario was also explored, with RA as the exposure variable and atherosclerotic variables as outcomes.

Based on the IVW approach, GlycA showed a significant causal association with RA, atherosclerosis, CAD, heart failure, heart attack/MI, HDL, LDL (p = 0.019), TGs, and TC (all $p < 0.001$ except LDL) (Table S3a). When RA was the exposure phenotype, a causal association was seen with atherosclerosis, CAD, heart failure, and heart attack/MI (all $p < 0.001$) (Table S3b).

Implementing MRE, where GlycA was the exposure variable, we found that only atherosclerosis (p = 0.017) and CAD (p = 0.029) were significantly causally associated with GlycA, without evidence of horizontal pleiotropy (MRE intercept was non-significant, Table 3a). Alternatively, testing the relationship between GlycA and RA, heart failure as well as heart attack/MI revealed significant intercept estimates (and non-significant regression coefficients), thus suggesting horizontal pleiotropy. However, the implementation of MRE in testing the GlycA/lipid factors relationship did not provide evidence of causal or horizontally pleiotropic relationships (Table 3a).

Table 3. Mendelian randomization, MR Egger approach. (**a**) GlycA as the exposure. (**b**) RA as the exposure. (**c**) MR PRESSO results from the Global Test.

(a)							
Outcome	**IVs**	**Estimate**	**95% Confidence Interval**	***p*-Value**	**MR Egger Intercept *p*-Value**	**I²Gx**	**Heterogeneity**
RA	40	0.019	−0.180, 0.217	0.854	0.001	0.9988	97.7%
Heart attack/MI	46	0.004	−0.001, 0.009	0.087	0.030	0.9940	94.3%
Heart failure	25	0.086	−0.074, 0.246	0.246	0.052	0.9341	94.2%
CAD	22	0.084	0.009, 0.160	0.029	0.061	0.3833	97.3%
Atherosclerosis	22	0.237	0.043, 0.431	0.017	0.757	0.8650	96.8%
HDL	9	−0.049	−0.114, 0.016	0.143	0.574	0.3526	99.4%
LDL	5	0.153	−0.196, 0.051	0.390	0.988	0.1189	97.5%
TC	9	−0.021	−0.180, 0.138	0.794	0.080	0.8227	98.2%
TGs	8	0.070	−0.022, 0.162	0.135	0.439	0.1620	99.1%

(b)							
Outcome	**IVs**	**Estimate**	**95% Confidence Interval**	***p*-Value**	**MR Egger Intercept *p*-Value**	**I²Gx**	**Heterogeneity**
Heart attack/MI	36	0.001	0.000, 0.001	0.171	0.004	0.9900	99.6%
Heart failure	38	0.016	−0.003, 0.034	0.094	0.062	0.9956	99.4%
CAD	30	0.008	−0.008, 0.023	0329	0.002	0.8684	99.1%
Atherosclerosis	40	0.005	−0.023, 0.034	0.716	<0.001	0.9656	99.3%

Table 3. *Cont.*

(c)		
Exposure→Outcome	**Global Test T-Value**	**Global Test *p*-Value**
GlycA → RA	4310.5	<0.001
GlycA → Atherosclerosis	781.2	<0.001
GlycA → CAD	1920.3	<0.001
GlycA → Heart Attack/MI	394.8	<0.001
GlycA → Heart Failure	232.0	<0.001
GlycA → HDL	4574.1	<0.001
GlycA → LDL	2464.9	<0.001
GlycA → TRIG	9001.9	<0.001
GlycA → TCH	4087.2	<0.001
RA → Atherosclerosis	113.5	0.003
RA → CAD	168.4	<0.001
RA → Heart Attack/MI	97.9	0.025
RA → Heart Failure	82.2	0.224

Significant results indicate the presence of horizontal pleiotropy.

In examining causality using MRE with RA as the exposure variable, the relationship between RA and atherosclerosis, CAD, and heart attack/MI may be described by horizontal pleiotropy ($p < 0.001$, 0.002, and 0.004, respectively), but not causally (Table 3b). A causal or pleiotropic relationship between RA and heart failure was not apparent (Table 3b).

Based on MR PRESSO, horizontal pleiotropy was suggested to explain nearly all relationships examined (Table 3c). For example, GlycA appeared to be horizontally pleiotropic with RA, all cardiovascular variables, and lipid variables ($p < 0.001$ for all, Table 3c). RA appeared to be horizontally pleiotropic with atherosclerosis and CAD only ($p = 0.003$ and <0.001, respectively; Table 3c).

2.4. Colocalization and Gene Enrichment Analyses

Colocalization analyses accompanied by FUMA aimed to identify shared genomic regions with SNPs associated with multiple phenotypes. We limited our colocalization results to those supporting hypothesis PP.H4 or PP.H3 with probability ≥75%. Nonsynonymous exonic SNPs or repeating genes associated with intronic SNPs are reported in Table 4. However, a detailed description of all the colocalization results and corresponding gene enrichment outcomes obtained with FUMA are provided in Supplementary Table S4.

GlycA and RA colocalization revealed six genomic regions significantly associated with both phenotypes (Table 4a). As expected, HLA regions were identified on chromosome 6, corresponding to the intergenic regions between *HLA-DRB1* and *HLA-DQA1* and also between *HLA-DQB2* and *HLA-DOB*, both with PP.H3 of 100%.

A summary of colocalization findings between GlycA and the atherosclerotic variables is provided in Table 4b. Several common genomic regions were found with each atherosclerotic phenotype, including six shared genomic regions between GlycA and atherosclerosis. On the other hand, several genomic regions were common for different atherosclerotic phenotypes. For instance, Chr6: 160580497–162169564, harboring lipoprotein (A) coding *gene* (LPA) was associated with all four phenotypes (Table 4). In the genomic regions shared by GlycA and atherosclerosis, five nonsynonymous exonic SNPs were mapped to genes *FGB*, *SLC22A1*, *LPL*, *SERPINA1*, and *ANGPTL4*, with the following high PPs, H3: 94.5%, H4: 96.8%, H4: 73.7%, H4: 97.2%, and H4: 100% (Table 4b). In addition, one intronic SNP (rs10455872) of interest was mapped to LPA, with strong evidence of PP of H4: 99.6%.

Evidence of the causal effect was similarly high (99.7–99.8%) for all the other atherosclerotic phenotypes (Table 4b).

Table 4. Colocalization Results. (**a**) GlycA and RA. (**b**) GlycA and atherosclerosis-related phenotypes. (**c**) GlycA and lipid factors. (**d**) RA and atherosclerosis-related phenotypes.

(a)

Phenotype in Colocalization with GlycA	Genomic Region Chromosome: Base Pairs	Gene (SNP) Function	GlycA *p*-Value	Other Phenotype *p*-Value	PP.H4 (Posterior Probability of Shared Causal SNP) or PP.H3 (of SNPs in the Same Region)
RA	Chr2: 110572432–113921856	*IL1F10/RNU6-1180P* (rs6734238) intergenic	4.00×10^{-9}	1.40×10^{-4}	H4: 79.9%
RA	Chr6: 28917608–29737971	*XXbac-BPG170G13.32/XXbac-BPG170G13.31* (rs2394164) intergenic	6.40×10^{-9}	8.60×10^{-44}	H3: 100%
RA	Chr6: 31571218–32682664	*HLA-DRB1/HLA-DQA1* (rs532965) intergenic	1.70×10^{-7}	1.00×10^{-250}	H3: 100%
RA	Chr6: 32682664–33236497	*HLA-DQB2/HLA-DOB* (rs34422230) intergenic	8.80×10^{-3}	7.20×10^{-235}	H3: 100%
RA	Chr6: 158218719–160580497	*RP1-111C20.3/RP11-13P5.1* (rs1994564) intergenic	1.50×10^{-3}	1.00×10^{-9}	H3: 100%
RA	Chr8: 11278998–13491775	*BLK* (rs2736345) intronic	3.70×10^{-6}	8.60×10^{-7}	H3: 99.9%

(b)

Phenotype in Colocalization with GlycA	Genomic Region Chromosome: Base Pairs	Gene (SNP) Function	GlycA *p*-Value	Other Phenotype *p*-Value	PP.H4 (Posterior Probability of Shared Causal SNP) or PP.H3 (of SNPs in Same Region)
Atherosclerosis	Chr4: 155056126–157485097	*FGB* (rs6054) Nonsynonymous SNV, exon3	1.80×10^{-9}	6.71×10^{-3}	H3: 94.5%
Atherosclerosis	Chr6: 158218719–160580497	*SLC22A1* (rs2282143) Nonsynonymous SNV, exon6	7.40×10^{-9}	6.73×10^{-20}	H4: 96.8%
Atherosclerosis	Chr6: 160580497–162169564	*LPA* (rs10455872) intronic	1.00×10^{-25}	3.52×10^{-75}	H4: 99.6%
Atherosclerosis	Chr8: 19469840–20060856	*LPL* (rs328) exon9 (stopagain)	7.90×10^{-36}	2.97×10^{-5}	H4: 73.7%
Atherosclerosis	Chr14: 94325285–95750867	*SERPINA1* (rs28929474) Nonsynonymous SNV, exon6	3.80×10^{-80}	5.90×10^{-5}	H4: 97.2%

Table 4. *Cont.*

(b)					
Phenotype in Colocalization with GlycA	**Genomic Region Chromosome: Base Pairs**	**Gene (SNP) Function**	**GlycA *p*-Value**	**Other Phenotype *p*-Value**	**PP.H4 (Posterior Probability of Shared Causal SNP) or PP.H3 (of SNPs in Same Region)**
Atherosclerosis	Chr19: 8347513–9238393	*ANGPTL4* (rs116843064) Nonsynonymous SNV, exon11	4.00×10^{-11}	4.94×10^{-11}	H4: 100%
CAD	Chr6: 158218719–160580497	*SLC22A1* (rs2282143) Nonsynonymous SNV, exon6	7.40×10^{-9}	7.35×10^{-42}	H4: 97.5%
CAD	Chr6: 160580497–162169564	*LPA* (rs10455872) intronic	1.00×10^{-25}	2.18×10^{-186}	H4: 99.8%
CAD	Chr8: 19492840–20060856	*LPL* (rs328) exon9 (stopagain)	7.90×10^{-36}	2.43×10^{-11}	H3: 100%
CAD	Chr11: 116383348–117747110	*ZNF259* (rs964184) UTR3	2.70×10^{-68}	4.41×10^{-17}	H4: 100%
CAD	Chr14: 943252885–95750867	*SERPINA1* (rs28929474) Nonsynonymous SNV, exon6	3.80×10^{-80}	5.23×10^{-10}	H4: 99.7%
CAD	Chr19: 8347513–9238393	*ANGPTL4* (rs116843064) Nonsynonymous SNV, exon11	4.00×10^{-11}	3.56×10^{-21}	H4: 100%
CAD	Chr22: 43714200–44995308	*PNPLA3* (rs738409) Nonsynonymous SNV, exon3	7.50×10^{-11}	1.13×10^{-5}	H4: 95.4%
Heart failure	Chr6: 160580497–162169564	*LPA* (rs10455872) intronic	1.00×10^{-25}	1.89×10^{-11}	H4: 99.7%
Heart failure	Chr9: 135298842–137041122	*ABO* (rs9411378) ncRNA_intronic	5.80×10^{-9}	4.11×10^{-9}	H4: 72.2%
Heart failure	Chr11: 116383348–117747110	*ZNF259* (rs964184) UTR3	2.70×10^{-68}	4.24×10^{-4}	H4: 70.1%
Heart attack/MI	Chr6: 158218719–160580497	*SLC22A1* (rs3798170) intronic	2.30×10^{-9}	1.67×10^{-8}	H4: 96.8%
Heart attack/MI	Chr6: 160580497–162169564	*LPA* (rs10455872) intronic	1.00×10^{-25}	2.44×10^{-29}	H4: 99.7%

Table 4. *Cont.*

(c)					
Cytokine in Colocalization with GlycA	**Genomic Region Chromosome: Base Pairs**	**Gene (SNP) Function**	**GlycA *p*-Value**	**Other Phenotype *p*-value**	**PP.H4 (Posterior Probability of Shared Causal SNP) or PP.H3 (of SNPs in Same Region)**
HDL	Chr1: 61922365–63445089	*DOCK7* (rs1167998) intronic	3.00×10^{-20}	4.90×10^{-5}	H4: 84.2%
HDL	Chr2: 21050490–23341383	*APOB* (rs676210) Nonsynonymous SNV, exon26	2.20×10^{-8}	4.17×10^{-88}	H4: 99.8%
HDL	Chr6: 30798168–31571218	*PPP1R18* (rs9262143) Nonsynonymous SNV, exon2	2.30×10^{-8}	1.65×10^{-9}	H3: 100%
HDL	Chr6: 158218719–160580497	*SLC22A1* (rs12208357) Nonsynonymous SNV, exon1	6.20×10^{-9}	7.53×10^{-7}	H4: 99.8%
HDL	Chr8: 9154694–9640787	*RP11-115J16.1* (rs4841132) ncRNA_exonic	3.90×10^{-22}	1.04×10^{-123}	H4: 97.6%
HDL	Chr8: 19492840–20060856	*LPL* (rs15825) UTR3	8.30×10^{-28}	9.88×10^{-324}	H3: 100%
HDL	Chr9: 135298842–137041122	*ABO* (rs687621) ncRNA_intronic	6.30×10^{-11}	4.92×10^{-8}	H4: 99.9%
HDL	Chr10: 63341695–65794114	*JMJD1C* (rs1935) Nonsynonymous SNV, exon26	8.90×10^{-11}	2.59×10^{-6}	H4: 98.7%
HDL	Chr11: 116383348–117747110	*ZNF259* (rs964184) UTR3	2.70×10^{-68}	2.60×10^{-217}	H4: 100%
HDL	Chr11: 124495528–126311320	*TIRAP* (rs8177399) Nonsynonymous SNV, exon4	1.80×10^{-4}	1.84×10^{-7}	H4: 96.9%
HDL	Chr15: 42776399–44198049	*MAP1A* (rs55707100) Nonsynonymous SNV, exon4	1.50×10^{-7}	2.26×10^{-34}	H4: 100%
HDL	Chr19: 8347513–9238393	*ANGPTL4* (rs116843064) Nonsynonymous SNV, exon1	4.00×10^{-11}	4.79×10^{-146}	H4: 100%
HDL	Chr22: 43714200–44995308	*PNPLA3* (rs738409) Nonsynonymous SNV, exon3	7.50×10^{-11}	6.99×10^{-5}	H4: 84.4%
LDL	Chr1: 61922365–63445089	*DOCK7* (rs2131925) intronic	1.10×10^{-19}	1.44×10^{-24}	H4: 99.2%

Table 4. *Cont.*

(c)					
Cytokine in Colocalization with GlycA	**Genomic Region Chromosome: Base Pairs**	**Gene (SNP) Function**	**GlycA *p*-Value**	**Other Phenotype *p*-value**	**PP.H4 (Posterior Probability of Shared Causal SNP) or PP.H3 (of SNPs in Same Region)**
LDL	Chr2: 26894985–28598777	*GCKR* (rs1260326) Nonsynonymous SNV, exon15	2.60×10^{-125}	7.77×10^{-17}	H4: 100%
LDL	Chr2: 110572432–113921856	*IL1F10/RNU6–1180P* (rs6734238) intergenic	4.00×10^{-9}	1.39×10^{-5}	H4: 95.7%
LDL	Chr4: 155056126–157485097	*FGB* (rs6054) Nonsynonymous SNV, exon3	1.80×10^{-9}	2.90×10^{-5}	H4: 98.7%
LDL	Chr6: 31571218–32682664	*SKIV2L* (rs437179) Nonsynonymous SNV, exon8	2.40×10^{-19}	8.16×10^{-6}	H3: 100%
LDL	Chr6: 32682664–33236497	*TAP12* (rs241447) Nonsynonymous SNV, exon12	6.80×10^{-5}	6.22×10^{-9}	H3: 75.5%
LDL	Chr6: 158218719–160580497	*SLC22A1* (rs15643438) intronic	9.80×10^{-6}	2.11×10^{-38}	H3: 88.0%
LDL	Chr6: 160580497–162169564	*LPA* (rs3798220) Nonsynonymous SNV, exon37	6.20×10^{-17}	5.53×10^{-27}	H4: 99.6%
LDL	Chr8: 10463197–11278998	*RP1L1* (rs35602868) Nonsynonymous SNV, exon4	6.70×10^{-7}	1.34×10^{-5}	H4: 75.7%
LDL	Chr10: 63341695–65794114	*JMJD1C* (rs1935) Nonsynonymous SNV, exon26	8.90×10^{-11}	6.95×10^{-12}	H4: 99.7%
LDL	Chr11: 116383348–117747110	*ZNF259* (rs964184) UTR3	2.70×10^{-68}	1.13×10^{-23}	H4: 100%
LDL	Chr14: 943252885–95750867	*SERPINA1* (rs28929474) Nonsynonymous SNV, exon6	3.80×10^{-80}	4.30×10^{-14}	H4: 100%
LDL	Chr19: 18409862–19877471	*TM6SF2* (rs58542926) Nonsynonymous SNV, exon6	7.80×10^{-13}	6.48×10^{-93}	H4: 100%
LDL	Chr22: 43714200–44995308	*PNPLA3* (rs738409) Nonsynonymous SNV, exon3	7.50×10^{-11}	1.00×10^{-8}	H4: 100%
TGs	Chr1: 25516845–27401867	*NR0B2* (rs6659176) Nonsynonymous SNV, exon1	1.30×10^{-6}	3.27×10^{-9}	H4: 99.8%

Table 4. *Cont.*

(c)					
Cytokine in Colocalization with GlycA	**Genomic Region Chromosome: Base Pairs**	**Gene (SNP) Function**	**GlycA *p*-Value**	**Other Phenotype *p*-value**	**PP.H4 (Posterior Probability of Shared Causal SNP) or PP.H3 (of SNPs in Same Region)**
TGs	Chr1: 61922365–63445089	*DOCK7* (rs10889353) intronic	2.10×10^{-19}	6.39×10^{-170}	H4: 99.2%
TGs	Chr2: 21050490–23341383	*APOB* (rs676210) Nonsynonymous SNV, exon26	2.20×10^{-8}	4.94×10^{-118}	H4: 99.8%
TGs	Chr2: 26894985–28598777	*GCKR* (rs1260326) Nonsynonymous SNV, exon15	2.60×10^{-125}	9.88×10^{-324}	H4: 100%
TGs	Chr2: 110572432–113921856	*IL1F10/RNU6-1180P* (rs6734238) intergenic	4.00×10^{-9}	1.06×10^{-4}	H4: 76.0%
TGs	Chr2: 201576284–202818637	*CASP8* (rs3769823) Nonsynonymous SNV, exon1	1.70×10^{-6}	1.36×10^{-9}	H4: 99.7%
TGs	Chr4: 155056126–157485097	*FGB* (rs6054) Nonsynonymous SNV, exon3	1.80×10^{-9}	2.53×10^{-11}	H4: 100%
TGs	Chr6: 31571218–32682664	*SKIV2L* (rs419788) intronic	3020×10^{-19}	5.49×10^{-14}	H3: 100%
TGs	Chr6: 158218719–160580497	*SLC22A1* (rs12208357) Nonsynonymous SNV, exon1	6.20×10^{-9}	3.87×10^{-9}	H4: 99.9%
TGs	Chr7: 71874885–73334602	*MLXIPL* (rs35332062) Nonsynonymous SNV, exon4	4.10×10^{-56}	5.22×10^{-205}	H3: 90.3%
TGs	Chr8: 9154694–9640787	*RP11-115J16.1* (rs4841132) ncRNA_exonic	3.90×10^{-22}	1.29×10^{-15}	H4: 97.7%
TGs	Chr8: 19492840–20060856	*LPL* (rs328) exon9 (stopagain)	7.90×10^{-36}	9.88×10^{-324}	H4: 100%
TGs	Chr10: 63341695–65794114	*JMJD1C* (rs12355784) intronic	1.00×10^{-10}	4.96×10^{-13}	H4: 99.6%
TGs	Chr11: 116383348–117747110	*ZNF259* (rs964184) UTR3	2.70×10^{-68}	9.88×10^{-324}	H4: 100%
TGs	Chr15: 42776399–44198049	*MAP1A* (rs55707100) Nonsynonymous SNV, exon4	1.50×10^{-7}	8.60×10^{-54}	H4: 100%

Table 4. *Cont.*

(c)

Cytokine in Colocalization with GlycA	Genomic Region Chromosome: Base Pairs	Gene (SNP) Function	GlycA p-Value	Other Phenotype p-value	PP.H4 (Posterior Probability of Shared Causal SNP) or PP.H3 (of SNPs in Same Region)
TGs	Chr19: 8347513–9238393	*ANGPTL4* (rs116843064) Nonsynonymous SNV, exon11	4.00×10^{-11}	4.19×10^{-175}	H4: 100%
TGs	Chr19: 18409862–19877471	*TM6SF2* (rs58542926) Nonsynonymous SNV, exon6	7.80×10^{-13}	3.75×10^{-125}	H4: 100%
TGs	Chr20: 39610856–40585689	*PLGC1* (rs738409) Nonsynonymous SNV, exon21	2.80×10^{-7}	1.12×10^{-5}	H4: 99.6%
TGs	Chr22: 43714200–44995308	*PNPLA3* (rs738409) Nonsynonymous SNV, exon3	7.50×10^{-11}	4.35×10^{-9}	H4: 100%
TC	Chr1: 61922365–63445089	*DOCK7* (rs10889353) intronic	2.10×10^{-19}	9.15×10^{-158}	H4: 99.2%
TC	Chr2: 26894985–28598777	*GCKR* (rs1260326) Nonsynonymous SNV, exon15	2.60×10^{-125}	5.25×10^{-102}	H4: 100%
TC	Chr3: 49316972–51832015	*GRM2* (rs116567227) Nonsynonymous SNV, exon2	7.70×10^{-4}	6.01×10^{-7}	H3: 83.2%
TC	Chr4: 155056126–157485097	*FGB* (rs6054) Nonsynonymous SNV, exon3	1.80×10^{-9}	4.79×10^{-12}	H4: 100%
TC	Chr6: 31571218–32682664	*SKIV2L* (rs437179) Nonsynonymous SNV, exon8	2.40×10^{-19}	5.03×10^{-14}	H3: 100%
TC	Chr6: 158218719–160580497	*SLC22A1* (rs15643438) intronic	9.80×10^{-6}	3.52×10^{-37}	H3: 88.0%
TC	Chr8: 9154694–9640787	*RP11-115J16.1* (rs4841132) ncRNA_exonic	3.90×10^{-22}	2.09×10^{-69}	H4: 98.1%
TC	Chr10: 63341695–65794114	*JMJD1C* (rs1935) Nonsynonymous SNV, exon26	8.90×10^{-11}	3.11×10^{-5}	H4: 81.2%
TC	Chr11: 116383348–117747110	*ZNF259* (rs964184) UTR3	2.70×10^{-68}	4.71×10^{-135}	H4: 100%

Table 4. *Cont.*

(c)					
Cytokine in Colocalization with GlycA	**Genomic Region Chromosome: Base Pairs**	**Gene (SNP) Function**	**GlycA *p*-Value**	**Other Phenotype *p*-value**	**PP.H4 (Posterior Probability of Shared Causal SNP) or PP.H3 (of SNPs in Same Region)**
TC	Chr14: 943252885–95750867	*SERPINA1* (rs28929474) Nonsynonymous SNV, exon6	3.80×10^{-80}	5.53×10^{-14}	H4: 100%
TC	Chr19: 18409862–19877471	*TM6SF2* (rs28929474) Nonsynonymous SNV, exon6	7.80×10^{-13}	7.03×10^{-155}	H4: 100%
TC	Chr20: 39610856–40585689	*PLCG1* (rs755381) Nonsynonymous SNV, exon21	2.80×10^{-7}	6.66×10^{-47}	H4: 99.9%
TC	Chr22: 43714200–44995308	*PNPLA3* (rs738409) Nonsynonymous SNV, exon3	7.50×10^{-11}	1.69×10^{-21}	H4: 100%

(d)					
Cytokine in Colocalization with RA	**Genomic Region Chromosome: Base Pairs**	**Gene (SNP) Function**	**RA *p*-Value**	**Other Phenotype *p*-Value**	**PP.H4 (Posterior Probability of Shared Causal SNP) or PP.H3 (of SNPs in Same Region)**
Atherosclerosis	Chr6: 158218719–160580497	*IGF2R* (rs2230044) Synonymous SNV, exon33	1.30×10^{-3}	2.14×10^{-19}	H3: 100%
CAD	Chr1: 1892607–3582736	*SKI/MORN1* (rs2643905) intergenic	4.00×10^{-4}	1.97×10^{-11}	H3: 100%
CAD	Chr1: 37549183–38731847	*INPP5B* (rs35267671) Nonsynonymous SNV, exon7	7.00×10^{-3}	2.90×10^{-11}	H3: 100%
CAD	Chr1: 113273306–114873845	*MAGI3* (rs183352775) intronic	4.10×10^{-50}	1.69×10^{-5}	H3: 100%
CAD	Chr6: 31571218–32682664	*HLA-DRB1/HLA-DQA1* (rs532965) intergenic	1.00×10^{-250}	1.37×10^{-2}	H3: 99.7%
CAD	Chr6: 158218719–160580497	*SLC22A1* (rs2282143) Nonsynonymous SNV, exon6	1.80×10^{-2}	7.35×10^{-42}	H3: 100%
CAD	Chr15: 38530777–40384132	*RASGRP1* (rs72727388) intronic	1.80×10^{-11}	2.70×10^{-6}	H4: 96.3%

Comparable results were obtained between GlycA and CAD and concerned the *SLC22A1*, *LPA*, *LPL*, *SERPINA1*, and *ANGPTL4* genes, with correspondingly high PPs (H4: 97.5%, H4: 99.8%, H3: 100%, H4: 99.7%, and H4: 100%; Table 4b). Two other common genomic regions were identified between GlycA and CAD; one mapped to the *ZNF259* gene (PP.H4: 100%) and the other to the *PNPLA3* gene (PP.H4: 95.4%; Table 4b).

Colocalization between GlycA and heart failure identified three genomic regions harboring the *LPA*, *ABO*, and *ZNF259* genes with PP.H4 values of: 99.7, 72.2%, and 70.1%, respectively (Table 4b). Lastly, two more genomic regions in chromosome 6, containing two intronic SNPs with PP.H4 values of 96.8% and 99.7%, were identified and mapped to genes *SLC22A1* and *LPA* (Table 4b). These genes were also noted in other colocalized observations between GlycA and other atherosclerotic phenotypes.

Next, colocalization was performed between GlycA and the four lipid factors. In all comparisons, several significant common genetic variants were detected and are summarized in Table 4c. The major results based on atherosclerotic phenotype were as follows:

GlycA and HDL shared 10 exonic SNPs mapped to specific genomic regions on chromosomes 2, 6, 8, 10, 11, 15, 19, and 22 with mostly very high PP.H4 values ranging between 96.9% and 100%. Of these, the most remarkable were rs15825 belonging to the untranslated region of the *LPL* gene and associated with $p = 8.30 \times 10^{-28}$ (GlycA) and $p = 9.88 \times 10^{-324}$ (HDL) and observed PP.H3 of 100% (distinct polymorphisms located at the same site) and rs4841132 mapped to the *RP11-115J16.1* gene, $p = 3.90 \times 10^{-22}$ $p = 1.04 \times 10^{-123}$, respectively) with PP.H4 of 97.6%.

GlycA and LDL. Consistent with the colocalization observations between GlycA and HDL, SNPs mapped to the *DOCK7*, *JMJD1C*, and *ZNF259* genes were also observed in these analyses, with strong support of PP.H4, i.e., between 99.2% and 100%. In addition, eight other exonic SNPs were found in several known genes including *GCKR*, *FGB*, *SKIV2L*, *TAP12*, *LPA*, *RP1L1*, *TM6SF2*, and *PNPLA3*, with evidence of colocalization in support of PP.H4 (75.7% to 100%), but also with probabilities of 75.5% and 100% for H3 in two analyses.

GlycA and TGs. Colocalization and enrichment analyses revealed similarity to LDL and HDL genomic regions, including the genes *DOCK7*, *APOB*, *GCKR*, *FGB*, *SLC22A1*, *RP11-115J16.1*, *JMJD1C*, *ZNF259*, *MAP1A*, *ANGPTL4*, *TM6SF2*, and *PNPLA3* with high PP.H4 (ranging between 99.2% and 100%) and the *SKIV2L* gene with PP.H3 100%. In addition, five other exonic SNPs specifically colocalized between GlycA and TGs were identified and mapped to the genes *NR0B2*, *CASP8*, *MLXIPL*, *LPL*, and *PLGC1*, with PP.H4 values ranging between 90.6% and 100%.

GlycA and TC. Here, we also detected several genomic regions common with other lipid factors, namely, *DOCK7*, *GCKR*, *FGBRP11-115J16.1*, *JMJD1C*, *ZNF259*, *SERPINA1*, *TM6SF2*, *PLCG1*, and *PNPLA3*, with strong support for PP.H4: from 81.2%, but mostly from 99.2% to 100%, Two colocalization results strongly supported PP.H3 (with 88.0% and 100% probability for *SLC22A1* and *SKIV2L*, respectively). Finally, an additional exonic SNP was colocalized on chromosome 3, mapped to *GRM2*, with PP.H3 of 83.2%.

Importantly, several genes, namely, *FGB*, *SKIV2L*, *SLC22A1*, *LPA*, *LPL*, *SERPINA1*, *ANGPTL4*, *PNPLA3*, *ABO*, and *ZNF259*, colocalized between GlycA and some lipid factors and colocalized between GlycA and several atherosclerotic phenotypes (Table 4b,c). Lastly, the intergenic region between *IL1F10* and *RNU6-1180P*, seen to be colocalized between GlycA and some lipid factors (Table 4c), was also colocalized between GlycA and RA (Table 4a).

Considering RA and atherosclerotic variables, two regions of interest were apparent on chromosome 6, specifically between RA and CAD (Table 4d). There was consistent colocalization between GlycA and RA involving the HLA region, annotated to the intergenic regions between *HLA-DRB1* and *HLA-DQA1*, with very strong evidence of PP.H3: 99.7%. Another remarkable result was an exonic SNP on chromosome 6 between base pairs 158218719 and 160580497 and mapped to *SLC22A1* with strong evidence of colocalization of the distinct causal variants (PP.H3: 100%) (Table 4d).

Additionally, several colocalization results were apparent between GlycA and atherosclerotic phenotypes and between GlycA and lipid factors that corresponded to the HLA region and are reported in the Supplementary Materials (Table S2).

2.5. ABN Analysis

ABN analysis was used to generate the most likely network describing the relationships among GlycA, RA, and the atherosclerotic variables (Figure 1 and Table S5, Supplementary Materials). The resulting model suggests that RA induces GlycA (β = 0.350, 95%CI = 0.327 to 0.373), and GlycA is subsequently associated with atherosclerosis (β = 0.370, 95%CI = 0.333 to 0.406), while RA is also significantly and independently associated with atherosclerosis (β = 0.479, 95%CI = 0.291 to 0.652). As suspected, RA and GlycA are both directly linked to lipid factors, in this case LDL (β = −0.250, 95%CI = −0.229 to −0.273 and β = 0.306, 95%CI = 0.302 to 0.309, respectively), which in turn are linked with the other lipid factors. As such, the relationship with LDL may uniquely contribute to the development of atherosclerosis (β = −0.441, 95%CI = −0.403 to −0.479). Not surprisingly, age is the facilitating variable among major phenotypes, RA, GlycA, and atherosclerosis (Figure 1).

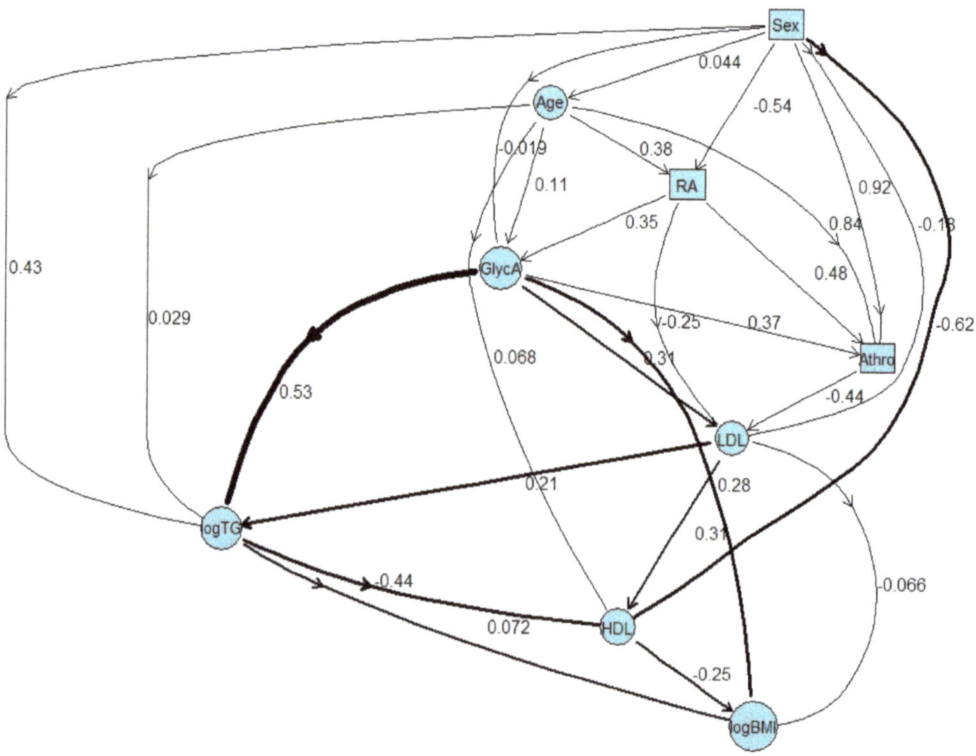

Figure 1. Additive Bayesian Network (ABN) Analysis. ABN analysis was used to create the statistical model describing pathways of risk factors contributing to RA, atherosclerosis, and GlycA. Arcs demonstrate the regression coefficients estimated by the model with corresponding 95% confidence intervals found in Table S5, Supplementary Materials.

3. Discussion

In this study we explored the genetic basis of the relationships between RA and its major comorbidity, atherosclerosis. Genetic correlations established that GlycA, an inflammation marker, plays a role in facilitating the relationship between RA and atherosclerosis. Two independent statistical analyses identified a pleiotropic relationship between GlycA and RA. GlycA appears to be causally related to atherosclerosis, further reinforcing the role of inflammation through a secondary approach/pathway. Lipid factors, known to be associated with the development of atherosclerosis, were previously shown to be pleiotropically associated with RA [20], further presenting another pathway that promotes the nature of the comorbidities. Lastly, colocalization and gene enrichment uncovered a series of genes that may partake in the complicated relationship between RA and atherosclerosis, through GlycA and other intermediatory forces, such as lipid factors.

While RA was previously reported to be in a causal genetic relationship with CRP [21], we find that RA appears to be in horizontal pleiotropy with GlycA. This difference suggests the presence of differing inflammatory pathways essentially induced by RA. Remarkably also, the genetic relationship between RA and atherosclerotic phenotypes appears to be described by horizontal pleiotropy, and yet, GlycA, or the inflammatory pathway in relation to GlycA, appears to serve as a mediator because it causally predicts atherosclerosis and CAD. Although the lipid contributions to cardiovascular complications are reportedly causal [22], our previous study [23] suggests a pleiotropic association between them. Our results from network analysis are in agreement with those of previous studies and shed further light on "the lipid paradox" in RA, i.e., the tendency for lower LDL and higher TG levels in RA individuals [24]. In addition, the lower LDL levels in association with atherosclerosis may be explained by the efficacy of therapy lowering LDL levels [25].

It is important to note that the IVW method suggested that GlycA showed a causal relationship with HDL and LDL, but no correlation or causation was demonstrated by the MRE method. In addition, the MR PRESSO method showed a correlation between GlycA and the lipid factors. IVW is a powerful and useful tool that considers that all selected instrumental variables are significant. However, IVW does not account for horizontal pleiotropy, which if present, falsely demonstrates a significantly causal relationship [26]. Thus, by implementing the MRE method, we are able to detect whether the significant MR estimate was indeed attributed to horizontal pleiotropy and not causally related. In examining the potential causal relationship between GlycA and HDL and LDL, a causal relationship seemed apparent through the IVW approach but was instead due to horizontal pleiotropy as suggested by the MR Egger approach. The MR PRESSO approach is a tool designed to calculate the presence of horizontal pleiotropy [27], and thus the global results significantly confirmed the presence of horizontal pleiotropy as was indicated in the results.

Here, we speculate that GlycA, a marker of systemic inflammation, predicts future CVD events [28] and may modulate the relationship between RA and atherosclerosis. Inflammatory pathways related to RA may attenuate CV complications as well as accelerate atherosclerosis arising from early-onset vascular deterioration [29]. Inflammation arising from atherosclerosis appears to contribute to plaque rupture, which is a typical complication of CVD, and may be influenced by cytokines and chemokines [11].

Several mechanisms may be involved in the genesis of atherosclerosis in RA [15]. One mechanism involves lipid level alterations, which elicit atherosclerotic tendencies, while another mechanism may include the escalation of the oxidative process triggered by RA [15]. While underlying genetic factors may induce these conditions pleiotropically, metabolic syndrome also appears to contribute to their joint manifestation [15]. Lipid factors further reinforce the relationship between RA and atherosclerosis, as the present analysis suggests. Similar observations have been recently reported and concluded that postprandial hyperlipidemia (TG levels > 220 mg/dL), was more common in patients with RA and was associated with inflammation and subclinical atherosclerosis [30].

Our study indicates that the inflammatory cascade in RA, as reflected by elevated GlycA levels, facilitates the development of atherosclerosis. GlycA appears to have a unique and pivotal role in this process, being strongly correlated with TG blood levels both phenotypically and genetically. These observations are well supported by the existing non-genetic data. GlycA coupled with triglyceride-rich lipoproteins was reportedly associated with the presence of subclinical myocardial dysfunction in subjects with type 1 diabetes mellitus [31]. Another study demonstrated that GlycA serum levels were high in RA subjects and associated with incident atherosclerosis, independent of cardiometabolic predictors [17]. The association between GlycA and subclinical CV was maintained after controlling for typical covariates including age, sex, dyslipidemia, smoking, BMI, and even CRP [17]. In addition, the early stages of RA generate high serum levels of GlycA, which appears to predict alterations in cholesterol levels such as lower LDL and higher TGs, in line with our findings [17].

3.1. Genes of Interest

This study revealed significant genetic correlations between GlycA, RA, and atherosclerosis-related phenotypes, which is supplemented by the colocalization analysis that pointed out several genes of interest. Of these, we believe the most significant are the following.

The *ILF10/RNU-1180P* genomic region consistently appeared in colocalization across lipid factors and GlycA but also between RA and GlycA. *ILF10/RNU-1180P* were implicated in a genome-wide meta-analysis conducted on IL6 in addition to the *HLA-DRB1/DRB5* loci [32]. These two regions may serve as major players in immunological and inflammatory pathways [32], while it is known that IL6 is a key cytokine involved in RA pathogenesis and the RA–atherosclerosis relationship [11].

Another gene of interest, *SLC22A1*, was noted across all phenotypes in colocalization to GlycA but also between RA and CAD. While this gene was not noted previously in the literature in relation to RA (or GlycA or lipids), its family member, *SLC22A4*, was associated with RA susceptibility in the Chinese population [33], and *SLC22A5* was suggested to be associated with extra-articular manifestations in RA subjects [34].

The HLA region, which may contribute to the cascade of events leading to inflammation [35] and which is strongly associated with RA [36], was observed to colocalize between all the variables examined. Importantly, glycoproteins demonstrated a relationship to HLA under heightened inflammatory conditions [37]. In addition, HLA was associated with the development of atherosclerosis [38] Moreover, HLA-DRB1 alleles were previously reported to define the shared genetic relationship between RA and atherosclerosis [15]. Our previous colocalization study revealed that HLA also participates in the pleiotropic relationship between RA and lipid factors [20].

Studies clarifying autoimmune disease and their genetic variation are of particular importance, as Ota et al. [39] clarifies and demonstrates that autoimmune GWAS findings reveal cell types involved and environmental influences, as they have produced an atlas containing these corresponding details.

3.2. Limitations

GWAS summary statistics were limited to participants of European ancestry; therefore, findings may not generalize to other populations. The sample sizes used were among the best available, yet LDSC genetic correlations were still underpowered, and some potentially meaningful correlations fell slightly below statistically significant. The presence of overlapping samples between the GWASs used for both the exposure and outcome in MR may cause inflated estimates, where the GlycA GWAS also included data from the UK Biobank, as well as the CAD phenotype.

4. Material and Methods

4.1. Dataset

Phenotypic data from the UK Biobank (UKBB) included 502,356 participants, of whom 13,514 had self-reported diagnosis RA, and 4532 were diagnosed with atherosclerosis. Furthermore, 499,249 participants had measured BMI, and 274,349 had lipid profiles.

Genome-wide association study (GWAS) summary statistics were acquired from several resources for GWAS-based analyses. RA summary statistics were collected from Okada et al. [40] and comprised 14,361 RA cases and 43,923 controls of European ancestry (18 data sources) subjected to meta-analysis using >8 million imputed genetic variants or single nucleotide polymorphisms (SNPs). Analysis of coronary atherosclerosis was based on 16,041 cases and 440,307 controls, with over 11 million genetic variants, carried out by

Jiang et al., using data from the UKBB [41]. Coronary artery disease (CAD) was analyzed by Aragam et al., based on 181,522 cases and 1,165,690 controls from 10 different data sources across Europe, with over 20 million genetic variants [42]. Heart failure was based on 47,039 cases and 903,014 controls compiled from 26 studies, including the UKBB, with over 8 million genetic variants [23]. Lastly, heart attack/MI was acquired from the Neale Lab website [43] and was based on 7735 cases and 329,424 controls with over 10 million genetic variants. The Global Lipids Genetics Consortium provided summary statistics for HDL, LDL, triglycerides (TGs), and total cholesterol (TC) [44]. The summary statistics came from meta-analysis of each lipid from 73 studies including 237,050 participants of European ancestry and nearly 250,000 genetic variants [44]. GWAS summary statistics for GlycA were based on 115,078 European participants and comprised over 12 million genetic variants. The full description of the GlycA GWAS, which is housed by Bristol University, was taken from 3 studies as detailed by Crick et al. [45].

The atherosclerotic phenotypes were defined as coronary atherosclerosis (CAD), heart failure, and heart attack/MI, whereas lipid factors included HDL, LDL, TGs, and TC.

4.2. Statistical Analysis

Basic statistical analyses were carried out using R 4.2.3 (https://www.R-project.org/, accessed on 27 April 2024). The *lm* and *glm* functions from R *stats* were used to conduct linear and logistic regression analyses, respectively. In general, a p-value ≤ 0.05 was considered significant in analyses executed throughout this study. GlycA was analyzed as the dependent variable, and RA or atherosclerotic phenotypes as independent variables, in addition to covariates age, sex, and BMI. Subsequently, the relationships between RA (as the dependent variable) and atherosclerotic variables, not including the lipid factors, as the independent variables, were examined.

4.3. Genetic Correlation

Genetic correlation was assessed between GlycA and RA along with atherosclerotic phenotypes, as well as between RA and atherosclerotic phenotypes, using cross-trait Linkage Disequilibrium Score Regression (LDSC) (https://github.com/bulik/ldsc, accessed on 27 April 2024) [46]. The LD reference panel was limited to the European subset from the 1000 Genomes Project.

4.4. Mendelian Randomization (MR)

To assess potential causal effects between two phenotypes, we conducted two-sample MR analyses using GWAS summary statistics and the *Mendelian Randomization* package in R (https://CRAN.R-project.org/package=MendelianRandomization, accessed on 27 April 2024) [47]. The principles of MR analysis have been extensively described elsewhere [48] Several MR approaches are available with the intent to satisfy different assumptions, including inverse variance weighted (IVW) and MR Egger (MRE). Except for MRE, most MR approaches correspond closely with IVW. Thus, we initially focused on MRE and IVW.

IVW, probably the most common method of MR, infers the existence and strength of the causal relation between an exposure and outcome variable [48]. The MRE approach is advantageous for its robustness and distinguishes between the pleiotropic and causal effects on pleiotropy [49]. The MRE approach can determine instrument validity using the I^2 sensitivity statistic, which measures instrumental variable dilution or bias [50], and is suggested to be at least 90% in a two-sample analysis [49].

In cases where MRE suggested the existence of pleiotropy, the MR PRESSO method was implemented to specifically test for horizontal pleiotropy (https://github.com/rondolab/MR-PRESSO, accessed on 27 April 2024) [27]. MR PRESSO is a robust outlier method, with the global test determining the presence of horizontal pleiotropy, assuming <50% of the chosen instrumental variants are horizontally pleiotropic [27].

4.5. Colocalization Analysis and Gene Enrichment

To confirm the presence of horizontal pleiotropy, colocalization analysis employed using the *coloc.abf* function in the *coloc* R package (https://github.com/chr1swallace/coloc, accessed on 27 April 2024), applicable to GWAS summary statistics [51,52]. Based on Bayesian statistical modeling, it generates five posterior probabilities corresponding to five hypotheses as described by Wallace et al. [51]. Of these, two alternative hypotheses, H3 and H4, were of interest to us:

Hypothesis 3 (H3). *Association to both traits detected but caused by distinct causal variants.*

Hypothesis 4 (H4). *Association to both traits detected and caused by a shared causal variant.*

H4 is essentially suggestive of horizontal pleiotropy. H3 may suggest spurious pleiotropy; however, it may also be suggestive of biological or horizontal pleiotropy in some cases. H3 becomes more evident than H4 when the genomic region examined contains a large number of SNPs. As a result, a high posterior probability (PP) of H3 might be evident although shared causal SNPs may instead appropriately explain the pleiotropic relationship [51]. Strong evidence of pleiotropy was defined as a PP > 75%, while 75% > PP > 50% is cautiously suggestive of the presence of significant SNPs, shared or distinct, mapped to the designated genomic region [52].

Colocalization analysis was carried out only between GlycA and all other variables and between RA and atherosclerotic variables, except for lipid factors, for which the results were reported elsewhere [20].

Genomic regions that revealed strong evidence of pleiotropy were subsequently examined to identify the corresponding genes of the apparent causal SNPs using gene enrichment analysis. The most likely SNP in the genomic region common to both traits under comparison was generated by colocalization analysis and was considered in the gene enrichment analysis. The latter was conducted using the Functional Mapping and Annotation (FUMA) GWAS platform (https://fuma.ctglab.nl/, accessed on 27 April 2024) [53].

4.6. Additive Bayesian Network (ABN) Modeling

ABN modeling, utilizing the *abn* R package (version 3.0.1) (https://r-bayesian-networks.org/, accessed on 27 April 2024) [54], employs a multidimensional approach to estimate the most likely network of relationships among selected phenotypes [54]. Bootstrapping is applied to control for over-fitting [54]. The correlations, or arcs, produced describe relationships between pairs of traits and are analogous to regression coefficients from multiple regression analysis. The following variables were considered for the analysis: GlycA, RA, coronary atherosclerosis, CAD, heart failure, heart attack/MI, HDL, LDL, TGs, TC with adjustment for age and sex, and BMI in all the analyses.

5. Conclusions

In this study, we present a potential metabolic pathway that describes the relationship between RA and atherosclerosis-related conditions, modeled by inflammation indicated by GlycA. RA is suggested to elicit inflammatory pathways leading to the development of atherosclerotic complications. GlycA causes atherosclerosis, and CAD and is therefore a potential pivotal marker in the early screening of cardiovascular complications in RA subjects. RA, concomitantly, induces lipid alteration through inflammatory pathways, but also through GlycA, suggesting that several pathways may be involved in the manifestation of atherosclerotic complications following the onset of RA. This study identified several genes likely involved directly in the association between RA and atherosclerotic phenotypes and indirectly through the mediator, GlycA. Interestingly, *SLC22A1* appeared in colocalization between GlycA and all tested atherosclerosis-related phenotypes as well as between RA and atherosclerotic phenotypes.

Supplementary Materials: The following supporting information can be downloaded at: https://www.mdpi.com/article/10.3390/ijms25115981/s1.

Author Contributions: All authors contributed to the study conception and design. BigData were acquired by M.K., G.L. and S.A. Statistical genetic analysis was performed by M.K., S.S.C., G.L. and M.B.F.; G.L., S.A. and F.M.K.W. supervised the entire project. The first draft of the manuscript was written by M.K., M.B.F., G.L. and F.M.K.W. All authors have read and agreed to the published version of the manuscript.

Funding: The study was supported by the Israel Science Foundation (grant #2054/19) and the Ariel University Research and Development Department (grant #RA2000000457).

Informed Consent Statement: Informed consent was obtained from all subjects involved in the study.

Data Availability Statement: Data is contained within the article (and Supplementary Materials).

Conflicts of Interest: The authors declare no conflicts of interest.

References

1. Chopra, A.; Abdel-Nasser, A. Epidemiology of Rheumatic Musculoskeletal Disorders in the Developing World. *Best Pract. Res. Clin. Rheumatol.* **2008**, *22*, 583–604. [CrossRef] [PubMed]
2. Venetsanopoulou, A.I.; Alamanos, Y.; Voulgari, P.V.; Drosos, A.A. Epidemiology and Risk Factors for Rheumatoid Arthritis Development. *Mediterr. J. Rheumatol.* **2023**, *34*, 404. [CrossRef] [PubMed]
3. Boots, A.M.H.; Maier, A.B.; Stinissen, P.; Masson, P.; Lories, R.J.; De Keyser, F. The Influence of Ageing on the Development and Management of Rheumatoid Arthritis. *Nat. Rev. Rheumatol.* **2013**, *9*, 604–613. [CrossRef] [PubMed]
4. Dadoun, S.; Zeboulon-Ktorza, N.; Combescure, C.; Elhai, M.; Rozenberg, S.; Gossec, L.; Fautrel, B. Mortality in Rheumatoid Arthritis over the Last Fifty Years: Systematic Review and Meta-Analysis. *Joint Bone Spine* **2013**, *80*, 29–33. [CrossRef] [PubMed]
5. Lee, Y.K.; Ahn, G.Y.; Lee, J.; Shin, J.M.; Lee, T.H.; Park, D.J.; Song, Y.J.; Kim, M.K.; Bae, S.C. Excess Mortality Persists in Patients with Rheumatoid Arthritis. *Int. J. Rheum. Dis.* **2021**, *24*, 364–372. [CrossRef] [PubMed]
6. Avina-Zubieta, J.A.; Thomas, J.; Sadatsafavi, M.; Lehman, A.J.; Lacaille, D. Risk of Incident Cardiovascular Events in Patients with Rheumatoid Arthritis: A Meta-Analysis of Observational Studies. *Ann. Rheum. Disease* **2012**, *71*, 1524–1529. [CrossRef] [PubMed]
7. Crowson, C.S.; Liao, K.P.; Davis, J.M., III; Solomon, D.H.; Matteson, E.L.; Knutson, K.L.; Hlatky, M.A.; Gabriel, S.E. Rheumatoid Arthritis and Cardiovascular Disease. *Am. Heart J.* **2013**, *166*, 622–628. [CrossRef] [PubMed]
8. Krüger, K.; Nüßlein, H. Cardiovascular Comorbidities in Rheumatoid Arthritis. *Z. Rheumatol.* **2019**, *78*, 221–227. [CrossRef]
9. Ruscitti, P.; Cipriani, P.; Liakouli, V.; Iacono, D.; Pantano, I.; Margiotta, D.P.E.; Navarini, L.; Destro Castaniti, G.M.; Maruotti, N.; Di Scala, G.; et al. Subclinical and Clinical Atherosclerosis in Rheumatoid Arthritis: Results from the 3-Year, Multicentre, Prospective, Observational GIRRCS (Gruppo Italiano Di Ricerca in Reumatologia Clinica e Sperimentale) Study. *Arthritis Res. Ther.* **2019**, *21*, 204. [CrossRef] [PubMed]
10. Jebari-Benslaiman, S.; Galicia-García, U.; Larrea-Sebal, A.; Olaetxea, J.R.; Alloza, I.; Vandenbroeck, K.; Benito-Vicente, A.; Martín, C. Pathophysiology of Atherosclerosis. *Int. J. Mol. Sci.* **2022**, *23*, 3346. [CrossRef]
11. Frostegård, J. Immunity, Atherosclerosis and Cardiovascular Disease. *BMC Med.* **2013**, *11*, 117. [CrossRef]
12. MacGregor, A.J.; Snieder, H.; Rigby, A.S.; Koskenvuo, M.; Kaprio, J.; Aho, K.; Silman, A.J. Characterizing the Quantitative Genetic Contribution to Rheumatoid Arthritis Using Data from Twins. *Arthritis Rheum.* **2000**, *43*, 30–37. [CrossRef] [PubMed]
13. Zdravkovic, S.; Wienke, A.; Pedersen, N.L.; Marenberg, M.E.; Yashin, A.I.; De Faire, U. Heritability of Death from Coronary Heart Disease: A 36-Year Follow-up of 20 966 Swedish Twins. *J. Intern. Med.* **2002**, *252*, 247–254. [CrossRef] [PubMed]
14. Rodríguez-Rodríguez, L.; López-Mejías, R.; García-Bermúdez, M.; González-Juanatey, C.; González-Gay, M.A.; Martín, J. Genetic Markers of Cardiovascular Disease in Rheumatoid Arthritis. *Mediat. Inflamm.* **2012**, *2012*, 574817. [CrossRef] [PubMed]
15. Cavagna, L.; Boffini, N.; Cagnotto, G.; Inverardi, F.; Grosso, V.; Caporali, R. Atherosclerosis and Rheumatoid Arthritis: More Than a Simple Association. *Mediat. Inflamm.* **2012**, *2012*, 147354. [CrossRef] [PubMed]
16. Connelly, M.A.; Otvos, J.D.; Shalaurova, I.; Playford, M.P.; Mehta, N.N. GlycA, a Novel Biomarker of Systemic Inflammation and Cardiovascular Disease Risk. *J. Transl. Med.* **2017**, *15*, 219. [CrossRef] [PubMed]
17. Rodríguez-Carrio, J.; Alperi-López, M.; López, P.; Pérez-álvarez, Á.I.; Gil-Serret, M.; Amigó, N.; Ulloa, C.; Benavente, L.; Ballina-García, F.J.; Suárez, A. GlycA Levels during the Earliest Stages of Rheumatoid Arthritis: Potential Use as a Biomarker of Subclinical Cardiovascular Disease. *J. Clin. Med.* **2020**, *9*, 2472. [CrossRef]
18. Raj, R.; Thomas, S.; Gorantla, V. Accelerated Atherosclerosis in Rheumatoid Arthritis: A Systematic Review. *F1000Res* **2022**, *11*, 466. [CrossRef] [PubMed]
19. Liu, Q.-P.; Du, H.-C.; Xie, P.-J.; Zhang, L.-X.; Gao, H.-Z.; Luo, J.-H.; Chai, S.-T.; Qi, O.; Liu, P. Causal Relationship between Rheumatoid Arthritis and Atherosclerosis Risk: A Mendelian Randomized Study. *medRxiv* **2024**. [CrossRef]
20. Kasher, M.; Cherny, S.S.; Livshits, G. Exploring Potential Shared Genetic Influences between Rheumatoid Arthritis and Blood Lipid Levels. *Atherosclerosis* **2022**, *363*, 48–56. [CrossRef]

21. Kasher, M.; Williams, F.M.K.; Freidin, M.B.; Malkin, I.; Cherny, S.S.; CHARGE Inflammation Working Group; Livshits, G. Understanding the Complex Genetic Architecture Connecting Rheumatoid Arthritis, Osteoporosis, and Inflammation: Discovering Causal Pathways. *Hum. Mol. Genet.* **2022**, *26*, 312–318. [CrossRef]
22. Hedayatnia, M.; Asadi, Z.; Zare-Feyzabadi, R.; Yaghooti-Khorasani, M.; Ghazizadeh, H.; Ghaffarian-Zirak, R.; Nosrati-Tirkani, A.; Mohammadi-Bajgiran, M.; Rohban, M.; Sadabadi, F.; et al. Dyslipidemia and Cardiovascular Disease Risk among the MASHAD Study Population. *Lipids Health Dis.* **2020**, *19*, 2810–2819. [CrossRef] [PubMed]
23. Shah, S.; Henry, A.; Roselli, C.; Lin, H.; Sveinbjörnsson, G.; Fatemifar, G.; Hedman, Å.K.; Wilk, J.B.; Morley, M.P.; Chaffin, M.D.; et al. Genome-Wide Association and Mendelian Randomisation Analysis Provide Insights into the Pathogenesis of Heart Failure. *Nat. Commun.* **2020**, *11*, 163. [CrossRef] [PubMed]
24. Myasoedova, E.; Crowson, C.S.; Kremers, H.M.; Roger, V.L.; Fitz-Gibbon, P.D.; Therneau, T.M.; Gabriel, S.E. Lipid Paradox In Rheumatoid Arthritis: The Impact of Serum Lipid Measures and Systemic Inflammation on the Risk of Cardiovascular Disease. *Ann. Rheum. Dis.* **2011**, *70*, 482. [CrossRef]
25. Chen, G.; Farris, M.S.; Cowling, T.; Colgan, S.M.; Xiang, P.; Pericleous, L.; Rogoza, R.M.; Tai, M.H.; Anderson, T. Treatment and Low-Density Lipoprotein Cholesterol Management in Patients Diagnosed With Clinical Atherosclerotic Cardiovascular Disease in Alberta. *Can. J. Cardiol.* **2019**, *35*, 884–891. [CrossRef]
26. Lin, Z.; Deng, Y.; Pan, W. Combining the Strengths of Inverse-Variance Weighting and Egger Regression in Mendelian Randomization Using a Mixture of Regressions Model. *PLoS Genet.* **2021**, *17*, e1009922. [CrossRef]
27. Verbanck, M.; Chen, C.Y.; Neale, B.; Do, R. Detection of Widespread Horizontal Pleiotropy in Causal Relationships Inferred from Mendelian Randomization between Complex Traits and Diseases. *Nat. Genet.* **2018**, *50*, 693–698. [CrossRef] [PubMed]
28. Akinkuolie, A.O.; Buring, J.E.; Ridker, P.M.; Mora, S. A Novel Protein Glycan Biomarker and Future Cardiovascular Disease Events. *J. Am. Heart Assoc.* **2014**, *3*, e001221. [CrossRef]
29. Kahlenberg, J.M.; Kaplan, M.J. Mechanisms of Premature Atherosclerosis in Rheumatoid Arthritis and Lupus. *Annu. Rev. Med.* **2013**, *64*, 249. [CrossRef]
30. Mena-Vázquez, N.; Redondo-Rodríguez, R.; Rioja, J.; Jimenez-Nuñez, F.G.; Manrique-Arija, S.; Lisbona-Montañez, J.M.; Cano-García, L.; Rojas-Gimenez, M.; Ureña, I.; Valdivielso, P.; et al. Postprandial Hyperlipidemia: Association with Inflammation and Subclinical Atherosclerosis in Patients with Rheumatoid Arthritis. *Biomedicines* **2022**, *10*, 133. [CrossRef]
31. Puig-Jové, C.; Julve, J.; Castelblanco, E.; Julián, M.T.; Amigó, N.; Andersen, H.U.; Ahluwalia, T.S.; Rossing, P.; Mauricio, D.; Jensen, M.T.; et al. The Novel Inflammatory Biomarker GlycA and Triglyceride-Rich Lipoproteins Are Associated with the Presence of Subclinical Myocardial Dysfunction in Subjects with Type 1 Diabetes Mellitus. *Cardiovasc. Diabetol.* **2022**, *21*, 257. [CrossRef] [PubMed]
32. Ahluwalia, T.S.; Prins, B.P.; Abdollahi, M.; Armstrong, N.J.; Aslibekyan, S.; Bain, L.; Jefferis, B.; Baumert, J.; Beekman, M.; Ben-Shlomo, Y.; et al. Genome-Wide Association Study of Circulating Interleukin 6 Levels Identifies Novel Loci. *Hum. Mol. Genet.* **2021**, *30*, 393. [CrossRef] [PubMed]
33. Ren, T.L.; Han, Z.J.; Yang, C.J.; Hang, Y.X.; Fang, D.Y.; Wang, K.; Zhu, X.; Ji, X.J.; Zhou, F.F. Association of SLC22A4 Gene Polymorphism with Rheumatoid Arthritis in the Chinese Population. *J. Biochem. Mol. Toxicol.* **2014**, *28*, 206–210. [CrossRef] [PubMed]
34. Pawlik, A.; Paradowska-Gorycka, A.; Safranow, K.; Dziedziejko, V.; Dutkiewicz, G.; Słucznowska-Głabowska, S.; Juzyszyn, Z.; Drozdzik, M. SLC22A5 Polymorphism Associated with Risk of Extra-Articular Manifestations in Rheumatoid Arthritis Patients. *Reumatologia* **2019**, *57*, 3. [CrossRef] [PubMed]
35. Perdaens, O.; van Pesch, V. Molecular Mechanisms of Immunosenescene and Inflammaging: Relevance to the Immunopathogenesis and Treatment of Multiple Sclerosis. *Front. Neurol.* **2021**, *12*, 811518. [CrossRef] [PubMed]
36. van Drongelen, V.; Holoshitz, J. HLA-Disease Associations in Rheumatoid Arthritis. *Rheum. Dis. Clin. N. Am.* **2017**, *43*, 363. [CrossRef] [PubMed]
37. Malo, A.I.; Peraire, J.; Ruiz-Mateos, E.; Masip, J.; Amigó, N.; Alcamí, J.; Moreno, S.; Girona, J.; García-Pardo, G.; Reig, R.; et al. Evolution of Serum Acute-Phase Glycoproteins Assessed by 1H-NMR in HIV Elite Controllers. *Front. Immunol.* **2021**, *12*, 730691. [CrossRef] [PubMed]
38. Fava, C.; Montagnana, M. Atherosclerosis Is an Inflammatory Disease Which Lacks a Common Anti-Inflammatory Therapy: How Human Genetics Can Help to This Issue. A Narrative Review. *Front. Pharmacol.* **2018**, *9*, 328994. [CrossRef]
39. Ota, M.; Nagafuchi, Y.; Hatano, H.; Ishigaki, K.; Terao, C.; Takeshima, Y.; Yanaoka, H.; Kobayashi, S.; Okubo, M.; Shirai, H.; et al. Dynamic Landscape of Immune Cell-Specific Gene Regulation in Immune-Mediated Diseases. *Cell* **2021**, *184*, 3006–3021.e17. [CrossRef]
40. Okada, Y.; Wu, D.; Trynka, G.; Raj, T.; Terao, C.; Ikari, K.; Kochi, Y.; Ohmura, K.; Suzuki, A.; Yoshida, S.; et al. Genetics of Rheumatoid Arthritis Contributes to Biology and Drug Discovery. *Nature* **2014**, *506*, 376–381. [CrossRef]
41. Jiang, L.; Zheng, Z.; Fang, H.; Yang, J. A Generalized Linear Mixed Model Association Tool for Biobank-Scale Data. *Nat. Genet.* **2021**, *53*, 1616–1621. [CrossRef] [PubMed]
42. Aragam, K.G.; Jiang, T.; Goel, A.; Kanoni, S.; Wolford, B.N.; Atri, D.S.; Weeks, E.M.; Wang, M.; Hindy, G.; Zhou, W.; et al. Discovery and Systematic Characterization of Risk Variants and Genes for Coronary Artery Disease in over a Million Participants. *Nat. Genet.* **2022**, *54*, 1803–1815. [CrossRef] [PubMed]

43. Rapid GWAS of Thousands of Phenotypes for 337,000 Samples in the UK Biobank—Neale Lab. Available online: http://www.nealelab.is/blog/2017/7/19/rapid-gwas-of-thousands-of-phenotypes-for-337000-samples-in-the-uk-biobank (accessed on 17 December 2020).
44. Zheng, H.F.; Forgetta, V.; Hsu, Y.H.; Estrada, K.; Rosello-Diez, A.; Leo, P.J.; Dahia, C.L.; Park-Min, K.H.; Tobias, J.H.; Kooperberg, C.; et al. Whole-Genome Sequencing Identifies EN1 as a Determinant of Bone Density and Fracture. *Nature* **2015**, *526*, 112–117. [CrossRef] [PubMed]
45. Crick, D.C.P.; Sanderson, E.; Jones, H.; Goulding, N.; Borges, M.C.; Clayton, G.; Carter, A.R.; Halligan, S.; Lawlor, D.A.; Khandaker, G.M.; et al. Glycoprotein Acetyls and Depression: Testing for Directionality and Potential Causality Using Longitudinal Data and Mendelian Randomization Analyses. *J. Affect. Disord.* **2023**, *335*, 431. [CrossRef] [PubMed]
46. Bulik-Sullivan, B.K.; Loh, P.-R.; Finucane, H.K.; Ripke, S.; Yang, J.; Patterson, N.; Daly, M.J.; Price, A.L.; Neale, B.M. LD Score Regression Distinguishes Confounding from Polygenicity in Genomewide Association Studies. *Nat. Genet.* **2015**, *47*, 291–295. [CrossRef] [PubMed]
47. Yavorska, O.O.; Burgess, S. MendelianRandomization: An R Package for Performing Mendelian Randomization Analyses Using Summarized Data. *Int. J. Epidemiol.* **2017**, *46*, 1734–1739. [CrossRef] [PubMed]
48. Burgess, S.; Davey Smith, G.; Davies, N.M.; Dudbridge, F.; Gill, D.; Glymour, M.M.; Hartwig, F.P.; Holmes, M.V.; Minelli, C.; Relton, C.L.; et al. Guidelines for Performing Mendelian Randomization Investigations. *Wellcome Open Res.* **2020**, *4*, 186. [CrossRef]
49. Bowden, J.; Fabiola Del Greco, M.; Minelli, C.; Smith, G.D.; Sheehan, N.A.; Thompson, J.R. Assessing the Suitability of Summary Data for Two-Sample Mendelian Randomization Analyses Using MR-Egger Regression: The Role of the I 2 Statistic. *Int. J. Epidemiol.* **2016**, *45*, 1961–1974. [CrossRef] [PubMed]
50. Burgess, S.; Davies, N.M.; Thompson, S.G. Bias Due to Participant Overlap in Two-Sample Mendelian Randomization. *Genet. Epidemiol.* **2016**, *40*, 597–608. [CrossRef]
51. Wallace, C. Eliciting Priors and Relaxing the Single Causal Variant Assumption in Colocalisation Analyses. *PLoS Genet.* **2020**, *16*, e1008720. [CrossRef]
52. Giambartolomei, C.; Vukcevic, D.; Schadt, E.E.; Franke, L.; Hingorani, A.D.; Wallace, C.; Plagnol, V. Bayesian Test for Colocalisation between Pairs of Genetic Association Studies Using Summary Statistics. *PLoS Genet.* **2014**, *10*, e1004383. [CrossRef] [PubMed]
53. Watanabe, K.; Taskesen, E.; Van Bochoven, A.; Posthuma, D. Functional Mapping and Annotation of Genetic Associations with FUMA. *Nat. Commun.* **2017**, *8*, 1826. [CrossRef] [PubMed]
54. Kratzer, G.; Lewis, F.I.; Comin, A.; Pittavino, M.; Furrer, R. Additive Bayesian Network Modelling with the R Package Abn. *arXiv* **2019**, arXiv:1911.09006.

International Journal of
Molecular Sciences

MDPI

Review

Insights from Murine Studies on the Site Specificity of Atherosclerosis

Godfrey S. Getz * and Catherine A. Reardon

Department of Pathology, University of Chicago, Chicago, IL 60637, USA; reardon@uchicago.edu
* Correspondence: getz@bsd.uchicago.edu; Tel.: +1-312-505-0499

Abstract: Atherosclerosis is an inflammatory reaction that develops at specific regions within the artery wall and at specific sites of the arterial tree over a varying time frame in response to a variety of risk factors. The mechanisms that account for the interaction of systemic factors and atherosclerosis-susceptible regions of the arterial tree to mediate this site-specific development of atherosclerosis are not clear. The dynamics of blood flow has a major influence on where in the arterial tree atherosclerosis develops, priming the site for interactions with atherosclerotic risk factors and inducing cellular and molecular participants in atherogenesis. But how this accounts for lesion development at various locations along the vascular tree across differing time frames still requires additional study. Currently, murine models are favored for the experimental study of atherogenesis and provide the most insight into the mechanisms that may contribute to the development of atherosclerosis. Based largely on these studies, in this review, we discuss the role of hemodynamic shear stress, SR-B1, and other factors that may contribute to the site-specific development of atherosclerosis.

Keywords: atherosclerosis; hemodynamics; site specificity; arterial tree; risk factors

1. Introduction

While there are many excellent reviews on the initiation, progression, and regression of atherosclerosis, relatively few papers or reviews have been devoted to the development of lesions at particular sites of the vascular tree. In the decades that have followed our 2004 review on site-selective atherosclerosis [1], our understanding of the cellular and molecular aspects of atherogenesis has advanced immensely. This merits analysis of the improved appreciation of the basis for the focality of atherosclerotic lesion development.

Atherosclerosis is an inflammatory reaction that develops at specific regions within the artery wall of large and medium-sized arteries and at specific sites of the arterial tree over a varying time frame, with some reactions occurring early after the initiation of an atherogenic stimulus and some appearing later. There are a number of risk factors that are associated with the development of atherosclerosis, most of which are systemic in nature and therefore cannot on their own account for the focal nature of lesion development. Among the risk factors are hyperlipidemia, hypertension, diabetes, and sex. An ignored but critical systemic risk factor is age, which was highlighted in a recent analysis of clonal hematopoiesis [2]. These expanded blood cell clones with somatic mutations increase with age and produce enhanced levels of proinflammatory cytokines. One of the few good examples of the site-selective action of risk factors is seen in the multidisciplinary Pathological Determinants of Atherosclerosis in Youth (PDAY) studies. In these studies, early atherosclerosis was examined at autopsy in approximately 3000 apparently healthy (asymptomatic) individuals between the ages of 15 and 34 and its association with smoking, hypertension, hyperlipidemia, impaired glucose homeostasis (glycohemoglobin), and sex determined. Females had more abdominal aortic lesions than males, while the reverse sex bias was found in the right coronary artery [3]. Subjects who were smokers in life had three times as many raised abdominal lesions as nonsmokers, but smoking had no significant impact on lesions in the right coronary artery [4]. On the other hand, elevated glycohemoglobin levels were associated with more extensive lesions in the right coronary artery but not with the extent of abdominal aorta lesions [5]. The basis for these selective effects on atherosclerosis is not clear. Other examples of the effects of risk factors on site-specific lesion development are seen in the increased prevalence of peripheral vascular disease in patients with type III hyperlipoproteinemia (apoE2/E2) [6,7] and diabetes [8].

The focal nature of atherosclerotic lesions is generally thought to be driven by the hemodynamic properties of blood flow. Disturbed or oscillatory flow leads to low wall shear stress and occurs at sites where atherosclerotic lesions develop, while regions of the aorta with laminar flow with high wall shear stress seldom develop atherosclerosis. The geometry of the blood vessel contributes to the blood flow pattern. Disturbed flow is observed at the curvatures, branches, and bifurcation of arteries, and laminar blood flow is observed at straight, non-branching regions of the artery. The hemodynamic drivers of lesion development have largely been inferred from our understanding of the flow pattern in areas where lesions appear in human specimens. A good example of this is seen in the asymmetry of lesion development in human carotid arteries, where one artery contains significant atherosclerosis while the contralateral carotid artery is relatively plaque-free. Carotid arteries with lesions generally manifest lower shear stress [9]. But it is not clear whether the hemodynamic profile alone can account for lesion development at various locations along the vascular tree across differing time frames.

Since it is difficult to undertake detailed experimentation in humans, investigators have turned to experimental animals, large and small, to approach the mechanisms that account for the development of lesions at atherosclerosis-susceptible regions of the arterial tree [10,11]. Murine models are currently favored for the experimental study of atherogenesis. In a valuable commentary, Peter Libby points out that mice offer unique advantages for the exploration of the mechanisms of atherogenesis. These advantages relate to the relative ease of experimentally manipulating genes and controlling genetics, the environment, and other experimental variables, which cannot be applied in humans. While there are limitations to mice in relation to the complex, multifaceted pathogenesis of human atherosclerosis [12], nonetheless, studies in mice have contributed to the identification of cells, cellular pathways, and proteins that participate in atherogenesis, for example, inflammation and efferocytosis, for which targeted therapeutics have been developed [13,14].

Therefore, in this review, we focus primarily on studies in murine models. Since atherosclerosis develops in large and medium-sized arteries, we first outline the structure and components of these arteries and then describe a prototypic lesion as a platform for further analysis of lesion development. As the basis for insights into the mechanisms that contribute to site selectivity rests on temporal–spatial lesion development, we will describe the commonly used atherogenic mouse models of apolipoprotein E (apoE) deficiency and low-density lipoprotein (LDL) receptor deficiency and studies of lesion development over time. Finally, we end with a detailed treatment of what is known of the mechanisms that can be said to contribute to selective lesion development.

2. Artery Walls

The walls of large and medium-size arteries consist of three major layers, the endothelium, the media, and the adventitia, each of which participates in lesion development and may contribute to site-selective responses. The endothelial cells represent the thin barrier layer separating the blood from the rest of the artery. This layer is the most important sensor of the blood flow dynamics and hence is critically involved in the initiation of plaque development. Endothelial cells detect these shear stresses via mechanosensitive proteins such as G-protein-coupled receptors, flow-sensitive ion channels, and adhesion junction proteins, leading to the activation of cell signaling pathways that alter endothelial cell function and morphology in distinct ways [15]. The endothelial cells in disturbed (atherosusceptible) and laminar (atheroresistant) flow regions of the aorta differ in cell shape, the organization of the cytoskeleton, and intercellular junctional proteins. In the atheroresistant regions with laminar flow, the endothelial cells are aligned in the direction of the flow. Transcriptional and epigenetic differences have been noted in endothelial cells isolated from atherosusceptible and atheroresistant aortic areas and in cultured endothelial cells subjected to different flow patterns (see Section 5.1). For the most part, there is good concordance between the in vivo and in vitro results [16,17]. In vivo, the endothelium at atherosusceptible and atheroresistant sites sees the same systemic risk factors.

Almost all the vascular smooth muscle cells of normal arteries are found in the media, where they contribute to the contractility and vascular tone of the vessel wall. Lineage mapping studies have shown that smooth muscle cells at various aortic sites along the arterial tree may originate from different embryological precursors [18,19]. The smooth muscle cells of the ascending aorta and the aortic arch and its branches are derived from neural crest cells, while the cells of the thoracic aorta are derived from somites, and cells in the abdominal aorta and those of its branches are derived from the serosal mesothelium. Not only do they arise from different sources but their postnatal signaling networks may also differ, which may contribute to differences in the response of the aorta sites to risk factors. For example, aortic homograft transplantation studies suggest that intrinsic differences in the aortic wall, including smooth muscle cells of different lineage sources, may contribute to the unique properties of the artery wall at different locations. In these studies, an atherosusceptible abdominal aortic segment was transplanted into the atheroresistant thoracic artery in canines, and vice versa (thoracic aortic section into the abdominal aorta) [18,20]. Following feeding them an atherogenic diet, the transplanted abdominal aorta segments developed severe atherosclerotic lesions despite being transplanted into an atheroresistant region of the aorta. Similarly, the transplanted thoracic artery segments developed minimal lesions when transplanted into the atherosusceptible abdominal aortic region.

The adventitia is the outermost layer of the artery wall and has received increased attention [21]. The arterial adventitia is made up of many cell types, including fibroblasts, microvascular endothelial cells, resident macrophages, T cells, B cells, adipocytes, and perivascular nerves, and contributes to vascular development, homeostasis, repair, and disease pathologies. In humans and large animals, it is also the site that regulates the vasa vasorum, a microvascular network that supplies oxygen and nutrients to the cells in the outer layers of the vessel wall and the intima of developing plaques and can serve as a route for leukocyte trafficking into the lesion. During atherosclerosis, the adventitia accumulates inflammatory cells and is thought to be an important area of immune surveillance. The adventitia also contains resident vascular progenitor cells that in mice express the stem cell antigen 1 marker (Sca-1) [22] and that can differentiate into smooth muscle cells, endothelial cells, and macrophages. Adventitial progenitor cells have also been observed in humans. These cells may exchange between the adventitia and the media and contribute to lesion development and healing [23]. Whether these progenitor cells differ in concentration or function in the adventitia at different arterial sites is not known.

3. The Prototypic Atherosclerotic Lesion

The prototypic atherosclerotic lesion represents various phases of the chronic inflammatory reaction in arteries. As mentioned, the sites at which lesions develop are largely determined by the interaction of blood flow characteristics with the underlying vessel wall, especially endothelial cells. Dysfunctional and inflamed endothelial cells are found in regions of disturbed flow, especially in the presence of atherosclerosis risk factors. The most common systemic risk factor that drives the blood vessel response is hyperlipidemia, usually characterized by elevated LDL. The low shear stress of disturbed flow permits a longer residence time for LDL interaction with the arterial wall than in regions of lamellar flow. LDL particles, especially when its levels are elevated, cross the endothelium into the intimal space, where they are retained according to charged-based interactions with matrix proteoglycans like biglycan (human) or perlecan (mouse) [24–26] and are modified enzymatically and by oxidation and may aggregate [27]. The interaction of modified LDL with the endothelial cells enhances the expression of cell surface adhesion molecules and chemotactic factors to promote the influx of immune cells into the intima [28]. Monocyte chemoattractant protein 1 (MCP-1) is a key chemokine that promotes the ingress of monocytes. Intimal monocytes differentiate into macrophages and may proliferate locally under the influence of macrophage colony-stimulating factor (M-CSF). Macrophages also secrete MCP-1 to further enhance the ingress of monocytes. Within the intima, the resident and monocyte-derived macrophages take up modified LDL by the scavenger receptor pathways, phagocytosis, and micropinocytosis, resulting in the formation of lipid-loaded foam cells [27]. If the concentration of LDL is high enough, even unmodified LDL is taken up by micropinocytosis. The activation of macrophages in the intima results in the secretion of a panoply of cytokines and chemokines that act on local cells, promoting the further ingress of immune cells, including cells of the adaptive immune system, such as T cells, B cells, and natural killer T (NKT) cells [29,30]. These cells also contribute to the local cytokine milieu. The modified LDLs may serve as neoantigens, eliciting an immune response, with the production of antibodies against components of the atheromatous plaque [31]. It should be borne in mind that single-cell RNA sequencing (scRNA-seq) and cytometry by time of flight (CyTOF) analysis of murine atherosclerotic lesions have demonstrated the presence of multiple subtypes of macrophages in the atherosclerotic plaque, including some having characteristics of foam cells and others of a non-foamy inflammatory phenotype [32]. These studies also shed light on the heterogeneity of other leukocytes in lesions.

Foam cells may undergo apoptosis. In the initial stages of atherogenesis, these apoptotic cells are efficiently phagocytosed by neighboring phagocytes, mostly macrophages, according to a process designated as efferocytosis [33]. As lesions progress, efferocytosis becomes less efficient, and the accumulating apoptotic cells may undergo secondary necrosis, which, if extensive enough, produces the necrotic core of the advanced plaque.

Growth factors secreted by cells in the developing lesion promote the migration of medial smooth muscle cells into the intima [34]. The intimal smooth muscle cells undergo transdifferentiation from a contractile to a synthetic phenotype and are a major source of matrix molecules, including collagen and the proteoglycans that play a role in retaining plasma lipoproteins in the intima [35,36]. The smooth muscle cells and collagen are major components of the fibrous cap that overlies the atherosclerotic plaque. An intact fibrous cap helps to stabilize the plaque, limiting its interaction with the blood coagulation system. However, the disruption of this cap by inflammatory macrophages may generate an unstable plaque, with the possibility of the formation of a thrombus, causing acute obstruction of the blood flow, with dire clinical consequences [34].

In addition, smooth muscle cells that migrate into the intima can contribute to the pool of lipid-loaded foam cells [37,38]. Indeed, lineage tracing studies have suggested that the proportion of smooth-muscle-derived foam cells may be equal to the proportion derived from macrophages [39]. However, smooth-muscle-cell-derived foam cells exhibit reduced phagocytic and efferocytic activity compared to macrophage-derived foam cells, which may contribute to the accumulation of apoptotic cells, with ensuing secondary necrosis in the lesions, indirectly contributing to necrotic core formation [40]. A recent scRNA-seq analysis of atherosclerotic lesions revealed the heterogeneity of the smooth muscle cells in the artery wall and also the expansion of various clones of smooth muscle cells [36,41]. This recalls the findings of Benditt that atherosclerotic atheromas are clonal expansions of smooth muscle cells [42].

The above is a broad overview of the typical process of atherogenesis, mediated by numerous molecules derived from local cell participants. However, the evolution of the atherogenic plaque is not a one-way pro-atherogenic process. It is balanced by counter-regulatory processes involved in lesion healing and resolution. This includes the removal of lipids from the plaque cells by reverse cholesterol transport [43], the emigration of macrophages from the lesions to draining lymph nodes [44], and the generation of resolving molecules, mostly from polyunsaturated fatty acids [45]. This may be promoted by the removal of pro-atherogenic stimuli such as hyperlipidemia and hypertension. The generation of alternatively activated macrophages, along with regulatory T cells, produces anti-inflammatory cytokines such as IL-10 and transforming growth factor-β (TGFβ), which can, in turn, stimulate the production of stabilizing matrix molecules [27,45,46].

The state of the atherosclerotic plaque represents a balance between pro- and anti-atherogenic processes, which may differ quantitatively from plaque to plaque and from site to site within the vascular tree. At any given time point, lesions at differing stages of evolution and resolution may be encountered. These considerations need to be borne in mind as we examine examples of apparent site-selective atherosclerosis in this review.

4. Murine Models of Atherosclerosis

The above brief review of atherogenic lesion formation reveals an extremely complex set of interactions, with most of these potential interactions illuminated by studies in animals, particularly mice. Aside from mice, pigs, especially minipigs, are valuable models for atherosclerosis studies [11]. Inducing atherosclerosis in mice requires significantly increasing the levels of apoB-containing lipoproteins. Among the most frequently used models to study the mechanisms underlying atherosclerosis are mice with germ-line deletion of the apoE gene (*Apoe*) or the LDL receptor gene (*Ldlr*).

The $Apoe^{-/-}$ mouse was first described in 1992 by Maeda and colleagues [47] and by Plump and Breslow [48]. ApoE is an important ligand for the clearance of remnant lipoproteins. In its absence, remnant particles accumulate, leading to hypercholesterolemia and atherosclerosis on a low-fat chow diet. The administration of a high-fat, high-cholesterol, Western-type diet exacerbates hyperlipidemia and atherosclerosis. An important paper by Nakashima et al. [49] contributed to our thinking about the temporal–spatial evolution of atherosclerosis. To follow the evolution of lesions over time, atherosclerosis was examined throughout the vascular tree in $Apoe^{-/-}$ mice maintained on chow or a Western-type diet for up to 40 weeks. Lesions were first noted in the aortic root, the lesser curvature of the aortic arch, the brachiocephalic artery (or innominate artery), and the right common carotid artery, followed by the carotid bifurcation, where lesions occurred on the outer wall of the bifurcation, while the flow dividers were spared [50]. Lesions were later observed in the branches of the superior mesenteric artery, the origins of the two renal arteries, and the aortic bifurcation and finally seen in the descending thoracic and common iliac arteries and the iliac bifurcation. The sites of lesion development were not different between the chow- and Western-type-diet-fed mice, but lesions developed more rapidly when the mice were fed the Western-type diet. In this study, sex did not influence the sites of lesion development. It is probably worth noting that these mice had a mixed C57BL/6 × 129 genetic background.

The $Ldlr^{-/-}$ mouse is a model of human familial hypercholesterolemia with elevated levels of LDL [51]. Humans with homozygous deficiency of the receptor develop xanthomatous lesions; widespread atherosclerosis, including in the aortic root; and often myocardial infarction and premature death [52,53]. In contrast to the $Apoe^{-/-}$ mice, the development of significant atherosclerosis in the $Ldlr^{-/-}$ mouse requires feeding them a high-fat diet [54,55]. This more readily allows us to study the initial stages of lesion development that occur after the initiation of a high-cholesterol diet. The two models also differ in their lipoprotein profile, with apoB100-containing LDL being the major lipoprotein in $Ldlr^{-/-}$ mice and apoB48-containing remnant lipoproteins being the major lipoproteins that accumulate in $Apoe^{-/-}$ mice. These two apoproteins differ in their binding affinity to intimal proteoglycans [56]. Due to these differences, the detailed early atherogenic mechanisms may well differ between the two models. Nonetheless, the distribution of atherosclerotic lesions is very similar for the two models as a function of age or duration of diet.

These murine models have been used extensively to study the mechanisms underlying atherosclerosis. These studies use inbred strains of these murine models in specific pathogen-free environments fed a closely defined diet. While these experimental conditions allow for the performance of well-controlled experiments, they are not readily translated to free-living human environments. The advantage of mice is that multiple genes can be manipulated at the same time and their impact on atherosclerosis studied in a reasonable time frame. However, this has its limitations. The choice of the gene(s) for study may introduce an inherent bias. Often, the genes chosen are eliminated (knocked out) or overexpressed (transgenic or viral-mediated expression). These are extreme changes in gene expression that are not usually encountered in human populations. To ground these findings in the human experience, where more subtle quantitative or structural genetic variations are seen, Genome-Wide Association Studies (GWAS) are often consulted for corresponding human genetic variations. The closest murine counterpart is the Hybrid Mouse Diversity Panel (HMDP), which represents a panel of 100 inbred mouse strains studied on a hyperlipidemic background (transgenic for human apoE3 Leiden and human cholesteryl ester transfer protein) to identify natural variations in mice that contribute to atherosclerosis [57]. There is a good deal of concordance between the risk factors and trait loci identified in humans and mice. However, there is a lack of concordance for two aspects: namely sex and the effects of obesity [58]. In humans, atherosclerosis develops earlier in males, whereas in mice, females often exhibit greater atherosclerosis. Obesity in humans is associated with increased atherosclerosis, but atherosclerosis is reduced in genetically obese mice.

However, not all studies examining the impact of specific genes or drugs on atherosclerosis in the *Apoe*$^{-/-}$ and *Ldlr*$^{-/-}$ models have produced the same phenotype [52]. This discordance may be related to mechanistic differences in the models, as mentioned above: the stage of atherogenesis at the time of sacrifice, the duration and nature of diet employed, the sex of the animals, or the housing conditions (e.g., microbiome complexity).

5. Factors Contributing to the Site-Selective Development of Atherosclerosis

In this section we will review what is known about the contribution of various factors listed in Figure 1 to the site specificity of atherosclerosis observed in murine atherosclerotic models.

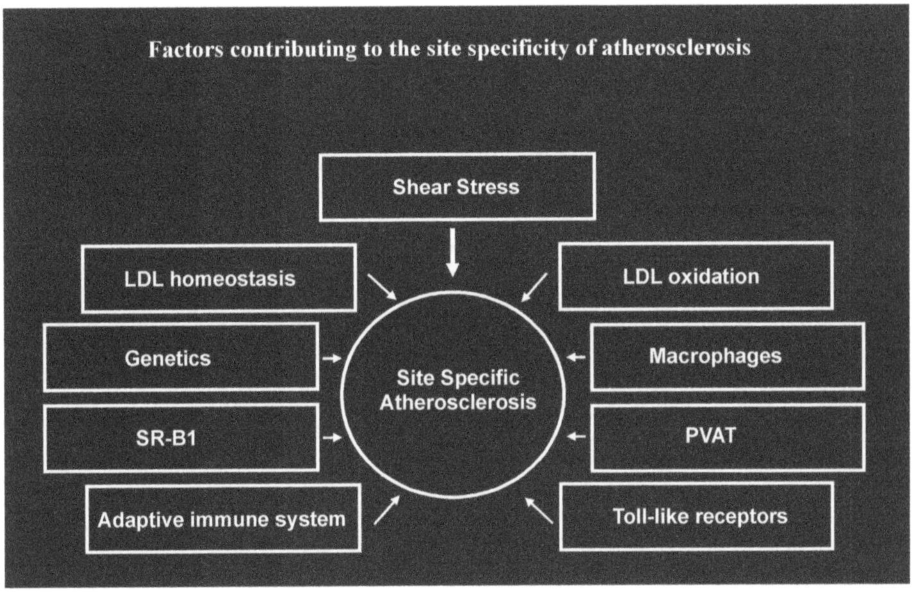

Figure 1. Factors contributing to site specificity of atherosclerosis. While shear stress induced by blood flow has an important role in priming cells in the artery wall for susceptibility or resistance to atherosclerosis, the response to risk factors at atherosusceptible sites may be differentially impacted by other factors that result in lesion initiation and progression proceeding at different rates at different sites along the artery wall. SR-B1, scavenger receptor B1, PVAT, perivascular adipose tissue.

5.1. Hemodynamics and Shear Stress

The progressive development of atherosclerotic lesions at different sites in the vascular tree might be a reflection of the extent of blood flow disruption, with it being greatest at the most rapidly developing sites. A strict quantitative comparison of flow dynamics with a propensity for lesion development through the vascular tree has not been reported, although a few attempts have been made. Giddens and colleagues [59] noted that the wall shear stress measured in the aortic arch and its principal branches is much higher in mice than in humans. The heart rate in mice is also much higher. The average flow velocity across the cardiac cycle (cm/s) in various aortic vessels in mice was measured, showing a progressive decline in flow velocity moving down from the suprarenal aorta to the infrarenal aorta and to the femoral artery [60]. This correlates with the relative temporal appearance of lesions in the mouse model, in which the suprarenal artery develops lesions sooner than the other sites. In another study, the flow pattern in the thoracic and abdominal aortas in Western-type-diet-fed *Ldlr*$^{-/-}$ mice was changed from atheroresistant laminar flow to disturbed (oscillatory) flow using catheter-induced aortic regurgitation. The lesion burden in the descending thoracic and abdominal aortas were drastically increased, while the lesion burden in the non-flow-modified ascending aorta and the proximal aortic arch in the control and aortic regurgitation mice was comparable [61]. An increased prevalence of atherosclerosis in the descending thoracic aorta in humans with aortic regurgitation has also been observed [62]. These results highlight the importance of flow disturbance in lesion development. The genetics of the aortic geometry also highlights the importance of hemodynamics. A study of atherosclerosis in *Apoe*$^{-/-}$ mouse strains with atheroresistant 129S6/SvEvTac (129) and atherosusceptible C57BL/6 genetic backgrounds found that the aortic root lesions were smaller in the 129 *Apoe*$^{-/-}$ strain, as expected, but the aortic arch lesions were significantly larger compared to the C57BL/6 *Apoe*$^{-/-}$ strain [63,64]. A possible contributor to the unexpected larger aortic arch lesions is that the aortic arch in the 129 strain has a sharper bend than in the C57BL/6 mice, which in modeling studies was associated with lower shear stress in the curvature of the aortic arch than in the C57BL/6 mice. Genetic crosses between these two strains show that the quantitative train locus (QTL) for aortic arch curvature and for atherosclerosis overlap [65].

Laminar shear stress upregulates mechanosensitive transcription factors (e.g., Krüppel-like factor (KLF)2, KLF4, nuclear factor-erythroid 2-related factor 2 (NRF2)) in endothelial cells. This leads to increased expression of endothelial nitric oxide synthase (eNOS) and bioavailable nitric oxide (NO), heme oxygenase 1, and thrombomodulin, among other genes, and KLF2-mediated inhibition of NF-kB to promote the anti-atherogenic, anti-inflammatory, and antithrombotic phenotype in the cells in laminar flow regions of the aorta [66,67]. The downregulation of KLF2 with the low shear stress of disturbed flow leads to the activation of NF-kB and the expression of inflammatory genes (e.g., vascular adhesion molecule (VCAM)-1, MCP-1, cytokines). Disturbed flow also leads to increased oxidative stress and endothelial–mesenchymal transition and induces metabolic reprogramming of the endothelial cells to increase glycolysis and reduce oxidative phosphorylation. Hypoxia-inducible factor 1α (HIF1α) appears to have an important role in this reprogramming. The induction of NAPDPH oxidase 4 (NOX4) and the subsequent increase in reactant oxidant species leads to the stabilization of HIF1α and subsequent induction of glycolytic enzymes such as hexokinase 2, (HK2), 6-phosphofructo-2-kinase/fructose-2,6-bisphosphatase 3 (PFKFB3), and 3-phosphoinosital-dependent kinase 1 (PDKI) (an inhibitor of pyruvate dehydrogenase) [68]. These metabolic changes also contribute to the increased inflammatory phenotype of endothelial cells subjected to disturbed flow. Additionally, the ATP-dependent purinergic receptor P2X7 may be implicated in the inflammatory phenotype of endothelial cells in regions with disturbed flow via increasing p38 signaling [69]. While this accounts for the location of atherosclerosis in particular regions of the aortic wall, whether differences in the expression levels of these proteins at different locations along the arterial tree account for site-specific atherosclerosis effects is not known.

5.2. Genetics

The susceptibility to atherosclerosis of inbred strains of mice differs vastly. Cross-breeding strains of differing susceptibility to lesion formation clearly indicates the impact of genetics on atherogenesis. As mentioned above, the interaction of genetics and hemodynamics may explain the differential atherogenic response of the aortic root and the aortic arch in C57BL/6 *Apoe*$^{-/-}$ mice and 129 *Apoe*$^{-/-}$ mice [65]. Another genetic example is seen in relation to lesion formation in the innominate artery in *Apoe*$^{-/-}$ mice with C57BL/6 and C3H/HeJ genetic backgrounds. The former strain is atherosusceptible, while the latter is atheroresistant, and this is reflected in the higher level of aortic root lesions in C57BL/6 *Apoe*$^{-/-}$ mice. Yet innominate artery atherosclerosis is very similar for these two strains [70], indicating that the genetic impact on lesion development may be site-specific. CD44 was identified as a candidate gene associated with innominate artery atherosclerosis.

The literature is full of suggestions that the temporal–spatial atherosclerosis developmental profile is driven by the hemodynamic profile of the low shear stress of disturbed flow, which permits a longer residence time for effector particles within the arterial wall and produces differences in gene expression in the endothelial cells compared to laminar shear stress. While this is the consensual view, it does not seem to be the case in all studies [71]. For example, in a comparison of the evolution of lesions in *Ldlr*$^{-/-}$ mice with C57BL/6 and FVB genetic backgrounds fed semi-synthetic diets with increasing levels of dietary cholesterol, ranging from 0% to 0.5%, there appeared to be more at play [72]. In the C57BL/6 *Ldlr*$^{-/-}$ mice, their VLDL, IDL, and LDL levels were much higher than in the FVB mice with the diets with a higher cholesterol content. The C57BL/6 mice also had much larger aortic roots and innominate artery lesions than the FVB mice. On the other hand, the lesion sizes in the thoracic and abdominal aortas were similar for the two strains. Since various regions of the arterial tree are subject to the same level of lipoproteins, the differential responses of the abdominal aorta and the more proximal regions cannot be accounted for by the plasma lipids or hemodynamics. It is likely that there is a more complex explanation, probably dependent on the selective gene expression profile in the abdominal aorta.

5.3. LDL Homeostasis

Hyperlipidemia is a major risk factor for human disease and is required for lesions to develop in mice. Lipoproteins accumulate in the intimal of lesion-prone areas even before there is any evidence of the influx of blood cells. This was demonstrated morphologically using electron microscopy analysis by Frank and Breslow [73], who showed lipid particles the sizes of LDL, intermediate-density lipoprotein (IDL), or their remnants aligned along the collagen fibrils of the matrix of lesion-prone areas beginning at 3 weeks of age in chow-fed *Apoe*$^{-/-}$ mice, while monocyte association with the endothelial cells was not observed until 5 weeks of age. Lipoprotein accumulation could be attributable to selective changes in lipoprotein permeability, influx, retention, or metabolism. Recent experiments have described an active transcellular transport pathway in endothelial cells that contributes to the accumulation of lipids in the artery wall. Caveolae and scavenger receptor class B, type 1 (SR-B1), which localizes to the caveolae, are more abundant in the endothelial cells in the atherosusceptible area of the aortic arch (lesser curvature) than in the atheroresistant area (greater curvature) [74]. LDL binding to SR-B1 promotes its interaction with dedicator of cytokine-like kinase 4 (DOCK4), leading to the activation of Rac1 and the transcytosis of LDL across the endothelial cells into the subendothelial intima [75]. The transcytosed LDL may be retained in the intima by binding to local proteoglycans [76]. Although most of the experiments by Huang et al. [75] were conducted with the aortic arch, SR-B1-dependent transcytosis is probably operative throughout the atherosusceptible areas of the aorta, as shown by the reduction in the en face staining of lesions in the whole aorta in *Apoe*$^{-/-}$ mice with endothelial-cell-specific *Srb1* deficiency. The inhibition of SR-B1-mediated transcytosis of LDL may be a mechanism contributing to the atheroprotective effect of estrogen. The estrogen receptor GPER (G-protein-coupled estrogen receptor) reduced LDL transcytosis in cultured endothelial cells by downregulating the expression of SR-B1 [77].

Increased lipoprotein permeability through the endothelial layer may also contribute. Permeability has been probed in several ways. Aortic areas of increased permeability to macromolecules are visualized using an injection of albumin–Evans blue, a probe that can be used in experimental models in the absence of hyperlipidemia to provide a measure of in vivo sites of intrinsic increased permeability. Uptake of Evans blue dye in Yorkshire pigs was seen in the coronary ostia, the intercostal ostia, and the iliac bifurcation, sites of lesion formation [78]. Young and mature pigs exhibited similar patterns of staining. The exposure of vessels to the Evans blue complex ex vivo did not yield the same pattern of staining, highlighting the importance of hemodynamic factors. The blue areas were also the preferential sites of labeling with radioactive cholesterol. As mentioned, lipoproteins accumulated and were associated with the matrix in atherosusceptible murine sites early, before monocytes were observed to associate with the endothelial cells [73]. These findings could be accounted for by changes in the influx of lipoproteins, changes in their retention, or changes in their degradation or removal. This was partially examined in rabbit aortas without measurable atherosclerosis by Schwenke and Carew using radiolabeled LDL to measure the accumulation of intact LDL and tyramine-cellobiose-radiolabeled LDL to measure degraded LDL [79]. They found that the intact LDL concentration and degradation rates (per gram of fresh tissue) were several times higher in the aortic arch than in the descending thoracic aorta and abdominal aorta, which develop lesions later than the aortic arch. Examination of the LDL accumulation and degradation in the branched and non-branched regions of the abdominal aorta showed that the branched regions had a higher LDL concentration than the unbranched areas. However, the LDL concentration in the highly atherosusceptible aortic arch was significantly higher than in the branched regions of the abdominal aorta. What these results suggest is that the temporal–spatial development of lesions could be related, at least in part, to differences in the uptake and metabolism of LDL in atherosusceptible regions. The extent of disturbed flow in atherosusceptible arterial sites may be a determinant, but quantitation of this flow parameter in susceptible arteries is needed. Many other aspects of LDL homeostasis will need to be examined to fully understand its contribution to the temporal–spatial atherosclerotic developmental profile. Among these is the extent of LDL retention in the intima by proteoglycans and the extent of LDL modification by, for example, sphingomyelinase or oxidation.

5.4. LDL Oxidation

The oxidation of LDL is thought to be an important modification of LDL that facilitates the activation of macrophages in the early stages of atherogenesis. Treatment with antioxidants has hinted at the importance of this initial activation of macrophages. Surprisingly, treatment of $Apoe^{-/-}$ mice with the antioxidant probucol led to an increase in the aortic root lesion area, though at other sites (i.e., the aortic arch, descending thoracic aorta, and abdominal aorta), there was a reduction in the lesion area [80]. The possibility that the oxidation of LDL is important at some arterial sites but not others has to be considered.

5.5. SR-B1

5.5.1. SR-B1 and HDL

While SR-B1-dependent LDL transcytosis across the endothelium is an important factor that contributes to the difference between atherosusceptible and atheroresistant sites, the function of endothelial SR-B1 in the process of atherosclerosis is complex [81]. High-density lipoprotein (HDL) has several atheroprotective functions. Among them is that the interaction of HDL with SR-B1 in endothelial cells triggers binding of the adaptor protein PDZ domain-containing 1 (PDZK1) and the activation of AKT serine/threonine kinase 1 (AKT1), resulting in the activation of eNOS and increased production of NO, which is anti-atherogenic [82]. In addition, one of the atheroprotective mechanisms of HDL might be to compete with LDL for SR-B1-dependent LDL transcytosis [75].

SR-B1-mediated transcytosis of HDL by the endothelial cells [75] may also enhance reverse cholesterol transport, in which the interaction of intimal HDL with ATP-binding cassette G1 (ABCG1) in macrophage foam cells promotes the efflux of cholesterol to HDL for its transport to the liver [83]. SR-B1 on hepatocytes mediates the selective uptake of cholesteryl esters from HDL and influences HDL composition [81].

5.5.2. SR-B1 and Coronary Artery Atherosclerosis

As valuable as the "mighty" mouse is for investigating the mechanisms involved in atherogenesis, this model does have important limitations in extrapolating its results to humans [12]. A major limitation is the absence of significant coronary artery lesions in most studies involving $Apoe^{-/-}$ and $Ldlr^{-/-}$ mice. Yet certain complex genetic models can elicit occlusive coronary disease accompanied by myocardial infarction. For example, in Western-type-diet-fed mice with combined *Apoe* and *Ldlr* deficiency [84] and with overexpression of the urokinase plasminogen activator in the macrophages in $Apoe^{-/-}$ mice fed a Western-type diet [85], the development of occlusive coronary arterial disease and myocardial infarction occurred. The most dramatic murine model for occlusive coronary artery atherosclerosis with myocardial infarction and notably premature mortality (mean age of 6 weeks) is seen with chow-fed mice with double knockout of the *Apoe* and *Srb1* genes [86]. $Ldlr^{-/-}Srb1^{-/-}$ mice fed a high cholesterol diet also develop coronary artery atherosclerosis and myocardial fibrosis [87]. Mortality is particularly premature when the diet is supplemented with sodium cholate. Interestingly, in contrast to what appears to be the response of the aortic root to probucol treatment [80], coronary artery atherosclerosis in $Apoe^{-/-}Srb1^{-/-}$ mice is rescued by probucol treatment [88]. Obstructive coronary artery disease being observed in mice with global deficiency of *Srb1* together with *Apoe* or *Ldlr* deficiency suggests that in the coronary arteries processes other than LDL transcytosis and eNOS activation may be at play [86,87]. Paracellular diffusion of LDL from the plasma may be one such process.

Individual global knockout of the pathway by which HDL binding to SR-B1 promotes NO production (*Pdzk1*, *Akt1*, or *eNOS*), accompanied by *Apoe* deficiency, also promotes occlusive coronary artery disease but only when the animals are fed atherogenic diets, with some requiring cholate in the diet [89–91]. Bone marrow transfer experiments indicate that it is the deficiency of *Akt1* in non-hemopoietic cells, probably the endothelial cells, that accounts for the coronary artery phenotype in $Akt1^{-/-}Apoe^{-/-}$ mice [90].

A related but valuable model for the study of coronary artery disease and myocardial infarction is $Srb1^{-/-}$ mice crossed with a hypomorphic apoE mutant (threonine 61 substituted with arginine), in which apoE is expressed at 5% of the wild-type levels and fed a high-fat, high-cholesterol, cholate-containing diet [92]. SR-B1 is expressed on endothelial cells, macrophages, and hepatocytes. The importance of SR-B1 outside of the endothelium is indicated by the observation that the transplantation of bone marrow from apoE hypomorphic mice expressing SR-B1 into $Srb1^{-/-}$ apoE hypomorphic mice protects against coronary artery disease [93]. The anti-atherogenic role of SR-B1 in the macrophages may be related to its role in promoting cholesterol efflux, reducing their inflammatory phenotype and maintaining efferocytotic activity [81].

But the transplantation of bone marrow deficient in *Srb1* into $Ldlr^{-/-}$ recipients suggests that the role of SR-B1 in bone-marrow-derived cells is complex. SR-B1-expressing bone marrow reduces very early atherosclerosis after 4 weeks of a Western-type diet, yet at longer periods on this diet, atherosclerosis is increased [94]. This suggests that SR-B1 on bone-marrow-derived cells, likely macrophages, can be pro-atherogenic or anti-atherogenic at different stages of atherogenesis. The expression of SR-B1 on macrophages is associated with reduced expression of the inflammatory cytokines IL-1, IL-6, and tumor necrosis factor-α (TNFα) [95].

In summary, SR-B1 is associated with pro- and anti-atherogenic pathways depending on context and the site of expression.

5.6. Macrophages

Intimal lipoproteins promoting atherosclerosis requires the participation of the macrophages. In the absence of M-CSF, which regulates the proliferation and survival of monocytes/macrophages, very little atherosclerosis is seen in *Apoe*$^{-/-}$ [96] and *Ldlr*$^{-/-}$ mice [97]. In the highly atherosusceptible, lesser curvature of the ascending aortic arch, intimal leukocytes, with markers of monocytes or dendritic cells, are present in normal arteries. In the first few days after the initiation of feeding a cholesterol-rich diet to *Ldlr*$^{-/-}$ mice, these cells become loaded with lipids [98]. These foam cells are not clearly evidenced in less atherosusceptible regions like the greater curvature of the ascending aortic arch, the descending thoracic aorta, or the abdominal aorta, even though the latter is a site of atherosclerosis after exposure to a cholesterol-rich diet for longer durations [99]. These cells have the characteristics of dendritic cells [100]. After the consumption of a cholesterol-rich diet for 2–12 weeks, foam cells are derived from monocytes recruited from the blood and from the local proliferation of macrophages [99].

The influx of monocytes into evolving lesions requires chemokines and their receptors. In the combined absence of CCL2, CCR5, and CX3CR1, very few lesions develop [101]. The absence of CX3CR1 in the *Apoe*-deficient background results in reduced atherosclerosis in the aortic root and aortic arch and reduced en face staining of lesions in the whole aorta [102,103]. In mice, there are two major monocyte subtypes, Ly6C^{hi} and Ly6C^{lo}. Ly6C^{hi} monocytes are more inflammatory and preferentially infiltrate the artery wall [104]. The monocyte subsets differentially employ the three receptors to enter the artery wall [105]. Ly6C^{hi} monocytes require all three receptors, while the influx of Ly6C^{lo} monocytes is much less dependent on CX3CR1 and partially dependent on CCR5. These chemokine/chemokine receptor pairs are not all equally involved in atherogenesis at all arterial sites. For example, in the absence of the ligand CX3CL1, lesions are preferentially reduced in the innominate artery in *Apoe*$^{-/-}$ mice [106].

5.7. Adaptive Immune System

The adaptive immune system embodies several subsets of B and T cells. We examined chow-fed male *Apoe*$^{-/-}$ mice lacking both B and T cells due to deficient of recombination activating gene 1 (*Rag*$^{-/-}$ mice) at 27 weeks of age. When adjusted for plasma cholesterol, aortic root lesions were reduced in the immune-deficient mice, though no differences were observed in the innominate artery [107]. This might be explained by the different balance between pro-atherogenic and anti-atherogenic immune cells (e.g., CD4+ Th cells vs. CD4+ regulatory T cells) at the two sites, at least at the time of monitoring. This suggestion has yet to be validated. These animals were fully backcrossed into the C57BL/6 background. In this background, Western-type-diet-fed *Ldlr*$^{-/-}$ mice showed similar results. However, in a strain that was only 93% C57BL/6, adaptive immune deficiency was associated with a reduction in lesions in the aortic root, as well as in the innominate artery [108]. This suggests that the genes expressed in the innominate artery may influence the state of regulatory T cells at this site.

Other cells of the immune system also have a site-specific impact on atherosclerosis. NKT cells exist as at least two subtypes [109]. Type I or invariant NKT cells express a semi-invariant T cell receptor (TCR) composed of the Vα14-Jα18 chain coupled with a limited number of TCRβ chains in mice. Type II NKT cells have more variable TCRs. Both recognize the lipid antigens presented by CD1d on antigen-presenting cells. *Ldlr*$^{-/-}$ mice transgenic for the Vα14-Jα18 TCRα chain with increased levels of type I NKT cells and mice lacking type I NKT cells due to deficiency of the Jα18 chain were fed a Western-type diet for 4 or 12 weeks [110]. The atherosclerosis response was quite complex. There was a selective decrease in atherosclerosis in the ascending aorta near the lesser curvature of the aortic arch in the absence of type I NKT cells after 4 weeks of the diet (early atherosclerosis) despite a noticeable increase in plasma lipids. But after 12 weeks of the diet, the lesions were similar at this site. The overexpression of Vα14 Jα18 resulted in a site-specific increase in innominate artery atherosclerosis after 12 weeks of feeding.

Lymphotoxin ligands are mainly expressed by lymphocytes and innate lymphoid cells and come in two forms [111]. Soluble homotrimers of lymphotoxin α ligands (LTα_3) are secreted mainly by lymphocytes and signal via TNF receptors, which are widely expressed. The heterotrimeric LT$\alpha_1\beta_2$ ligand is bound to the cell surface of lymphocytes and signals through interaction with the lymphotoxin β receptor (LTβR), expressed on the cell surface of many cell types. Female *Ldlr*$^{-/-}$ *Lta*$^{-/-}$ animals that lacked both lymphotoxin ligands were compared with mice with T-cell-specific lymphotoxin β deficiency, lacking LT$\alpha_1\beta_2$ on their T cells, and mice deficient in the LTβR. The animals were fed a Western-type diet for either 6 or 12 weeks. Atherosclerosis in the innominate artery was not impacted by the manipulation of this ligand–receptor pathway at either time point. There was a selective reduction in aortic arch lesions with global deficiency of *Lta* or T-cell-specific deficiency of *Ltb* at the 12 week time point. The aortic root lesion responses were quite complex. Aortic root lesions were reduced in *Lta* deficiency, associated mainly with reduced atherosclerosis in the left-coronary-artery-associated sinus, which is the sinus that carries the major burden of lesion development compared to the right-coronary-artery-associated sinus and the sinus not associated with a coronary artery. However, in T-cell-specific *Ltb* deficiency, the aortic root lesions were increased, especially in the non-coronary-artery-associated sinus. In contrast, compared to the *Ldlr*$^{-/-}$ mice, the *Ltbr*$^{-/-}$*Ldlr*$^{-/-}$ mice exhibited no lesion differences at any arterial site examined. In the *Apoe*$^{-/-}$ background with Western-type diet feeding, the absence of the LTβR was associated with a reduction in lesions in the aortic root and reduced en face staining of the whole aorta [112]. Bone marrow transplantation studies suggest that the expression of the receptor on hematopoietic cells, likely monocytes, is determinative. Clearly, this is a very complex system, and much further experimentation is required to unravel the intricacies of the observed findings.

In aged chow-fed *Apoe*$^{-/-}$ mice, a tertiary lymphoid organ develops in the adventitia surrounding abdominal aortas with atherosclerotic lesions [113]. The lymphoid organs are rich in B cells and T cells, including regulatory T cells. The tertiary lymphoid organs begin to appear at 32 weeks of age, being obvious at 52 weeks and peaking at 78 weeks. Their development is dependent on signaling via the LTβR on the smooth muscle cells, resulting in the secretion of the lymphorganogenic chemokines CXCL13 and CCL21 [114]. Vascular smooth muscle cell depletion of *Ltbr* suggests that the signaling via the receptor is age-dependent, initially having no impact on atherosclerosis in young mice and then being atheroprotective in aged mice, especially in the abdominal aorta [115]. Intriguing is the territoriality of these tertiary lymphoid organs, which are particularly found around the abdominal aorta, a site that develops lesions later in the temporal progression of atherosclerosis in the vascular tree. The basis for this specific location is yet to be clarified.

5.8. Toll-Like Receptors (TLRs) and Lesion Localization

Many TLRs have been implicated in atherogenesis. In relation to differential lesion localization, TLR2 is particularly relevant. TLR2 is widely expressed among the cells involved in atherogenesis, including endothelial cells, monocytes and macrophages, smooth muscle cells, and lymphocytes [116]. TLR2 is upregulated in the endothelium by disturbed flow and hyperlipidemia [117]. TLR2 can be activated by both endogenous and exogenous activators of bacterial origin [118]. Among the endogenous activators are oxidized LDL, apoCIII, biglycan, versican, decorin, and hyaluronan fragments. The synthetic TLR2 activator PAM3CSK4, in a dose- and TLR2-dependent fashion, was shown to enhance atherosclerosis in an *Ldlr*$^{-/-}$ model fed a Western-type diet, particularly in the abdominal aorta [119]. The basis for the almost unique impact at this site is unclear. However, it is in part dependent on the expression of TLR2 in bone-marrow-derived cells. Among the effects of TLR2 activation is the proliferation of regulatory T cells, which is accompanied by temporary inhibition of their suppressive activity [120].

5.9. Perivascular Adipose Tissue (PVAT)

Recent work has indicated the potential importance of PVAT in the evolution of atherosclerosis. PVAT is located adjacent to the adventitia of most of the major arteries, with the cerebral and pulmonary arteries being notable exceptions, and is functionally distinct from other adipose depots [121]. It is composed of adipocytes, nerves, monocytes, endothelial cells, macrophages, and T and B cells. PVAT regulates vasomotor tone and vascular homeostasis through the secretion of relaxing and contracting factors and inflammatory status through the secretion of pro- and anti-inflammatory factors. The regional phenotypic heterogeneity of perivascular adipocytes has been noted among different PVAT arterial sites. In rodents, thoracic aorta PVAT is composed of mostly brown adipocytes, abdominal aorta PVAT contains predominately white adipocytes with some brown adipocytes, and mesenteric PVAT is largely white adipocytes [121,122]. In humans, the perivascular fat contains mostly white adipocytes. Interestingly, TLR2 is upregulated in brown adipose non-PVAT tissue in obese mice [123].

The potential contribution of PVAT may differ depending on the vascular bed it surrounds. A recent study has explored this complexity in the thoracic aorta in mice. The anterior thoracic and lateral thoracic artery PVAT pads differ in their developmental pathways and transcriptional profiles and are associated with different effects on vascular function [124].

6. Conclusions and Future Directions

From this review, it is clear that atherosclerosis and its site specificity is extremely complex and that the basis for the temporal–spatial lesion localization in *Apoe*- and *Ldlr*-deficient mice is incompletely understood. While most studies of regionalization have been made in mice, there is also evidence that this occurs in humans too, as evidenced by the PDAY studies [1]. In a great deal of the research on the mechanisms of atherosclerosis using mouse models, the emphasis is on the lesions in the aortic root, a site not often developing lesions in humans, and on en face analysis of lesions over the entire aorta and principal branches, without specific analysis of discrete aortic regions. To achieve a better understanding of the mechanisms of these localizations, further studies are necessary at appropriately selected sites at various stages of atherogenesis. These include a more accurate measurement of the flow patterns along the extent of the aorta and its branches, a detailed analysis of transcytosis, and the distribution of proteoglycans along the vasculature to determine the basis for lipoprotein retention at these sites. In addition, the application of evolving single-cell technologies, such as scRNA-seq, CITE-seq (cellular indexing of transcriptomes and epitopes), scATAC-seq (single-cell transposase-accessible chromatin with sequencing), and CyTOF, to analysis of atherosclerosis at different sites in the vascular tree should provide insight into the cellular and molecular heterogeneity that may contribute to the site-specific development of atherosclerosis [125]. This is a tall order, but this will be required to understand the patterns of lesion initiation and progression along the vasculature.

Author Contributions: All the authors participated in the research and writing of the review. All the authors have read and agreed to the published version of the manuscript.

Funding: This research received no external funding.

Conflicts of Interest: The authors declare no conflicts of interest.

Abbreviations

ABCG1	ATP-binding cassette G1
AKT1	AKT serine/threonine kinase 1
ApoE	Apolipoprotein E
CITE-seq	cellular indexing of transcriptomes and epitopes
CyTOF	cytometry by time of flight
DOCK4	dedicator of cytokine-like kinase 4
eNOS	endothelial nitric oxide synthase
GPER	G-protein-coupled estrogen receptor
GWAS	Genome-Wide Association Studies
HDL	high-density lipoprotein
HIF1	hypoxia-inducible factor 1
HK2	hexokinase 2
HMDP	Hybrid Mouse Diversity Panel
IDL	intermediate-density lipoprotein
KLF	Krüppel-like factor
LDL	low-density lipoprotein
LDLR	low-density lipoprotein receptor
LT	lymphotoxin
LTβR	lymphotoxin β receptor
M-CSF	macrophage colony-stimulating factor
MCP-1	monocyte chemoattractant protein 1
NKT	natural killer T cell
NO	nitric oxide
NOX4	NADPH oxidase 4
NRF2	nuclear factor-erythroid 2 related factor 2
PDAY	Pathological Determination of Atherosclerosis in Youth
PDH	pyruvate dehydrogenase
PDK1	3-phosphoinosital-dependent kinase 1
PDZK1	PDZ domain-containing 1
PFKFB3	6-phosphofructo-2-kinase/fructose-2,6-bisphosphatase 3
PVAT	perivascular adipose tissue
QTL	quantitative trait locus
RAG	recombination activating gene
Sca-1	stem cell antigen 1 marker
scATAC-seq	single-cell transposase-accessible chromatin with sequencing
scRNA-seq	single-cell RNA sequencing
SR-B1	scavenger receptor class B, type 1
TCR	T cell receptor
TGFβ	Transforming growth factor-β
TLR	toll-like receptor
TNF	tumor necrosis factor
VCAM1	vascular adhesion molecule 1

References

1. VanderLaan, P.A.; Reardon, C.A.; Getz, G.S. Site specificity of atherosclerosis: Site-selective responses to atherosclerotic modulators. *Arter. Thromb. Vasc. Biol.* **2004**, *24*, 12–22. [CrossRef] [PubMed]
2. Jaiswal, S.; Libby, P. Clonal haematopoiesis: Connecting ageing and inflammation in cardiovascular disease. *Nat. Rev. Cardiol.* **2020**, *17*, 137–144. [CrossRef] [PubMed]
3. McGill, H.C., Jr.; McMahan, C.A.; Herderick, E.E.; Tracy, R.E.; Malcom, G.T.; Zieske, A.W.; Strong, J.P. Effects of coronary heart disease risk factors on atherosclerosis of selected regions of the aorta and right coronary artery. PDAY Research Group. Pathobiological Determinants of Atherosclerosis in Youth. *Arter. Thromb. Vasc. Biol.* **2000**, *20*, 836–845. [CrossRef] [PubMed]
4. McGill, H.C., Jr.; McMahan, C.A. Determinants of atherosclerosis in the young. Pathobiological Determinants of Atherosclerosis in Youth (PDAY) Research Group. *Am. J. Cardiol.* **1998**, *82*, 30t–36t. [CrossRef] [PubMed]

5. McGill, H.C., Jr.; McMahan, C.A.; Zieske, A.W.; Sloop, G.D.; Walcott, J.V.; Troxclair, D.A.; Malcom, G.T.; Tracy, R.E.; Oalmann, M.C.; Strong, J.P. Associations of coronary heart disease risk factors with the intermediate lesion of atherosclerosis in youth. The Pathobiological Determinants of Atherosclerosis in Youth (PDAY) Research Group. *Arter. Thromb. Vasc. Biol.* **2000**, *20*, 1998–2004. [CrossRef]
6. Morganroth, J.; Levy, R.I.; Fredrickson, D.S. The biochemical, clinical, and genetic features of type III hyperlipoproteinemia. *Ann. Intern. Med.* **1975**, *82*, 158–174. [CrossRef] [PubMed]
7. Mahley, R.W.; Weisgraber, K.H.; Huang, Y. Apolipoprotein E: Structure determines function, from atherosclerosis to Alzheimer's disease to AIDS. *J. Lipid Res.* **2009**, *50*, S183–S188. [CrossRef] [PubMed]
8. Leibson, C.L.; Ransom, J.E.; Olson, W.; Zimmerman, B.R.; O'Fallon, M.W.; Palumbo, P.J. Peripheral arterial disease, diabetes, and mortality. *Diabetes Care* **2004**, *27*, 2843–2849. [CrossRef]
9. Gnasso, A.; Irace, C.; Carallo, C.; De Franceschi, M.S.; Motti, C.; Mattioli, P.L.; Pujia, A. In vivo association between low wall shear stress and plaque in subjects with asymmetrical carotid atherosclerosis. *Stroke* **1997**, *28*, 993–998. [CrossRef]
10. Getz, G.S.; Reardon, C.A. Animal models of atherosclerosis. *Arter. Thromb. Vasc. Biol.* **2012**, *32*, 1104–1115. [CrossRef]
11. Getz, G.S.; Reardon, C.A. Pig and Mouse Models of Hyperlipidemia and Atherosclerosis. *Methods Mol. Biol.* **2022**, *2419*, 379–411. [CrossRef] [PubMed]
12. Libby, P. Murine "model" monotheism: An iconoclast at the altar of mouse. *Circ. Res.* **2015**, *117*, 921–925. [CrossRef] [PubMed]
13. Engelen, S.E.; Robinson, A.J.B.; Zurke, Y.X.; Monaco, C. Therapeutic strategies targeting inflammation and immunity in atherosclerosis: How to proceed? *Nat. Rev. Cardiol.* **2022**, *19*, 522–542. [CrossRef] [PubMed]
14. Adkar, S.S.; Leeper, N.J. Efferocytosis in atherosclerosis. *Nat. Rev. Cardiol.* 2024; *Online ahead of print*. [CrossRef]
15. Fang, Y.; Wu, D.; Birukov, K.G. Mechanosensing and Mechanoregulation of Endothelial Cell Functions. *Compr. Physiol.* **2019**, *9*, 873–904. [CrossRef] [PubMed]
16. Gimbrone, M.A., Jr.; García-Cardeña, G. Endothelial Cell Dysfunction and the Pathobiology of Atherosclerosis. *Circ. Res.* **2016**, *118*, 620–636. [CrossRef] [PubMed]
17. Davies, P.F. Hemodynamic shear stress and the endothelium in cardiovascular pathophysiology. *Nat. Clin. Pr. Cardiovasc. Med.* **2009**, *6*, 16–26. [CrossRef] [PubMed]
18. Majesky, M.W. Developmental basis of vascular smooth muscle diversity. *Arter. Thromb. Vasc. Biol.* **2007**, *27*, 1248–1258. [CrossRef] [PubMed]
19. Wilm, B.; Ipenberg, A.; Hastie, N.D.; Burch, J.B.; Bader, D.M. The serosal mesothelium is a major source of smooth muscle cells of the gut vasculature. *Development* **2005**, *132*, 5317–5328. [CrossRef]
20. Haimovici, H.; Maier, N. Fate of aortic homografts in canine atherosclerosis. 3. study of fresh abdominal and thoracic aortic implants into thoracic aorta: Role of tissue susceptibility in atherogenesis. *Arch. Surg.* **1964**, *89*, 961–969. [CrossRef]
21. Majesky, M.W.; Weiser-Evans, M.C.M. The adventitia in arterial development, remodeling, and hypertension. *Biochem. Pharmacol.* **2022**, *205*, 115259. [CrossRef]
22. Hu, Y.; Zhang, Z.; Torsney, E.; Afzal, A.R.; Davison, F.; Metzler, B.; Xu, Q. Abundant progenitor cells in the adventitia contribute to atherosclerosis of vein grafts in ApoE-deficient mice. *J. Clin. Investig.* **2004**, *113*, 1258–1265. [CrossRef] [PubMed]
23. Psaltis, P.J.; Puranik, A.S.; Spoon, D.B.; Chue, C.D.; Hoffman, S.J.; Witt, T.A.; Delacroix, S.; Kleppe, L.S.; Mueske, C.S.; Pan, S.; et al. Characterization of a resident population of adventitial macrophage progenitor cells in postnatal vasculature. *Circ. Res.* **2014**, *115*, 364–375. [CrossRef] [PubMed]
24. Williams, K.J.; Tabas, I. The response-to-retention hypothesis of atherogenesis reinforced. *Curr. Opin. Lipidol.* **1998**, *9*, 471–474. [CrossRef] [PubMed]
25. Allahverdian, S.; Ortega, C.; Francis, G.A. Smooth Muscle Cell-Proteoglycan-Lipoprotein Interactions as Drivers of Atherosclerosis. *Handb. Exp. Pharmacol.* **2022**, *270*, 335–358. [CrossRef] [PubMed]
26. Tannock, L.R.; King, V.L. Proteoglycan mediated lipoprotein retention: A mechanism of diabetic atherosclerosis. *Rev. Endocr. Metab. Disord.* **2008**, *9*, 289–300. [CrossRef]
27. Moore, K.J.; Sheedy, F.J.; Fisher, E.A. Macrophages in atherosclerosis: A dynamic balance. *Nat. Rev. Immunol.* **2013**, *13*, 709–721. [CrossRef] [PubMed]
28. Glass, C.K.; Witztum, J.L. Atherosclerosis. the road ahead. *Cell* **2001**, *104*, 503–516. [CrossRef] [PubMed]
29. Hansson, G.K.; Hermansson, A. The immune system in atherosclerosis. *Nat. Immunol.* **2011**, *12*, 204–212. [CrossRef] [PubMed]
30. Witztum, J.L.; Lichtman, A.H. The influence of innate and adaptive immune responses on atherosclerosis. *Annu. Rev. Pathol.* **2014**, *9*, 73–102. [CrossRef]
31. Porsch, F.; Mallat, Z.; Binder, C.J. Humoral immunity in atherosclerosis and myocardial infarction: From B cells to antibodies. *Cardiovasc. Res.* **2021**, *117*, 2544–2562. [CrossRef]
32. Zernecke, A.; Winkels, H.; Cochain, C.; Williams, J.W.; Wolf, D.; Soehnlein, O.; Robbins, C.S.; Monaco, C.; Park, I.; McNamara, C.A.; et al. Meta-Analysis of Leukocyte Diversity in Atherosclerotic Mouse Aortas. *Circ. Res.* **2020**, *127*, 402–426. [CrossRef] [PubMed]
33. Yurdagul, A., Jr.; Doran, A.C.; Cai, B.; Fredman, G.; Tabas, I.A. Mechanisms and Consequences of Defective Efferocytosis in Atherosclerosis. *Front. Cardiovasc. Med.* **2017**, *4*, 86. [CrossRef] [PubMed]
34. Basatemur, G.L.; Jørgensen, H.F.; Clarke, M.C.H.; Bennett, M.R.; Mallat, Z. Vascular smooth muscle cells in atherosclerosis. *Nat. Rev. Cardiol.* **2019**, *16*, 727–744. [CrossRef] [PubMed]

35. Bennett, M.R.; Sinha, S.; Owens, G.K. Vascular Smooth Muscle Cells in Atherosclerosis. *Circ. Res.* **2016**, *118*, 692–702. [CrossRef] [PubMed]
36. Jacobsen, K.; Lund, M.B.; Shim, J.; Gunnersen, S.; Füchtbauer, E.M.; Kjolby, M.; Carramolino, L.; Bentzon, J.F. Diverse cellular architecture of atherosclerotic plaque derives from clonal expansion of a few medial SMCs. *JCI Insight* **2017**, *2*, e95890. [CrossRef] [PubMed]
37. Feil, S.; Fehrenbacher, B.; Lukowski, R.; Essmann, F.; Schulze-Osthoff, K.; Schaller, M.; Feil, R. Transdifferentiation of vascular smooth muscle cells to macrophage-like cells during atherogenesis. *Circ. Res.* **2014**, *115*, 662–667. [CrossRef] [PubMed]
38. Shankman, L.S.; Gomez, D.; Cherepanova, O.A.; Salmon, M.; Alencar, G.F.; Haskins, R.M.; Swiatlowska, P.; Newman, A.A.; Greene, E.S.; Straub, A.C.; et al. KLF4-dependent phenotypic modulation of smooth muscle cells has a key role in atherosclerotic plaque pathogenesis. *Nat. Med.* **2015**, *21*, 628–637. [CrossRef] [PubMed]
39. Wang, Y.; Dubland, J.A.; Allahverdian, S.; Asonye, E.; Sahin, B.; Jaw, J.E.; Sin, D.D.; Seidman, M.A.; Leeper, N.J.; Francis, G.A. Smooth Muscle Cells Contribute the Majority of Foam Cells in ApoE (Apolipoprotein E)-Deficient Mouse Atherosclerosis. *Arter. Thromb. Vasc. Biol.* **2019**, *39*, 876–887. [CrossRef] [PubMed]
40. Vengrenyuk, Y.; Nishi, H.; Long, X.; Ouimet, M.; Savji, N.; Martinez, F.O.; Cassella, C.P.; Moore, K.J.; Ramsey, S.A.; Miano, J.M.; et al. Cholesterol loading reprograms the microRNA-143/145-myocardin axis to convert aortic smooth muscle cells to a dysfunctional macrophage-like phenotype. *Arter. Thromb. Vasc. Biol.* **2015**, *35*, 535–546. [CrossRef]
41. Miano, J.M.; Fisher, E.A.; Majesky, M.W. Fate and State of Vascular Smooth Muscle Cells in Atherosclerosis. *Circulation* **2021**, *143*, 2110–2116. [CrossRef]
42. Benditt, E.P.; Benditt, J.M. Evidence for a monoclonal origin of human atherosclerotic plaques. *Proc. Natl. Acad. Sci. USA* **1973**, *70*, 1753–1756. [CrossRef] [PubMed]
43. Rosenson, R.S.; Brewer, H.B., Jr.; Davidson, W.S.; Fayad, Z.A.; Fuster, V.; Goldstein, J.; Hellerstein, M.; Jiang, X.C.; Phillips, M.C.; Rader, D.J.; et al. Cholesterol efflux and atheroprotection: Advancing the concept of reverse cholesterol transport. *Circulation* **2012**, *125*, 1905–1919. [CrossRef] [PubMed]
44. Moore, K.J.; Koplev, S.; Fisher, E.A.; Tabas, I.; Björkegren, J.L.M.; Doran, A.C.; Kovacic, J.C. Macrophage Trafficking, Inflammatory Resolution, and Genomics in Atherosclerosis: JACC Macrophage in CVD Series (Part 2). *J. Am. Coll. Cardiol.* **2018**, *72*, 2181–2197. [CrossRef] [PubMed]
45. Bäck, M.; Yurdagul, A., Jr.; Tabas, I.; Öörni, K.; Kovanen, P.T. Inflammation and its resolution in atherosclerosis: Mediators and therapeutic opportunities. *Nat. Rev. Cardiol.* **2019**, *16*, 389–406. [CrossRef] [PubMed]
46. Spitz, C.; Winkels, H.; Bürger, C.; Weber, C.; Lutgens, E.; Hansson, G.K.; Gerdes, N. Regulatory T cells in atherosclerosis: Critical immune regulatory function and therapeutic potential. *Cell Mol. Life Sci.* **2016**, *73*, 901–922. [CrossRef] [PubMed]
47. Zhang, S.H.; Reddick, R.L.; Piedrahita, J.A.; Maeda, N. Spontaneous hypercholesterolemia and arterial lesions in mice lacking apolipoprotein E. *Science* **1992**, *258*, 468–471. [CrossRef] [PubMed]
48. Plump, A.S.; Smith, J.D.; Hayek, T.; Aalto-Setälä, K.; Walsh, A.; Verstuyft, J.G.; Rubin, E.M.; Breslow, J.L. Severe hypercholesterolemia and atherosclerosis in apolipoprotein E-deficient mice created by homologous recombination in ES cells. *Cell* **1992**, *71*, 343–353. [CrossRef] [PubMed]
49. Nakashima, Y.; Plump, A.S.; Raines, E.W.; Breslow, J.L.; Ross, R. ApoE-deficient mice develop lesions of all phases of atherosclerosis throughout the arterial tree. *Arter. Thromb.* **1994**, *14*, 133–140. [CrossRef] [PubMed]
50. Dhawan, S.S.; Avati Nanjundappa, R.P.; Branch, J.R.; Taylor, W.R.; Quyyumi, A.A.; Jo, H.; McDaniel, M.C.; Suo, J.; Giddens, D.; Samady, H. Shear stress and plaque development. *Expert. Rev. Cardiovasc. Ther.* **2010**, *8*, 545–556. [CrossRef]
51. Ishibashi, S.; Brown, M.S.; Goldstein, J.L.; Gerard, R.D.; Hammer, R.E.; Herz, J. Hypercholesterolemia in low density lipoprotein receptor knockout mice and its reversal by adenovirus-mediated gene delivery. *J. Clin. Investig.* **1993**, *92*, 883–893. [CrossRef]
52. Getz, G.S.; Reardon, C.A. Do the Apoe-/- and Ldlr-/- Mice Yield the Same Insight on Atherogenesis? *Arter. Thromb. Vasc. Biol.* **2016**, *36*, 1734–1741. [CrossRef] [PubMed]
53. Rallidis, L.; Naoumova, R.P.; Thompson, G.R.; Nihoyannopoulos, P. Extent and severity of atherosclerotic involvement of the aortic valve and root in familial hypercholesterolaemia. *Heart* **1998**, *80*, 583–590. [CrossRef] [PubMed]
54. Ishibashi, S.; Goldstein, J.L.; Brown, M.S.; Herz, J.; Burns, D.K. Massive xanthomatosis and atherosclerosis in cholesterol-fed low density lipoprotein receptor-negative mice. *J. Clin. Investig.* **1994**, *93*, 1885–1893. [CrossRef] [PubMed]
55. Du, W.; Wong, C.; Song, Y.; Shen, H.; Mori, D.; Rotllan, N.; Price, N.; Dobrian, A.D.; Meng, H.; Kleinstein, S.H.; et al. Age-associated vascular inflammation promotes monocytosis during atherogenesis. *Aging Cell* **2016**, *15*, 766–777. [CrossRef] [PubMed]
56. Flood, C.; Gustafsson, M.; Richardson, P.E.; Harvey, S.C.; Segrest, J.P.; Borén, J. Identification of the proteoglycan binding site in apolipoprotein B48. *J. Biol. Chem.* **2002**, *277*, 32228–32233. [CrossRef] [PubMed]
57. Bennett, B.J.; Davis, R.C.; Civelek, M.; Orozco, L.; Wu, J.; Qi, H.; Pan, C.; Packard, R.R.; Eskin, E.; Yan, M.; et al. Genetic Architecture of Atherosclerosis in Mice: A Systems Genetics Analysis of Common Inbred Strains. *PLoS Genet.* **2015**, *11*, e1005711. [CrossRef] [PubMed]
58. von Scheidt, M.; Zhao, Y.; Kurt, Z.; Pan, C.; Zeng, L.; Yang, X.; Schunkert, H.; Lusis, A.J. Applications and Limitations of Mouse Models for Understanding Human Atherosclerosis. *Cell Metab.* **2017**, *25*, 248–261. [CrossRef] [PubMed]
59. Suo, J.; Ferrara, D.E.; Sorescu, D.; Guldberg, R.E.; Taylor, W.R.; Giddens, D.P. Hemodynamic shear stresses in mouse aortas: Implications for atherogenesis. *Arter. Thromb. Vasc. Biol.* **2007**, *27*, 346–351. [CrossRef]

60. Crouch, A.C.; Cao, A.A.; Scheven, U.M.; Greve, J.M. In Vivo MRI Assessment of Blood Flow in Arteries and Veins from Head-to-Toe Across Age and Sex in C57BL/6 Mice. *Ann. Biomed. Eng.* **2020**, *48*, 329–341. [CrossRef]
61. Zhou, Y.Q.; Zhu, S.N.; Foster, F.S.; Cybulsky, M.I.; Henkelman, R.M. Aortic regurgitation dramatically alters the distribution of atherosclerotic lesions and enhances atherogenesis in mice. *Arter. Thromb. Vasc. Biol.* **2010**, *30*, 1181–1188. [CrossRef]
62. Shimoni, S.; Zilberman, L.; Edri, O.; Bar, I.; Goland, S.; Gendelman, G.; Swissa, M.; Livshitz, S.; Paz, O.; Ayzenberg, O.; et al. Thoracic aortic atherosclerosis in patients with aortic regurgitation. *Atherosclerosis* **2011**, *218*, 107–109. [CrossRef] [PubMed]
63. Maeda, N.; Johnson, L.; Kim, S.; Hagaman, J.; Friedman, M.; Reddick, R. Anatomical differences and atherosclerosis in apolipoprotein E-deficient mice with 129/SvEv and C57BL/6 genetic backgrounds. *Atherosclerosis* **2007**, *195*, 75–82. [CrossRef] [PubMed]
64. Zhu, H.; Zhang, J.; Shih, J.; Lopez-Bertoni, F.; Hagaman, J.R.; Maeda, N.; Friedman, M.H. Differences in aortic arch geometry, hemodynamics, and plaque patterns between C57BL/6 and 129/SvEv mice. *J. Biomech. Eng.* **2009**, *131*, 121005. [CrossRef] [PubMed]
65. Tomita, H.; Zhilicheva, S.; Kim, S.; Maeda, N. Aortic arch curvature and atherosclerosis have overlapping quantitative trait loci in a cross between 129S6/SvEvTac and C57BL/6J apolipoprotein E-null mice. *Circ. Res.* **2010**, *106*, 1052–1060. [CrossRef] [PubMed]
66. Niu, N.; Xu, S.; Xu, Y.; Little, P.J.; Jin, Z.G. Targeting Mechanosensitive Transcription Factors in Atherosclerosis. *Trends Pharmacol. Sci.* **2019**, *40*, 253–266. [CrossRef] [PubMed]
67. Tamargo, I.A.; Baek, K.I.; Kim, Y.; Park, C.; Jo, H. Flow-induced reprogramming of endothelial cells in atherosclerosis. *Nat. Rev. Cardiol.* **2023**, *20*, 738–753. [CrossRef] [PubMed]
68. Wu, D.; Huang, R.T.; Hamanaka, R.B.; Krause, M.; Oh, M.J.; Kuo, C.H.; Nigdelioglu, R.; Meliton, A.Y.; Witt, L.; Dai, G.; et al. HIF-1α is required for disturbed flow-induced metabolic reprogramming in human and porcine vascular endothelium. *Elife* **2017**, *6*, e25217. [CrossRef] [PubMed]
69. Green, J.P.; Souilhol, C.; Xanthis, I.; Martinez-Campesino, L.; Bowden, N.P.; Evans, P.C.; Wilson, H.L. Atheroprone flow activates inflammation via endothelial ATP-dependent P2X7-p38 signalling. *Cardiovasc. Res.* **2018**, *114*, 324–335. [CrossRef] [PubMed]
70. Bennett, B.J.; Wang, S.S.; Wang, X.; Wu, X.; Lusis, A.J. Genetic regulation of atherosclerotic plaque size and morphology in the innominate artery of hyperlipidemic mice. *Arter. Thromb. Vasc. Biol.* **2009**, *29*, 348–355. [CrossRef]
71. Kandangwa, P.; Torii, R.; Gatehouse, P.D.; Sherwin, S.J.; Weinberg, P.D. Influence of right coronary artery motion, flow pulsatility and non-Newtonian rheology on wall shear stress metrics. *Front. Bioeng. Biotechnol.* **2022**, *10*, 962687. [CrossRef]
72. Teupser, D.; Persky, A.D.; Breslow, J.L. Induction of atherosclerosis by low-fat, semisynthetic diets in LDL receptor-deficient C57BL/6J and FVB/NJ mice: Comparison of lesions of the aortic root, brachiocephalic artery, and whole aorta (en face measurement). *Arter. Thromb. Vasc. Biol.* **2003**, *23*, 1907–1913. [CrossRef] [PubMed]
73. Tamminen, M.; Mottino, G.; Qiao, J.H.; Breslow, J.L.; Frank, J.S. Ultrastructure of early lipid accumulation in ApoE-deficient mice. *Arter. Thromb. Vasc. Biol.* **1999**, *19*, 847–853. [CrossRef]
74. Zhang, X.; Fernández-Hernando, C. Transport of LDLs into the arterial wall: Impact in atherosclerosis. *Curr. Opin. Lipidol.* **2020**, *31*, 279–285. [CrossRef]
75. Huang, L.; Chambliss, K.L.; Gao, X.; Yuhanna, I.S.; Behling-Kelly, E.; Bergaya, S.; Ahmed, M.; Michaely, P.; Luby-Phelps, K.; Darehshouri, A.; et al. SR-B1 drives endothelial cell LDL transcytosis via DOCK4 to promote atherosclerosis. *Nature* **2019**, *569*, 565–569. [CrossRef]
76. Yurdagul, A., Jr.; Finney, A.C.; Woolard, M.D.; Orr, A.W. The arterial microenvironment: The where and why of atherosclerosis. *Biochem. J.* **2016**, *473*, 1281–1295. [CrossRef] [PubMed]
77. Ghaffari, S.; Naderi Nabi, F.; Sugiyama, M.G.; Lee, W.L. Estrogen Inhibits LDL (Low-Density Lipoprotein) Transcytosis by Human Coronary Artery Endothelial Cells via GPER (G-Protein-Coupled Estrogen Receptor) and SR-BI (Scavenger Receptor Class B Type 1). *Arter. Thromb. Vasc. Biol.* **2018**, *38*, 2283–2294. [CrossRef] [PubMed]
78. Bell, F.P.; Somer, J.B.; Craig, I.H.; Schwartz, C.J. Patterns of aortic Evans blue uptake in vivo and in vitro. *Atherosclerosis* **1972**, *16*, 369–375. [CrossRef]
79. Schwenke, D.C.; Carew, T.E. Quantification in vivo of increased LDL content and rate of LDL degradation in normal rabbit aorta occurring at sites susceptible to early atherosclerotic lesions. *Circ. Res.* **1988**, *62*, 699–710. [CrossRef] [PubMed]
80. Witting, P.K.; Pettersson, K.; Letters, J.; Stocker, R. Site-specific antiatherogenic effect of probucol in apolipoprotein E-deficient mice. *Arter. Thromb. Vasc. Biol.* **2000**, *20*, E26–E33. [CrossRef]
81. Mineo, C. Lipoprotein receptor signalling in atherosclerosis. *Cardiovasc. Res.* **2020**, *116*, 1254–1274. [CrossRef]
82. Saddar, S.; Mineo, C.; Shaul, P.W. Signaling by the high-affinity HDL receptor scavenger receptor B type I. *Arter. Thromb. Vasc. Biol.* **2010**, *30*, 144–150. [CrossRef] [PubMed]
83. Zhang, X.; Sessa, W.C.; Fernández-Hernando, C. Endothelial Transcytosis of Lipoproteins in Atherosclerosis. *Front. Cardiovasc. Med.* **2018**, *5*, 130. [CrossRef] [PubMed]
84. Caligiuri, G.; Levy, B.; Pernow, J.; Thorén, P.; Hansson, G.K. Myocardial infarction mediated by endothelin receptor signaling in hypercholesterolemic mice. *Proc. Natl. Acad. Sci. USA* **1999**, *96*, 6920–6924. [CrossRef] [PubMed]
85. Cozen, A.E.; Moriwaki, H.; Kremen, M.; DeYoung, M.B.; Dichek, H.L.; Slezicki, K.I.; Young, S.G.; Véniant, M.; Dichek, D.A. Macrophage-targeted overexpression of urokinase causes accelerated atherosclerosis, coronary artery occlusions, and premature death. *Circulation* **2004**, *109*, 2129–2135. [CrossRef] [PubMed]

86. Braun, A.; Trigatti, B.L.; Post, M.J.; Sato, K.; Simons, M.; Edelberg, J.M.; Rosenberg, R.D.; Schrenzel, M.; Krieger, M. Loss of SR-BI expression leads to the early onset of occlusive atherosclerotic coronary artery disease, spontaneous myocardial infarctions, severe cardiac dysfunction, and premature death in apolipoprotein E-deficient mice. *Circ. Res.* **2002**, *90*, 270–276. [CrossRef] [PubMed]
87. Fuller, M.; Dadoo, O.; Serkis, V.; Abutouk, D.; MacDonald, M.; Dhingani, N.; Macri, J.; Igdoura, S.A.; Trigatti, B.L. The effects of diet on occlusive coronary artery atherosclerosis and myocardial infarction in scavenger receptor class B, type 1/low-density lipoprotein receptor double knockout mice. *Arter. Thromb. Vasc. Biol.* **2014**, *34*, 2394–2403. [CrossRef] [PubMed]
88. Braun, A.; Zhang, S.; Miettinen, H.E.; Ebrahim, S.; Holm, T.M.; Vasile, E.; Post, M.J.; Yoerger, D.M.; Picard, M.H.; Krieger, J.L.; et al. Probucol prevents early coronary heart disease and death in the high-density lipoprotein receptor SR-BI/apolipoprotein E double knockout mouse. *Proc. Natl. Acad. Sci. USA* **2003**, *100*, 7283–7288. [CrossRef]
89. Yesilaltay, A.; Daniels, K.; Pal, R.; Krieger, M.; Kocher, O. Loss of PDZK1 causes coronary artery occlusion and myocardial infarction in Paigen diet-fed apolipoprotein E deficient mice. *PLoS ONE* **2009**, *4*, e8103. [CrossRef]
90. Fernández-Hernando, C.; Ackah, E.; Yu, J.; Suárez, Y.; Murata, T.; Iwakiri, Y.; Prendergast, J.; Miao, R.Q.; Birnbaum, M.J.; Sessa, W.C. Loss of Akt1 leads to severe atherosclerosis and occlusive coronary artery disease. *Cell Metab.* **2007**, *6*, 446–457. [CrossRef]
91. Kuhlencordt, P.J.; Gyurko, R.; Han, F.; Scherrer-Crosbie, M.; Aretz, T.H.; Hajjar, R.; Picard, M.H.; Huang, P.L. Accelerated atherosclerosis, aortic aneurysm formation, and ischemic heart disease in apolipoprotein E/endothelial nitric oxide synthase double-knockout mice. *Circulation* **2001**, *104*, 448–454. [CrossRef]
92. Zhang, S.; Picard, M.H.; Vasile, E.; Zhu, Y.; Raffai, R.L.; Weisgraber, K.H.; Krieger, M. Diet-induced occlusive coronary atherosclerosis, myocardial infarction, cardiac dysfunction, and premature death in scavenger receptor class B type I-deficient, hypomorphic apolipoprotein ER61 mice. *Circulation* **2005**, *111*, 3457–3464. [CrossRef]
93. Pei, Y.; Chen, X.; Aboutouk, D.; Fuller, M.T.; Dadoo, O.; Yu, P.; White, E.J.; Igdoura, S.A.; Trigatti, B.L. SR-BI in bone marrow derived cells protects mice from diet induced coronary artery atherosclerosis and myocardial infarction. *PLoS ONE* **2013**, *8*, e72492. [CrossRef]
94. Van Eck, M.; Bos, I.S.; Hildebrand, R.B.; Van Rij, B.T.; Van Berkel, T.J. Dual role for scavenger receptor class B, type I on bone marrow-derived cells in atherosclerotic lesion development. *Am. J. Pathol.* **2004**, *165*, 785–794. [CrossRef] [PubMed]
95. Mineo, C.; Shaul, P.W. Functions of scavenger receptor class B, type I in atherosclerosis. *Curr. Opin. Lipidol.* **2012**, *23*, 487–493. [CrossRef]
96. Smith, J.D.; Trogan, E.; Ginsberg, M.; Grigaux, C.; Tian, J.; Miyata, M. Decreased atherosclerosis in mice deficient in both macrophage colony-stimulating factor (op) and apolipoprotein E. *Proc. Natl. Acad. Sci. USA* **1995**, *92*, 8264–8268. [CrossRef] [PubMed]
97. Rajavashisth, T.; Qiao, J.H.; Tripathi, S.; Tripathi, J.; Mishra, N.; Hua, M.; Wang, X.P.; Loussararian, A.; Clinton, S.; Libby, P.; et al. Heterozygous osteopetrotic (op) mutation reduces atherosclerosis in LDL receptor- deficient mice. *J. Clin. Investig.* **1998**, *101*, 2702–2710. [CrossRef]
98. Paulson, K.E.; Zhu, S.N.; Chen, M.; Nurmohamed, S.; Jongstra-Bilen, J.; Cybulsky, M.I. Resident intimal dendritic cells accumulate lipid and contribute to the initiation of atherosclerosis. *Circ. Res.* **2010**, *106*, 383–390. [CrossRef] [PubMed]
99. Cybulsky, M.I.; Cheong, C.; Robbins, C.S. Macrophages and Dendritic Cells: Partners in Atherogenesis. *Circ. Res.* **2016**, *118*, 637–652. [CrossRef]
100. Zhu, S.N.; Chen, M.; Jongstra-Bilen, J.; Cybulsky, M.I. GM-CSF regulates intimal cell proliferation in nascent atherosclerotic lesions. *J. Exp. Med.* **2009**, *206*, 2141–2149. [CrossRef]
101. Combadière, C.; Potteaux, S.; Rodero, M.; Simon, T.; Pezard, A.; Esposito, B.; Merval, R.; Proudfoot, A.; Tedgui, A.; Mallat, Z. Combined inhibition of CCL2, CX3CR1, and CCR5 abrogates Ly6C(hi) and Ly6C(lo) monocytosis and almost abolishes atherosclerosis in hypercholesterolemic mice. *Circulation* **2008**, *117*, 1649–1657. [CrossRef]
102. Combadière, C.; Potteaux, S.; Gao, J.L.; Esposito, B.; Casanova, S.; Lee, E.J.; Debré, P.; Tedgui, A.; Murphy, P.M.; Mallat, Z. Decreased atherosclerotic lesion formation in CX3CR1/apolipoprotein E double knockout mice. *Circulation* **2003**, *107*, 1009–1016. [CrossRef] [PubMed]
103. Lesnik, P.; Haskell, C.A.; Charo, I.F. Decreased atherosclerosis in CX3CR1-/- mice reveals a role for fractalkine in atherogenesis. *J. Clin. Investig.* **2003**, *111*, 333–340. [CrossRef] [PubMed]
104. Swirski, F.K.; Libby, P.; Aikawa, E.; Alcaide, P.; Luscinskas, F.W.; Weissleder, R.; Pittet, M.J. Ly-6Chi monocytes dominate hypercholesterolemia-associated monocytosis and give rise to macrophages in atheromata. *J. Clin. Investig.* **2007**, *117*, 195–205. [CrossRef] [PubMed]
105. Tacke, F.; Alvarez, D.; Kaplan, T.J.; Jakubzick, C.; Spanbroek, R.; Llodra, J.; Garin, A.; Liu, J.; Mack, M.; van Rooijen, N.; et al. Monocyte subsets differentially employ CCR2, CCR5, and CX3CR1 to accumulate within atherosclerotic plaques. *J. Clin. Investig.* **2007**, *117*, 185–194. [CrossRef] [PubMed]
106. Teupser, D.; Pavlides, S.; Tan, M.; Gutierrez-Ramos, J.C.; Kolbeck, R.; Breslow, J.L. Major reduction of atherosclerosis in fractalkine (CX3CL1)-deficient mice is at the brachiocephalic artery, not the aortic root. *Proc. Natl. Acad. Sci. USA* **2004**, *101*, 17795–17800. [CrossRef] [PubMed]
107. Reardon, C.A.; Blachowicz, L.; White, T.; Cabana, V.; Wang, Y.; Lukens, J.; Bluestone, J.; Getz, G.S. Effect of immune deficiency on lipoproteins and atherosclerosis in male apolipoprotein E-deficient mice. *Arter. Thromb. Vasc. Biol.* **2001**, *21*, 1011–1016. [CrossRef] [PubMed]

108. Reardon, C.A.; Blachowicz, L.; Lukens, J.; Nissenbaum, M.; Getz, G.S. Genetic background selectively influences innominate artery atherosclerosis: Immune system deficiency as a probe. *Arter. Thromb. Vasc. Biol.* **2003**, *23*, 1449–1454. [CrossRef] [PubMed]
109. Getz, G.S.; Reardon, C.A. Natural killer T cells in atherosclerosis. *Nat. Rev. Cardiol.* **2017**, *14*, 304–314. [CrossRef] [PubMed]
110. VanderLaan, P.A.; Reardon, C.A.; Cabana, V.G.; Wang, C.R.; Getz, G.S. Invariant Natural Killer T-Cells and Total CD1d Restricted Cells Differentially Influence Lipid Metabolism and Atherosclerosis in Low Density Receptor Deficient Mice. *Int. J. Mol. Sci.* **2019**, *20*, 4566. [CrossRef]
111. Šedý, J.; Bekiaris, V.; Ware, C.F. Tumor necrosis factor superfamily in innate immunity and inflammation. *Cold Spring Harb. Perspect. Biol.* **2014**, *7*, a016279. [CrossRef]
112. Grandoch, M.; Feldmann, K.; Göthert, J.R.; Dick, L.S.; Homann, S.; Klatt, C.; Bayer, J.K.; Waldheim, J.N.; Rabausch, B.; Nagy, N.; et al. Deficiency in lymphotoxin β receptor protects from atherosclerosis in apoE-deficient mice. *Circ. Res.* **2015**, *116*, e57–e68. [CrossRef] [PubMed]
113. Gräbner, R.; Lötzer, K.; Döpping, S.; Hildner, M.; Radke, D.; Beer, M.; Spanbroek, R.; Lippert, B.; Reardon, C.A.; Getz, G.S.; et al. Lymphotoxin beta receptor signaling promotes tertiary lymphoid organogenesis in the aorta adventitia of aged ApoE-/- mice. *J. Exp. Med.* **2009**, *206*, 233–248. [CrossRef] [PubMed]
114. Hu, D.; Yin, C.; Luo, S.; Habenicht, A.J.R.; Mohanta, S.K. Vascular Smooth Muscle Cells Contribute to Atherosclerosis Immunity. *Front. Immunol.* **2019**, *10*, 1101. [CrossRef] [PubMed]
115. Hu, D.; Mohanta, S.K.; Yin, C.; Peng, L.; Ma, Z.; Srikakulapu, P.; Grassia, G.; MacRitchie, N.; Dever, G.; Gordon, P.; et al. Artery Tertiary Lymphoid Organs Control Aorta Immunity and Protect against Atherosclerosis via Vascular Smooth Muscle Cell Lymphotoxin β Receptors. *Immunity* **2015**, *42*, 1100–1115. [CrossRef] [PubMed]
116. Cole, J.E.; Georgiou, E.; Monaco, C. The expression and functions of toll-like receptors in atherosclerosis. *Mediat. Inflamm.* **2010**, *2010*, 393946. [CrossRef] [PubMed]
117. Mullick, A.E.; Soldau, K.; Kiosses, W.B.; Bell, T.A., 3rd; Tobias, P.S.; Curtiss, L.K. Increased endothelial expression of Toll-like receptor 2 at sites of disturbed blood flow exacerbates early atherogenic events. *J. Exp. Med.* **2008**, *205*, 373–383. [CrossRef] [PubMed]
118. Goulopoulou, S.; McCarthy, C.G.; Webb, R.C. Toll-like Receptors in the Vascular System: Sensing the Dangers Within. *Pharmacol. Rev.* **2016**, *68*, 142–167. [CrossRef] [PubMed]
119. Mullick, A.E.; Tobias, P.S.; Curtiss, L.K. Modulation of atherosclerosis in mice by Toll-like receptor 2. *J. Clin. Investig.* **2005**, *115*, 3149–3156. [CrossRef] [PubMed]
120. Sutmuller, R.P.; den Brok, M.H.; Kramer, M.; Bennink, E.J.; Toonen, L.W.; Kullberg, B.J.; Joosten, L.A.; Akira, S.; Netea, M.G.; Adema, G.J. Toll-like receptor 2 controls expansion and function of regulatory T cells. *J. Clin. Investig.* **2006**, *116*, 485–494. [CrossRef]
121. Li, X.; Ma, Z.; Zhu, Y.Z. Regional Heterogeneity of Perivascular Adipose Tissue: Morphology, Origin, and Secretome. *Front. Pharmacol.* **2021**, *12*, 697720. [CrossRef]
122. Kim, H.W.; Belin de Chantemèle, E.J.; Weintraub, N.L. Perivascular Adipocytes in Vascular Disease. *Arter. Thromb. Vasc. Biol.* **2019**, *39*, 2220–2227. [CrossRef] [PubMed]
123. Bae, J.; Ricciardi, C.J.; Esposito, D.; Komarnytsky, S.; Hu, P.; Curry, B.J.; Brown, P.L.; Gao, Z.; Biggerstaff, J.P.; Chen, J.; et al. Activation of pattern recognition receptors in brown adipocytes induces inflammation and suppresses uncoupling protein 1 expression and mitochondrial respiration. *Am. J. Physiol. Cell Physiol.* **2014**, *306*, C918–C930. [CrossRef] [PubMed]
124. Ye, M.; Ruan, C.C.; Fu, M.; Xu, L.; Chen, D.; Zhu, M.; Zhu, D.; Gao, P. Developmental and functional characteristics of the thoracic aorta perivascular adipocyte. *Cell Mol. Life Sci.* **2019**, *76*, 777–789. [CrossRef] [PubMed]
125. Eberhardt, N.; Giannarelli, C. How Single-Cell Technologies Have Provided New Insights Into Atherosclerosis. *Arter. Thromb. Vasc. Biol.* **2022**, *42*, 243–252. [CrossRef]

MDPI AG
Grosspeteranlage 5
4052 Basel
Switzerland
Tel.: +41 61 683 77 34

International Journal of Molecular Sciences Editorial Office
E-mail: ijms@mdpi.com
www.mdpi.com/journal/ijms

www.ingramcontent.com/pod-product-compliance
Lightning Source LLC
Chambersburg PA
CBHW061453210926
51850CB00008B/1701

* 9 7 8 3 7 2 5 8 7 1 5 2 0 *